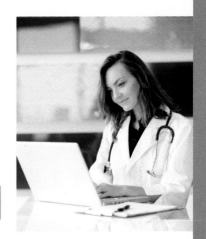

Obesity Medicine

Editors

SCOTT KAHAN
ROBERT F. KUSHNER

MEDICAL CLINICS
OF NORTH AMERICA

www.medical.theclinics.com

Consulting Editor
BIMAL H. ASHAR

January 2018 • Volume 102 • Number 1

ELSEVIER

1600 John F. Kennedy Boulevard • Suite 1800 • Philadelphia, Pennsylvania, 19103-2899

http://www.theclinics.com

MEDICAL CLINICS OF NORTH AMERICA Volume 102, Number 1
January 2018 ISSN 0025-7125, ISBN-13: 978-0-323-56643-8

Editor: Jessica McCool
Developmental Editor: Kristen Helm

Medical Clinics of North America (ISSN 0025-7125) is published bimonthly by Elsevier Inc., 360 Park Avenue South, New York, NY 10010-1710. Months of publication are January, March, May, July, September, and November. Business and editorial offices: 1600 John F. Kennedy Boulevard, Suite 1800, Philadelphia, PA 19103-2899. Periodicals postage paid at New York, NY, and additional mailing offices. Subscription prices are USD $273.00 per year (US individuals), $574.00 per year (US institutions), $100.00 per year (US Students), $336.00 per year (Canadian individuals), $746.00 per year (Canadian institutions), $200.00 per year (Canadian and foreign students), $402.00 per year (foreign individuals), and $746.00 per year (foreign institutions). To receive student/resident rate, orders must be accompanied by name of affiliated institution, date of term, and the signature of program/residency coordinator on institution letterhead. Orders will be billed at individual rate until proof of status is received. Foreign air speed delivery is included in all Clinics' subscription prices. All prices are subject to change without notice. **POSTMASTER:** Send address changes to *Medical Clinics of North America*, Elsevier Health Sciences Division, Subscription Customer Service, 3251 Riverport Lane, Maryland Heights, MO 63043. **Customer Service: Telephone: 1-800-654-2452** (U.S. and Canada); **1-314-447-8871** (outside U.S. and Canada). **Fax:** 314-447-8029. **E-mail: journalscustomerserviceusa@elsevier.com** (for print support); **journalsonlinesupport-usa@elsevier.com** (for online support).

Reprints. For copies of 100 or more of articles in this publication, please contact the Commercial Reprints Department, Elsevier Inc., 360 Park Avenue South, New York, NY 10010-1710. Tel.: 212-633-3874; Fax: 212-633-3820; E-mail: reprints@elsevier.com.

Medical Clinics of North America is also published in Spanish by McGraw-Hill Interamericana Editores S. A., P.O. Box 5-237, 06500 Mexico, D.F., Mexico.

Medical Clinics of North America is covered in *MEDLINE/PubMed (Index Medicus), Current Contents, ASCA, Excerpta Medica, Science Citation Index, and ISI/BIOMED.*

Printed in the United States of America.

PROGRAM OBJECTIVE
The goal of the *Medical Clinics of North America* is to keep practicing physicians up to date with current clinical practice by providing timely articles reviewing the state of the art in patient care.

TARGET AUDIENCE
All practicing physicians and other healthcare professionals.

LEARNING OBJECTIVES
Upon completion of this activity, participants will be able to:
1. Review updates and recommendations for the treatment of obesity.
2. Discuss obesity in special populations such as aging and pregnant patients.
3. Recognize management options for obesity such as medical devices and surgery.

ACCREDITATION
The Elsevier Office of Continuing Medical Education (EOCME) is accredited by the Accreditation Council for Continuing Medical Education (ACCME) to provide continuing medical education for physicians.

The EOCME designates this enduring material for a maximum of 15 *AMA PRA Category 1 Credit*(s)™. Physicians should claim only the credit commensurate with the extent of their participation in the activity.

All other healthcare professionals requesting continuing education credit for this enduring material will be issued a certificate of participation.

DISCLOSURE OF CONFLICTS OF INTEREST
The EOCME assesses conflict of interest with its instructors, faculty, planners, and other individuals who are in a position to control the content of CME activities. All relevant conflicts of interest that are identified are thoroughly vetted by EOCME for fair balance, scientific objectivity, and patient care recommendations. EOCME is committed to providing its learners with CME activities that promote improvements or quality in healthcare and not a specific proprietary business or a commercial interest.

The planning committee, staff, authors and editors listed below have identified no financial relationships or relationships to products or devices they or their spouse/life partner have with commercial interest related to the content of this CME activity:
Bimal H. Ashar, MD, MBA, FACP; Linda A. Barbour, MD, MSPH; John A. Batsis, MD, AGSF; Fateh Bazerbachi, MD; Sarah Jean Borengasser, PhD; Meghan L. Butryn, PhD; Heidi Dutton, MD; Olivia Farr, PhD; Anjali Fortna; Laura Marie Gaudet, MD, MSc; Wael Ghaly, MD; Kevin D. Hall, PhD; Helen M. Heneghan, MD, PhD; Leon I. Igel, MD, FACP, DABOM; Scott Kahan, MD, MPH; Erin Joanne Keely, MD; Leah Logan; Christos Mantzoros, MD, PhD; Jessica McCool; Nikolaos Perakakis, MD, PhD; Jocelyn E. Remmert, BA; Monika Rizk, BS; Katherine H. Saunders, MD, DABOM; Alissa D. Smethers, MS, RD; Jeyanthi Surendrakumar; Allison M. Sweeney, PhD; Adam G. Tsai, MD, MSCE; Devika Umashanker, MD, MBA; Jagriti Upadhyay, MD; Eric J. Vargas, MD; Thomas A. Wadden, PhD; Dawn K. Wilson, PhD; Alexandra B. Zagari, BA.

The planning committee, staff, authors and editors listed below have identified financial relationships or relationships to products or devices they or their spouse/life partner have with commercial interest related to the content of this CME activity:
Barham K. Abu Dayyeh, MD, MPH is a consultant/advisor for Apollo Endosurgery, Inc; Boston Scientific Corporation; Olympus Corporation of the Americas; and Metamodix, and has research support from Aspire Bariatrics; Medtronic, Apollo Endosurgery, Inc; and GI Dynamics.
Louis J. Aronne, MD, FACP, DABOM, FTOS is a consultant/advisor for Jamieson Laboratories; Pfizer Inc; Novo Nordisk; Eisai Co., LTD; GI Dynamics; Real Appeal, Inc; Janssen Global Services, LLC; United-Health Group; and Gelesis, has stock ownership in BMIQ; Zafgen; Gelesis; MYOS RENS Technology Inc; Jamieson Laboratories, and has research support from Aspire Bariatrics; AstraZeneca; and Eisai Co., LTD.
Rekha B. Kumar, MD, MS, DABOM is on the speakers' bureau for Janssen Global Services, LLC and Novo Nordisk, has stock ownership in VIVUS Inc and Zafgen, and his spouse/partner has stock ownership in VIVUS Inc and Zafgen.
Robert F. Kushner, MD, MS is a consutlant/advisor at Novo Nordisk; Weight Watchers International, Inc; and Retrofit.
Barbara J. Rolls, PhD receives royalties/patents from the Volumetrics books published by HarperTorch.
Carel W. le Roux, MD, PhD is on the speakers' bureau for Novo Nordisk; Ethicon US, LLC; Medtronic; Orexigen Therapeutics, Inc.; and Boehringer Ingelheim GmbH, is a consultant/advisor for Novo Nordisk; Ethicon; Herbalife; GI Dynamics; and Boehringer Ingelheim GmbH.

Donna H. Ryan, MD is on the speakers' bureau for Novo Nordisk; Orexigen Therapeutics, Inc.; and Eisai Co., LTD., is a consultant/advisor for Novo Nordisk; Orexigen Therapeutics, Inc.; Eisai Co., LTD.; Scientific Intake; Gila Thereapeutics, Inc; and Baro Novo, and has stock ownership in Scientific Intake and Gila Therapeutics, Inc.

UNAPPROVED/OFF-LABEL USE DISCLOSURE

The EOCME requires CME faculty to disclose to the participants:

1. When products or procedures being discussed are off-label, unlabelled, experimental, and/or investigational (not US Food and Drug Administration [FDA] approved); and
2. Any limitations on the information presented, such as data that are preliminary or that represent ongoing research, interim analyses, and/or unsupported opinions. Faculty may discuss information about pharmaceutical agents that is outside of FDA-approved labelling. This information is intended solely for CME and is not intended to promote off-label use of these medications. If you have any questions, contact the medical affairs department of the manufacturer for the most recent prescribing information.

TO ENROLL

To enroll in the *Medical Clinics of North America* Continuing Medical Education program, call customer service at 1-800-654-2452 or sign up online at http://www.theclinics.com/home/cme. The CME program is available to subscribers for an additional annual fee of USD $295.

METHOD OF PARTICIPATION

In order to claim credit, participants must complete the following:

1. Complete enrolment as indicated above.
2. Read the activity.
3. Complete the CME Test and Evaluation. Participants must achieve a score of 70% on the test. All CME Tests and Evaluations must be completed online.

CME INQUIRIES/SPECIAL NEEDS

For all CME inquiries or special needs, please contact elsevierCME@elsevier.com.

MEDICAL CLINICS OF NORTH AMERICA

FORTHCOMING ISSUES

March 2018
Urology
Robert E. Brannigan, *Editor*

May 2018
Clinical Examination
Brian T. Garibaldi, *Editor*

July 2018
Substance Use and Addiction Medicine
Jeffrey H. Samet, Patrick O'Connor, and
Michael Stein, *Editors*

RECENT ISSUES

November 2017
Care of Cancer Survivors
Kimberly S. Peairs, *Editor*

September 2017
Complementary and Integrative Medicine
Robert B. Saper, *Editor*

July 2017
Disease Prevention
Michael P. Pignone and
Kirsten Bibbins-Domingo, *Editors*

ISSUE OF RELATED INTEREST

Physician Assistant Clinics, January 2017 (Vol. 2, No. 1)
Endocrinology
Ji Hyun Chun, *Editor*
Available at: http://www.physicianassistant.theclinics.com/

Contributors

CONSULTING EDITOR

BIMAL H. ASHAR, MD, MBA, FACP
Associate Professor of Medicine, Division of General Internal Medicine, The Johns Hopkins University School of Medicine, Baltimore, Maryland, USA

EDITORS

SCOTT KAHAN, MD, MPH
Director, National Center for Weight and Wellness, Medical Director, Strategies To Overcome and Prevent (STOP) Obesity Alliance, The George Washington University Milken Institute School of Public Health, The George Washington University School of Medicine, Chair, Clinical Committee, The Obesity Society, Washington, DC, USA; Johns Hopkins Bloomberg School of Public Health, Baltimore, Maryland, USA

ROBERT F. KUSHNER, MD
Professor in Medicine-Endocrinology, Northwestern University Feinberg School of Medicine, Northwestern Center on Obesity, Chicago, Illinois, USA

AUTHORS

BARHAM K. ABU DAYYEH, MD, MPH
Division of Gastroenterology and Hepatology, Mayo Clinic, Rochester, Minnesota, USA

LOUIS J. ARONNE, MD, FACP, DABOM, FTOS
Sanford I. Weill Professor of Metabolic Research, Comprehensive Weight Control Center, Division of Endocrinology, Diabetes and Metabolism, Weill Cornell Medicine, New York, New York, USA

LINDA A. BARBOUR, MD, MSPH
Professor of Endocrinology and Maternal-Fetal Medicine, University of Colorado School of Medicine, Aurora, Colorado, USA

JOHN A. BATSIS, MD, FACP, AGSF
Associate Professor of Medicine and of The Dartmouth Institute for Health Policy and Clinical Practice, Geisel School of Medicine at Dartmouth, Section of General Internal Medicine, Dartmouth-Hitchcock Medical Center, Lebanon, New Hampshire, USA

FATEH BAZERBACHI, MD
Division of Gastroenterology and Hepatology, Mayo Clinic, Rochester, Minnesota, USA

SARAH JEAN BORENGASSER, PhD
University of Colorado School of Medicine, Aurora, Colorado, USA

MEGHAN L. BUTRYN, PhD
Associate Professor, Department of Psychology, Drexel University, Philadelphia, Pennsylvania, USA

HEIDI DUTTON, MD
Lecturer, Department of Medicine, University of Ottawa, Ottawa, Ontario, Canada

OLIVIA FARR, PhD
Division of Endocrinology, Diabetes and Metabolism, Department of Internal Medicine, Beth Israel Deaconess Medical Center, Harvard Medical School, Boston, Massachusetts, USA

LAURA MARIE GAUDET, MD, MSc
Assistant Professor, Department of Obstetrics/Gynecology, University of Ottawa, Ottawa, Ontario, Canada

WAEL GHALY, MD
Division of Endocrinology, Diabetes and Metabolism, Department of Internal Medicine, Beth Israel Deaconess Medical Center, Harvard Medical School, Boston, Massachusetts, USA

KEVIN D. HALL, PhD
National Institute of Diabetes and Digestive and Kidney Diseases, Bethesda, Maryland, USA

HELEN M. HENEGHAN, MD, PhD
Department of Surgery, St. Vincent's University Hospital, University College Dublin, Elm Park, Dublin, Ireland

LEON I. IGEL, MD, FACP, DABOM
Assistant Professor of Clinical Medicine, Comprehensive Weight Control Center, Division of Endocrinology, Diabetes and Metabolism, Weill Cornell Medicine, New York, New York, USA

SCOTT KAHAN, MD, MPH
Director, National Center for Weight and Wellness, Medical Director, Strategies To Overcome and Prevent (STOP) Obesity Alliance, The George Washington University Milken Institute School of Public Health, The George Washington University School of Medicine, Chair, Clinical Committee, The Obesity Society, Washington, DC, USA; Johns Hopkins Bloomberg School of Public Health, Baltimore, Maryland, USA

ERIN JOANNE KEELY, MD
Professor, Department of Medicine, University of Ottawa, Ottawa, Ontario, Canada

REKHA B. KUMAR, MD, MS, DABOM
Assistant Professor of Medicine, Comprehensive Weight Control Center, Division of Endocrinology, Diabetes and Metabolism, Weill Cornell Medicine, New York, New York, USA

ROBERT F. KUSHNER, MD
Professor in Medicine-Endocrinology, Northwestern University Feinberg School of Medicine, Northwestern Center on Obesity, Chicago, Illinois, USA

CAREL W. LE ROUX, MD, PhD
Diabetes Complication Research Centre, UCD Conway Institute, School of Medicine and Medical Science, University College Dublin, Dublin, Ireland

CHRISTOS MANTZOROS, MD, PhD
Section of Endocrinology, Diabetes and Metabolism, Boston VA Healthcare System, Division of Endocrinology, Diabetes and Metabolism, Department of Internal Medicine, Beth Israel Deaconess Medical Center, Harvard Medical School, Boston, Massachusetts, USA

NIKOLAOS PERAKAKIS, MD, PhD
Division of Endocrinology, Diabetes and Metabolism, Department of Internal Medicine, Beth Israel Deaconess Medical Center, Harvard Medical School, Boston, Massachusetts, USA

JOCELYN E. REMMERT, BA
PhD Candidate, Department of Psychology, Drexel University, Philadelphia, Pennsylvania, USA

MONIKA RIZK, BS
Division of Gastroenterology and Hepatology, Mayo Clinic, Rochester, Minnesota, USA

BARBARA J. ROLLS, PhD
Professor and Guthrie Chair in Nutrition, Department of Nutritional Sciences, The Pennsylvania State University, University Park, Pennsylvania, USA

DONNA H. RYAN, MD
Professor Emerita, Pennington Biomedical Research Center, Baton Rouge, Louisiana, USA

KATHERINE H. SAUNDERS, MD, DABOM
Assistant Professor of Clinical Medicine, Comprehensive Weight Control Center, Division of Endocrinology, Diabetes and Metabolism, Weill Cornell Medicine, New York, New York, USA

ALISSA D. SMETHERS, MS, RD
Doctoral Student, Department of Nutritional Sciences, The Pennsylvania State University, University Park, Pennsylvania, USA

ALLISON M. SWEENEY, PhD
Department of Psychology, University of South Carolina, Columbia, South Carolina, USA

ADAM G. TSAI, MD, MSCE
Kaiser Permanente, Denver, Colorado; University of Colorado School of Medicine, Aurora, Colorado, USA

DEVIKA UMASHANKER, MD, MBA
Clinical Fellow of Obesity Medicine, Comprehensive Weight Control Center, Division of Endocrinology, Diabetes and Metabolism, Weill Cornell Medicine, New York, New York, USA

JAGRITI UPADHYAY, MD
Section of Endocrinology, Diabetes and Metabolism, Boston VA Healthcare System, Division of Endocrinology, Diabetes and Metabolism, Department of Internal Medicine, Beth Israel Deaconess Medical Center, Harvard Medical School, Massachusetts, USA

ERIC J. VARGAS, MD
Division of Gastroenterology and Hepatology, Mayo Clinic, Rochester, Minnesota, USA

THOMAS A. WADDEN, PhD
Albert J. Stunkard Professor of Psychology in Psychiatry and Director Emeritus, Center for Weight and Eating Disorders, Perelman School of Medicine University of Pennsylvania, Philadelphia, Pennsylvania, USA

DAWN K. WILSON, PhD
Department of Psychology, University of South Carolina, Columbia, South Carolina, USA

ALEXANDRA B. ZAGARIA, BA
Associate Professor of Medicine and of The Dartmouth Institute for Health Policy and Clinical Practice, Geisel School of Medicine at Dartmouth, Section of General Internal Medicine, Dartmouth-Hitchcock Medical Center, Lebanon, New Hampshire, USA

Contents

Foreword: In Search of the 70-kg Man   xv

Bimal H. Ashar

Preface: Obesity Medicine: A Core Competency for Primary Care Providers   xvii

Scott Kahan and Robert F. Kushner

Introduction: The State of Obesity in 2017   1

Robert F. Kushner and Scott Kahan

> Obesity continues to be a major national and global health challenge and a risk factor for an expanding set of chronic diseases. In 2015, high body mass index contributed to 4.0 million deaths globally, which represented 7.1% of the deaths from any cause. Obesity is now regarded as a disease, and multiple health care societies have begun to tackle obesity as a discrete target for assessment and treatment that is supported by several position statements and guidelines. Nonetheless, a perception and treatment gap continues to exist between health care providers and patients regarding the provision of obesity care.

Obesity as a Disease   13

Jagriti Upadhyay, Olivia Farr, Nikolaos Perakakis, Wael Ghaly, and Christos Mantzoros

> Obesity is a complex disease with many causal factors, associated with multiple comorbidities that contribute to significant morbidity and mortality. It is a highly prevalent disease that poses an enormous health and economic burden to society. This article reviews the mechanisms of obesity and its related comorbidities.

Treatment of Obesity in Primary Care   35

Adam G. Tsai, Jocelyn E. Remmert, Meghan L. Butryn, and Thomas A. Wadden

> This article outlines some of the behavioral, pharmacologic, and surgical interventions available to primary care physicians (PCPs) to help their patients with weight management. Studies on lifestyle modification, commercial weight loss programs, and medical and surgical options are reviewed. Several clinical suggestions on obesity management that PCPs can take back and use immediately in office practice are offered.

Guideline Recommendations for Obesity Management   49

Donna H. Ryan and Scott Kahan

> It is an obligation for all health care providers to participate in obesity management. This article discusses obesity guidelines from The Obesity Society, the Endocrine Society, and the American Association of Clinical

Endocrinologists. It reviews and compares findings and recommendations across these guidelines, identifies areas of controversy and concordance, and suggests how primary care practices may make use of the most appropriate recommendations for their circumstances.

Addressing Obesity in Aging Patients

65

John A. Batsis and Alexandra B. Zagaria

Obesity in older adults affects not only morbidity and mortality but also quality of life and the risk of institutionalization. Weight loss interventions can effectively lead to improved physical function. Diet-alone interventions can detrimentally affect muscle and bone physiology and, without interventions to affect these elements, can lead to adverse outcomes. Understanding social and nutritional issues facing older adults is of utmost importance to primary care providers. This article also discusses the insufficient evidence related to pharmacotherapy as well as providing an overview of using physiologic rather than chronologic age for identifying suitable candidates for bariatric surgery.

Obesity in Pregnancy: Optimizing Outcomes for Mom and Baby

87

Heidi Dutton, Sarah Jean Borengasser, Laura Marie Gaudet, Linda A. Barbour, and Erin Joanne Keely

Obesity is common in women of childbearing age, and management of this population around the time of pregnancy involves specific challenges. Weight and medical comorbidities should be optimized both before and during pregnancy. During pregnancy, gestational weight gain should be limited, comorbidities should be appropriately screened for and managed, and fetal health should be monitored. Consideration should be given to the optimal timing of delivery and to reducing surgical and anesthetic complications. In the postpartum period, breastfeeding and weight loss should be promoted. Maternal obesity is associated with adverse metabolic effects in offspring, promoting an intergenerational cycle of obesity.

Dietary Management of Obesity: Cornerstones of Healthy Eating Patterns

107

Alissa D. Smethers and Barbara J. Rolls

Several dietary patterns, both macronutrient and food based, can lead to weight loss. A key strategy for weight management that can be applied across dietary patterns is to reduce energy density. Clinical trials show that reducing energy density is effective for weight loss and weight loss maintenance. A variety of practical strategies and tools can help facilitate successful weight management by reducing energy density, providing portion control, and improving diet quality. The flexibility of energy density gives patients options to tailor and personalize their dietary pattern to reduce energy intake for sustainable weight loss.

The Role of Behavioral Medicine in the Treatment of Obesity in Primary Care

125

Scott Kahan, Dawn K. Wilson, and Allison M. Sweeney

Behavioral medicine provides a framework for supporting patients to achieve changes in target health behaviors, such as dietary and physical activity changes. Behavioral medicine fits alongside traditional medical treatments, can minimize the need for more intensive medical treatments, improves outcomes of these treatments, and improves adherence to medication prescriptions or postsurgical recommendations. This article provides an overview of behavioral medicine counseling for obesity in primary care, rooted in the "5 As" approach to health behavior change, and the basic outline of behavioral skills interventions in which health care providers use self-regulatory and behavioral strategies to improve health-related behaviors among patients with obesity.

Obesity Pharmacotherapy   135

Katherine H. Saunders, Devika Umashanker, Leon I. Igel, Rekha B. Kumar, and Louis J. Aronne

Although diet, physical activity, and behavioral modifications are the cornerstones of weight management, weight loss achieved by lifestyle modifications alone is often limited and difficult to maintain. Pharmacotherapy for obesity can be considered if patients have a body mass index (BMI) of 30 kg/m^2 or greater or BMI of 27 kg/m^2 or greater with weight-related comorbidities. The 6 most commonly used antiobesity medications are phentermine, orlistat, phentermine/topiramate extended release, lorcaserin, naltrexone sustained release (SR)/bupropion SR, and liraglutide, 3.0 mg. Successful pharmacotherapy for obesity depends on tailoring treatment to patients' behaviors and comorbidities and monitoring of efficacy, safety, and tolerability.

Medical Devices for Obesity Treatment: Endoscopic Bariatric Therapies   149

Eric J. Vargas, Monika Rizk, Fateh Bazerbachi, and Barham K. Abu Dayyeh

Endoscopic bariatric therapies (EBTs) are effective tools for the management of obesity. By mimicking restrictive and bypass surgery physiology, they provide a safe and effective treatment option with the added capabilities of reaching a broader population. Multiple efficacious medical devices, such as intragastric balloons, endoscopic suturing or plication devices, and bypass liners, at various stages of development are available in the United States. EBTs represent the newest addition to a multidisciplinary approach in obesity management. This article reviews several devices' safety and efficacy for primary care providers in the era of evolving obesity treatment.

Bariatric Surgery for Obesity   165

Carel W. le Roux and Helen M. Heneghan

In this review, the authors discuss the indications for and the published outcomes of commonly performed bariatric procedures, including weight loss, perioperative morbidity and mortality, late complications, as well as the impact of bariatric surgery on comorbidities, cardiovascular risk, and mortality. They also briefly discuss the mechanisms by which bariatric and metabolic surgery causes such significant weight loss and health gain.

Maintenance of Lost Weight and Long-Term Management of Obesity 183

Kevin D. Hall and Scott Kahan

Weight loss can be achieved through a variety of modalities, but long-term maintenance of lost weight is much more challenging. Obesity interventions typically result in early weight loss followed by a weight plateau and progressive regain. This article describes current understanding of the biological, behavioral, and environmental factors driving this near-ubiquitous body weight trajectory and the implications for long-term weight management. Treatment of obesity requires ongoing clinical attention and weight maintenance–specific counseling to support sustainable healthful behaviors and positive weight regulation.

Foreword

In Search of the 70-kg Man

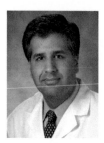

Bimal H. Ashar, MD, MBA, FACP
Consulting Editor

I remember only a small portion of what I was taught in medical school. The principles of pharmacology are a mere blur at this stage of my career. I have no recollection of how to calculate the volume of distribution of a drug after administration. Yet, I do remember that the 70-kg man was used as a reference for many such calculations. Interestingly, the concept of the "Reference Man" was developed by the International Commission on Radiological Protection in 1974 to assist in estimation and standardization of radiation exposure to individuals. A "standard man" was described as weighing 70 kg (154 pounds) and being 170 cm tall (5′7″). This individual would end up with a calculated body mass index (BMI) of 24.1 kg/m^2.

More than forty years have gone by since the "standard man" was defined. Over those four-plus decades, finding individuals (men or women) who conform to those measurements has become increasingly difficult. In the United States, individuals have become taller but their weight has increased much more dramatically. The Centers for Disease Control and Prevention estimates that on average men and women weigh 196 pounds and 169 pounds, respectively. More than 70% of adults in the United States are overweight (BMI $\geq$25-29 kg/m^2), whereas nearly 40% of adults are obese (BMI $\geq$30 kg/m^2).

In this issue of the *Medical Clinics of North America*, Drs Kahan and Kushner have enlisted experts from around the country to discuss the importance of recognizing obesity and its health consequences. The emphasis of this issue is on multimodality approaches to this highly prevalent chronic disease. It is hopeful that through this

Med Clin N Am 102 (2018) xv–xvi
https://doi.org/10.1016/j.mcna.2017.09.004
0025-7125/18/© 2017 Published by Elsevier Inc.

medical.theclinics.com

multimodal approach, the population as a whole will be able to break the trends in obesity rates and make the "standard man" appear more realistic.

Bimal H. Ashar, MD, MBA, FACP
Division of General Internal Medicine
The Johns Hopkins University School of Medicine
601 North Caroline Street
#7143
Baltimore, MD 21287, USA

E-mail address:
Bashar1@jhmi.edu

Preface

Obesity Medicine: A Core Competency for Primary Care Providers

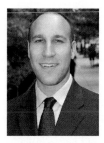 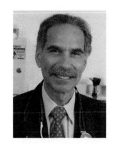

Scott Kahan, MD, MPH   Robert F. Kushner, MD
Editors

Few medical topics are more important to be addressed in primary care than obesity. Nearly 40% of American adults have clinical obesity; 70% have a body mass index greater than 25 kg/m^2.[1] Obesity increases the risk for hundreds of diseases, disability, impaired quality of life, and premature mortality, and strikingly increases health care costs.[2–6] With such a large proportion of Americans being affected by obesity and its associated conditions, the primary care workforce is best positioned to lead the way toward progress. Unfortunately, that has not been the case. Primary care providers have minimal training and confidence in addressing obesity, and medical credentialing examinations do not sufficiently include questions testing obesity knowledge.[7–9] Few patients with obesity receive screening and documentation of obesity in primary care, let alone receive counseling or evidence-based treatment for obesity.[10–12]

For these reasons, this issue of *Medical Clinics of North America* focuses on obesity medicine in primary care, offering health care providers guidance on addressing the range of issues surrounding obesity. The initial articles in this issue describe the current state of obesity in 2017, including updated information on the national and international burden of obesity, staging of obesity, models of care, and the (relatively) newly formed specialty of obesity medicine; why obesity should be treated as a disease, including an updated review of causes and mechanisms of obesity and pathways through which obesity leads to comorbidities; and overviews of principles of obesity treatment in primary care and published obesity treatment guidelines. We then review management of obesity in two special populations: older adults and pregnancy, reviewing patient assessment, goals of treatment, and nuances of treatment for each unique patient population. From there, several articles review a range of treatment modalities from

Med Clin N Am 102 (2018) xvii–xix
https://doi.org/10.1016/j.mcna.2017.09.003
0025-7125/18/© 2017 Published by Elsevier Inc.

the perspective of the primary care provider: nutrition and lifestyle management, behavioral counseling for obesity, obesity pharmacotherapy, medical devices for obesity treatment, and bariatric surgery. Finally, we conclude with an offering on weight maintenance and long-term management, offering perspectives of both physiology and behavior.

We hope this issue of *Medical Clinics of North America* will be a valuable resource for primary care clinicians, and we hope to see many more publications on this important topic in the future.

Scott Kahan, MD, MPH
National Center for Weight and Wellness
Strategies To Overcome and Prevent (STOP)
Obesity Alliance
George Washington University
Milken Institute School of Public Health
The Obesity Society
1020 19th Street NW, Suite 450
Washington, DC 20036, USA

Robert F. Kushner, MD
Northwestern University
Feinberg School of Medicine
Northwestern Center on Obesity
750 North Lake Shore Drive
Rubloff 9-976
Chicago, IL 60611, USA

E-mail addresses:
kahan@gwu.edu (S. Kahan)
rkushner@northwestern.edu (R.F. Kushner)

REFERENCES

1. Flegal KM, Knuszon-Moran D, Carroll MD, et al. Trends in obesity among adults in the United States, 2005-2014. J Am Med Assoc 2016;315(20):2284–91.

2. Yuen M, Earle R, Kadambi N, et al. A systematic review and evaluation of current evidence reveals 236 obesity-associated disorders. New Orleans (LA): The Obesity Society; 2016. p. T-P-3166.

3. Batsis JA, Zbehlik AJ, Barre LK, et al. Impact of obesity on disability, function, and physical activity: data from the Osteoarthritis Initiative. Scand J Rheumatol 2015;44:495–502.

4. Kushner RF, Foster GD. Obesity and quality of life. Nutrition 2000;16:947–52.

5. Kitahara CM, Flint AJ, Berrington de Gonzalez A, et al. Association between class III obesity and mortality (BMI of 40-59 kg/m2): a pooled analysis of 20 prospective studies. PLoS Med 2014;11(7):e1001673.

6. Withrow D, Alter DA. The economic burden of obesity worldwide: a systematic review of the direct costs of obesity. Obes Rev 2011;12(2):131–41.

7. Petrin C, Kahan S, Turner M, et al. Current attitudes and practices of obesity counselling by health care providers. Obes Res Clin Pract 2016;11(3):352–9.

8. Gunther S, Guo F, Sinfield P, et al. Barriers and enablers to managing obesity in general practice: a practical approach for use in implementation activities. Qual Prim Care 2012;20(2):93–103.

9. Kushner RF, Butsch WS, Kahan S, et al. Obesity coverage on medical licensing examinations in the United States. What is being tested? Teach Learn Med 2017; 29(2):123–8.
10. Post RE, Mainous AG 3rd, Gregorie SH, et al. The influence of physician acknowledgment of patients' weight status on patient perceptions of overweight and obesity in the United States. Arch Intern Med 2011;171(4):316–21.
11. Bardia A, Holtan SG, Slezak JM, et al. Diagnosis of obesity by primary care physicians and impact on obesity management. Mayo Clin Proc 2007;82(8):927–32.
12. Kraschnewski JL, Sciamanna CN, Stuckey HL, et al. A silent response to the obesity epidemic: decline in US physician weight counseling. Med Care 2013; 51(2):186–92.

Introduction
The State of Obesity in 2017

 CrossMark

Robert F. Kushner, MD, MS[a],*, Scott Kahan, MD, MPH[b,c]

KEYWORDS

- Obesity • Prevalence • Disease • Morbidity • Models of care

KEY POINTS

- Obesity is now included among the global noncommunicable disease targets identified by the World Health Organization and is a risk factor for an expanding set of chronic diseases.
- The global burden of obesity is related to the association between body mass index (BMI) and increased morbidity and mortality.
- Several position papers and guidelines have recently been published that provide recommendations for assessment and treatment of patients with obesity.
- A redesign of the health care environment to provide more effective and efficient obesity care is needed.
- The American Board of Obesity Medicine was founded facilitate increased competency and recognition for physicians to provide better-quality obesity care.

INTRODUCTION

Assessing where we stand in 2017 is an interesting exercise, now that we are several decades into the US obesity epidemic. On the one hand, there are several areas of progress, including increased awareness, increased political and social will to address obesity, new treatment options, and greatly expanded evidence base for prevention and intervention strategies. In contrast, prevalence rates have not declined, and severe obesity rates are still growing rapidly, and global obesity rates are steadily rising, now nearly 2 decades since the first Surgeon General's report on obesity,[1] with prevalence in many Western and non-Western countries now catching up with the United States. It will be important to continue current progress as well as significantly expand the scope and intensity of focus to make further gains at managing this chronic disease.

Disclosure Statement: R.F. Kushner has no disclosures.
[a] Northwestern University Feinberg School of Medicine, 750 North Lake Shore Drive, Rubloff 9-976, Chicago, IL 60611, USA; [b] Johns Hopkins Bloomberg School of Public Health, Baltimore, MD, USA; [c] Department of Health Policy and Management, 1020 19th Street NW #450, Washington, DC 20036, USA
* Corresponding author.
E-mail address: rkushner@northwestern.edu

Med Clin N Am 102 (2018) 1–11
http://dx.doi.org/10.1016/j.mcna.2017.08.003
0025-7125/18/© 2017 Elsevier Inc. All rights reserved.

medical.theclinics.com

THE BURDEN OF OBESITY

Obesity continues to be a major national and global health challenge and a risk factor for an expanding set of chronic diseases, including cardiovascular disease (CVD), diabetes, chronic kidney disease, nonalcoholic fatty liver disease, metabolic syndrome, and many cancers, among other comorbid conditions. Along with its increased global prevalence over the past decades, obesity is now included among the global noncommunicable disease targets identified by the World Health Organization.[2] A recent update of the Global Burden of Diseases (GBD) study quantified the burden of diseases related to high body mass index (BMI) during the period from 1990 through 2015.[3] Burden of disease was assessed by deaths and disability-adjusted life-years (DALYs), a composite metric defined as the sum of years lived with disability due to premature mortality and years lived with disability. In 2015, high BMI contributed to 4.0 million deaths globally, which represented 7.1% of the deaths from any cause. It also contributed to 120 million DALYs, which represented 4.9% of DALYs from any cause among adults. CVD was the leading cause of death and DALYs related to high BMI, followed by chronic kidney disease.

In 2014, the McKinsey Global Institute issued a report titled, "Overcoming obesity: an initial economic analysis," that contextualized the economic burden of obesity.[4] The report assessed the current impact to society of 14 major problems that are caused by humans, that is, those that are the result of human decisions, are amplified by human or societal behavior, or depend on societal, legal, or infrastructural environments created by humans. They estimated that the global economic impact of obesity is roughly $2 trillion, or 2.8% of global GDP. Among the sources of cost that were assessed, lost productivity was the most significant seen in their analysis, accounting for nearly 70% of the total global cost of obesity. The most striking finding was that obesity is one of the top 3 global social burdens, only being surpassed by smoking, armed violence, war, and terrorism. An additional analysis by the Milken Foundation estimates costs of more than $1 trillion in the United States alone, when taking into account direct and indirect medical and nonmedical costs of obesity.[5] Obesity can be considered a "syndemic," a new term defined as a condition in which biology, behavior, and social factors create the conditions in which several health conditions cluster and affect the health burden of the population.[6]

In addition to the burden caused by obesity, its prevalence rates are astounding. In 2015, a total of 107.7 million children and 603.7 million adults had obesity worldwide.[3] The overall prevalence of obesity was 5.0% among children and 12.0% among adults, a rapid increase in recent decades. Whereas the prevalence of underweight was more than double that of obesity 4 decades ago, the trend has now reversed: more people have obesity than underweight, both globally and in essentially all regions of the world.[7] The prevalence of obesity in the United States and Canada is among the highest in the world. According to the National Health and Nutrition Examination Survey (NHANES) 2013 to 2014 dataset, 36.5% of US adults and 17.0% of youth aged 2 to 19 years had obesity.[8] These data translates into 82.7 million adults and 12.7 million children and youth, respectively. More women (38.3%) than men (34.3%) were obese, with non-Hispanic black women (48.1%) showing the highest prevalence rates. Obesity prevalence has been steady among youth since 2003 to 2004 and overall among adults since 2011 to 2012.[9] However, prevalence rates in certain subpopulations continues to increase, and in particular, the rate of severe obesity (BMI $\geq$40 kg/m^2) continues to increase steadily.[10] The overall prevalence rates remain significantly above the Healthy People 2020 targets. The corresponding adult obesity prevalence rate among Canadians in 2014 was 20.2%, or roughly 5.3 million individuals.

ASSOCIATION WITH INCREASED MORBIDITY AND MORTALITY

The global burden of obesity is related to the association between BMI and increased morbidity and mortality. BMI provides the most useful population-level measurement of overweight and obesity, and its utility as an estimate of risk has been demonstrated in multiple large population studies across multiple continents.[11,12] The increased obesity-related morbidity was recently demonstrated in the Patient Outcome Research to Advance Learning study of more than 12 million US individuals who were overweight or had obesity and assessed for the prevalence of cardiometabolic risk factors (CRFs): elevated blood pressure, elevated triglycerides, low high-density lipoprotein–cholesterol, and prediabetes. Compared with overweight, obesity classes I (BMI 25–29.9), II (BMI 30–39.9), and III (BMI $\geq$40) were associated with a nearly 2-fold, 3-fold, and 4-fold greater probability of having at least 1 CRF.[13] Among those with obesity, only 9.6% had none of the CRFs.

The "J-shaped dose-response curve" for BMI and mortality has recently been confirmed in a large meta-analysis[14] and systematic review.[15] In the first study, data from 239 prospective studies involving 10.6 million participants from 32 countries were followed for a median of 13.7 years. All-cause mortality was minimal at 20 to 25 kg/m^2 with mortalities associated with increasing grades of overweight and obesity. The population-attributable fraction for all-cause mortality due to overweight or obesity was 19% in North America, the highest among the countries studied. In the second study, 228 cohort studies involving 30 million participants were reviewed for the relationship between BMI and all-cause mortality. A J-shaped association was seen among healthy people who had never smoked, with the lowest mortality observed at a BMI of 20 to 22 kg/m^2 with longer durations of follow-up. These 2 studies confirm that both overweight and obesity increases the risk of all-cause mortality and should be prioritized on a population level. Another publication that combined 3 prospective cohort studies totaling more than 225,000 men and women highlighted the importance of the weight history in identifying increased mortality risk.[16] In this analysis, maximum BMI over 16 years of weight history (as opposed to weight at a given point in time) in the overweight or obesity categories demonstrated an elevated risk for all-cause and cardiovascular death. This study supports that clinical practice of asking patients to report their maximum weight when taking a medical history. In addition, prospectively monitoring body weight trajectories and patterns of obesity shows promise in identifying phenotypes that may be at increased risk for developing comorbid conditions.[17–19] A recent systematic review identified 195 comorbid conditions associated with obesity.[20] The mechanisms whereby increased BMI is linked to increased morbidity and mortality vary by disease state and are more fully addressed in Jagriti Upadhyay and colleagues' article, "Obesity as a Disease," in this issue.

OBESITY AS A DISEASE, CLINICAL GUIDELINES, AND STAGING SYSTEMS

Based on the complexity of body weight regulation, the increased morbidity and mortality associated with obesity, and the substantial public health burden, obesity was officially recognized as a disease by the American Medical Association in 2013, along with multiple other organizations since, most recently by the World Obesity Federation.[21] Furthermore, identifying the impact of excess weight on multiple organ systems, wide-ranging health care societies have begun to tackle obesity as a discrete target for assessment and treatment. For example, in 2014, the American Society of Clinical Oncology issued a Position Statement on obesity and cancer in order to increase education and awareness, provide tools and resources, and build research opportunities.[22] Two recent review articles highlight the association between obesity (adiposity) and increased cancer risk.[23,24] In 2017, the American Gastroenterological Association issued a practice guide on obesity and weight management, education, and resources that emphasized a comprehensive approach to assessment, treatment, and prevention.[25] This guideline is particularly important for the increasing number of gastroenterologists who are performing endoscopic procedures for the treatment of obesity that include placement of intragastric balloons, plications and suturing of the stomach, and insertion of a duodenal-jejunal bypass liner among other procedures.[26] These novel therapies are further explored in Eric J. Vargas and colleagues article, "Medical Devices for Obesity Treatment – Endoscopic Bariatric Therapies (EBTs)," in this issue. Several other obesity treatment guidelines have been recently published as a resource for clinicians. Most notable are the American Heart Association/American College of Cardiology/The Obesity Society *Guideline for the Management of Overweight and Obesity in Adults*,[27] The American Society of Clinical Endocrinologists (AACE) and the American College of Endocrinology (ACE) *Clinical Practice Guidelines for Comprehensive Care of Patients with Obesity*,[28] the American Obesity Association Obesity Management Algorithm,[29] and the *Pharmacologic Management of Obesity* guidelines from the Endocrine Society.[30] A more expansive discussion of the guidelines is found in Donna H. Ryan and Scott Kahan's article, "Guideline Recommendations for Obesity Management," in this issue.

Efforts are also underway to develop more practical and useful assessments to identify patients who require increased medical attention. Analogous to other staging systems commonly used for congestive heart failure or chronic kidney disease, a cardiometabolic disease staging system was developed that assigns patients to 1 of 5 risk categories using quantitative parameters readily available to the clinician without regard to BMI.[31] With advancement from stage 0 to stage 4, there are significant increments in risk and adjusted hazard ratio for diabetes, all-cause mortality, and CVD-related mortality. A refinement of the staging system was incorporated in the recently released AACE/ACE guideline.[28] Using this guideline, obesity disease stage is based on ethnic-specific BMI cutoffs along with assessment for adiposity-related complications. Stage 0 is assigned to individuals who are overweight or obese by BMI classification but have no complications, whereas stage 1 and 2 are defined as individuals who are overweight or obese by BMI classification and having 1 or more mild to moderate complications (stage 1) or at least 1 severe complication (stage 2). Building off of this complications-centric approach to obesity care, AACE/ACE recently proposed a new diagnostic term for obesity using the abbreviation "ABCD": adiposity-based chronic disease.[32] Last, a different functional staging system for obesity was proposed by Sharma and Kushner.[33] Using a risk-stratification construct, called the Edmonton Obesity Staging System, individuals with obesity are classified into 5 graded categories, based on their morbidity and health-risk profile along 3 domains: medical, functional, and mental. The staging system was shown to predict increased mortality among 2 large population cohorts.[34,35]

PROVISION OF OBESITY TREATMENT

Despite the impact of obesity on morbidity and mortality, treatment continues to be difficult for primary care providers. Cited factors include lack of comfort with providing effective counseling, insufficient time, and limited resources among other barriers. In 2008, the National Cancer Institute conducted the National Survey of Energy Balance-Related Care among primary care physicians (EB-PCP) to assess the practice of delivering obesity care.[36,37] Results of the national survey were recently published and provide insight to physicians' personal beliefs and practice characteristics.

Ninety-seven percent of PCPs thought that physicians have a responsibility to promote healthy weight behaviors to their patients, and 80% thought they needed to be a role model. In contrast, only 63% thought they were able to deliver effective strategies for weight control, and 53% thought they were personally effective in changing patient behavior. Although most PCPs provided specific guidance on physical activity or diet, only 26% reported comprehensively providing obesity care by regularly assessing BMI, providing counseling on weight control, and systematically tracking patients over time. In a more recent survey conducted among 1501 health care providers (HCPs), 97% of respondents indicated some level of responsibility to counsel patients about obesity.[38] Most commonly cited barriers included lack of time, insufficient training, lack of reimbursement, and lack of access to patient education tools.

These studies show that clinicians recognize their role in treating obesity but do not have the resources or clinical environment to do so. Furthermore, rather than focusing on obesity as a discrete medical problem, PCPs are more likely to address obesity as a risk factor for another chronic condition, such as hypertension, hyperlipidemia, or diabetes. Data from the 2012 National Ambulatory Medical Care Survey bear this out.[39] In this study, hypertension, hyperlipidemia, diabetes, and depression were listed at a higher percentage of visits for obesity than at visits for other diagnoses. The tendency to embed weight-loss counseling within other types of medical visits rather than tackling it as a discrete medical problem is a common occurrence.[40] This observation may explain, in part, the modest weight loss outcomes that are achieved in primary care practice and discussed in Adam G. Tsai and colleagues' article, "Treatment of Obesity in Primary Care," in this issue.

Patient perspectives on obesity also need to be considered when rendering treatment. A recently released nationally representative survey of 1509 adults conducted by National Opinion Research Center (NORC) at the University of Chicago and the American Society for Metabolic and Bariatric Surgery show some conflicting views for HCPs to consider.[41] Although obesity ties with cancer as the most serious issue for Americans and 94% agree that obesity increases a person's risk of dying early even if they do not have any other health conditions, only 38% consider obesity in and of itself to be a disease. Lack of individual willpower is cited as the biggest barrier to weight loss, and 95% of Americans are trying to lose weight on their own through diet or exercise. Only 42% of those with obesity are seeking help with a doctor; 25% are seeing a dietitian, and 10% are using a prescription medication. Thus, there is a "perception and treatment gap" between HCPs and patients regarding obesity care that needs to be addressed when rendering obesity care.

PHARMACOTHERAPY

One of the resources available for the treatment of obesity is antiobesity medication (AOM). Use of medication is well defined in the obesity treatment guidelines based on their demonstrated weight loss efficacy and associated metabolic improvements. Four medications have been approved by the US Food and Drug Administration since 2012: phentermine/topiramate, lorcaserin, naltrexone/bupropion, and liraglutide 3.0 mg.[42] However, unlike other medical diseases, AOMs are infrequently prescribed by HCPs, even when clear indicators for use are present. Data from the 2007 to 2008 NHANES survey showed that only 2.2% of eligible respondents took prescription drugs for weight control.[43] Another retrospective analysis using information from the GE Centricity database from 2002 to 2011 and covering 1.8 million patients with overweight or obesity was recently published.[44] In this study, only 0.7% of patients received pharmacotherapy, and fewer than 2% of patients with severe obesity received pharmacotherapy. Although these surveys covered a period of time before approval of the 4 new medications, there is little evidence that prescription rates have increased dramatically. The low utilization rates are due to multiple factors, including lack of education and familiarity among HCPs, cost and limited insurance coverage, and concerns about sufficient efficacy and long-term risks. Practical use of pharmacotherapy is reviewed in Katherine H. Saunders and colleagues article, "Obesity Pharmacotherapy," in this issue.

MODELS OF CARE

Redesigning the health care environment to provide more effective and efficient obesity and chronic disease care is challenging. The chronic care model initially described a reengineering of the health care organization to include changes in decision support, development of clinical informatics, using well-designed delivery systems, involvement of community resources, and enhanced self-management.[45] This model has recently been updated into a new framework that integrates clinical and community systems to prevent and manage obesity.[46,47] The clinical system is envisioned as an interdisciplinary mix of HCPs, such as dietitians, nurse practitioners, social workers, and psychologists, who can facilitate long-term behavior change. The 5A2 Team (5AsT) intervention in Canada is currently applying this practice redesign to create clinic-based multidisciplinary teams to support of obesity care.[48,49] The complementary community component includes health workers, community leaders, programs, and organizations that provide a healthy and supportive environment that fosters healthy behaviors. Two models: the Patient-Centered Medical Homes, which is designed to improve quality of care through team-based coordination of care, and Affordable Care Organizations, which are groups of doctors, hospitals, and other HCPs, who come together to give coordinated high-quality care, have incorporated many of these components. An additional novel chronic care model was proposed by Milani and Lavie,[50] in which they describe integrated practice units that employ nonphysician personnel who are dedicated to a specific disease condition for the full cycle of care. In this model, patients are connected to the health delivery system using apps as well as home-based and wearable devices, with communication at regular intervals between the care team and the patient. This proposed model leverages the advances in technology that are currently underway and well suited for obesity care.

A newly proposed practice-based integrated model for provision of obesity care is shown in **Fig. 1**. In this model, comorbid conditions, such as hypertension, diabetes, and obstructive sleep apnea, are assessed and treated. In addition, patients are assessed for their readiness to engage in active obesity care using shared decision making. Depending on the practice setting, the HCP and patient can follow 1 of 4 treatment pathways. In the first scenario, HCPs provide weight management themselves, using lifestyle counseling and pharmacotherapy when indicated. In the second scenario, HCPs refer to resources outside of their practice to implement obesity treatment, such as commercial or Internet-based programs, registered dietitians, or disease management consultants. The third scenario depicts a multidisciplinary team approach whereby HCPs coordinate care with other professionals within their practice or health care setting and provide a range of treatments, including lifestyle counseling, pharmacotherapy, and behavioral therapy. In the fourth scenario, the patient is referred to an obesity medicine specialist for more intensive therapy that may include comprehensive lifestyle treatment, pharmacotherapy, very-low calorie diets, bariatric surgery, or placement of a gastrointestinal

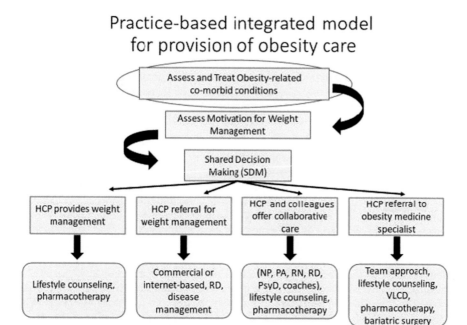

Fig. 1. The integrated model depicts 4 treatment scenarios among primary care providers for the provision of obesity care. HCP, health care provider; NP, nurse practitioner; PA, physician assistant; PsyD, psychologist; RD, registered dietitian; VLCD, very-low calorie diet.

device (see Eric J. Vargas and colleagues' article, "Medical Devices for Obesity Treatment: Endoscopic Bariatric Therapies (EBTs);" and Carel W. le Roux and Helen M. Heneghan's article, "Bariatric Surgery for Obesity," in this issue). All 4 scenarios are reasonable and focus on obesity as a discrete medical problem.

OBESITY MEDICINE SPECIALIST

The practice-based integrated model for provision of obesity care discussed above requires an increased competency among physicians to provide obesity care. This can be accomplished through continuing medical education (CME), promulgation of recommendations and clinical guidelines, and health care quality improvement initiatives. However, based on the increased prevalence and burden of overweight and obesity among US adults and children, need for more advanced competency in the field of obesity among some providers, and anticipated advances in obesity care over the next decade, there is rationale for developing a certification in obesity medicine. Thus, The American Board of Obesity Medicine (ABOM) was established in 2011 (www.abom.org). Certification as an ABOM diplomate signifies specialized knowledge in the practice of obesity medicine and distinguishes a physician as having achieved competency in obesity care. The ABOM board describes an obesity medicine physician as follows:

- A physician with expertise in the field of obesity medicine. This field requires competency in and a thorough understanding of the treatment of obesity and the genetic, biologic, environmental, social, and behavioral factors that contribute to obesity.

- The obesity medicine physician uses therapeutic interventions, including diet, physical activity, behavioral change, and pharmacotherapy.
- The obesity medicine physician uses a comprehensive approach and may include additional resources such as nutritionists, exercise physiologists, psychologists, and bariatric surgeons as indicated to achieve optimal results.
- In addition, the obesity medicine physician maintains competency in providing presurgical, perisurgical, and postsurgical care of bariatric surgery patients, promotes the prevention of obesity, and advocates for those who suffer from obesity.

In lieu of the paucity of fellowships available in obesity medicine, candidates for the ABOM examination are expected to gain knowledge about obesity through CME activities and self-directed practice experience. Since provision of the first certifying examination in 2012, the number of candidates enrolling in the examination has steadily increased.[51] As of 2017, there are 2068 certified Diplomats of which 53% are women. As an indication of a new specialty, 64% of Diplomats have spent less than 5 years in the practice of obesity medicine. Time spent devoted to obesity medicine varies among the Diplomats: 38% spend less than a quarter of time focused on obesity care; another third allocate 25% to 50% of time; and nearly 1 in 5 dedicate more than 75% of time exclusively to obesity medicine. The first group is represented by Internal Medicine or Family Medicine PCPs (66% of total Diplomats) who designate the equivalent of 1 day a week to obesity care. In contrast, the group that devotes greater than three-quarters of their time to obesity is primarily represented by physicians who practice in a specialty care setting. Overall, 57.4% of Diplomats participate in the care of patients who have undergone bariatric surgery. As of this time, the ABOM is not a member board of the American Board of Medical Specialties.

SUMMARY

Obesity continues to be a highly prevalent condition that poses a serious health and economic burden. It is generally considered to be a disease by both the public and HCPs, and multiple guidelines have been developed to aid the assessment and treatment process. However, because of demands placed on the primary care provider and the current structure of health care, obesity is seldom addressed as a discrete medical problem. Rather, it is often embedded in the care of other chronic diseases. Newly proposed models for the provision of obesity have been suggested that would incorporate a multidisciplinary team and coordinate care between the clinical and community environment. To meet the demands for creating a more competent work force, the ABOM was established and continues to grow as more physicians seek recognition as a specialist in this emerging field.

REFERENCES

1. The Surgeon General's Call to Action to Prevent and Decrease Overweight and Obesity 2001. Available at: https://www.cdc.gov/nccdphp/dnpa/pdf/calltoaction.pdf. Accessed August 2, 2017.
2. Kontis V, Mathers CD, Rehm J, et al. Contribution of six risk factors to achieving the 25×25 non-communicable disease mortality reduction target: a modelling study. Lancet 2014;384:427.
3. GBD 2015 Obesity Collaborators. Health effects of overweight and obesity in 195 countries over 25 years. N Engl J Med 2017;377:13–27.

4. McKinsey Global Institute. Overcoming obesity: an initial economic analysis, McKinsey and company. 2014. Available at: file:///C:/Users/Robert%20Kushner/Downloads/MGI_Overcoming_obesity_Full_report%20(1).pdf. Accessed July 30, 2017.

5. Weighing Down America: the health and economic impact of obesity. Available at: http://www.milkeninstitute.org/publications/view/833. Accessed August 2, 2017.

6. Singer M, Bulled N, Ostrach B, et al. Syndemics and the biosocial conception of health. Lancet 2017;389:941–50.

7. NCD Risk Factor Collaboration. Trends in adult body-mass index in 200 countries from 1975 to 21014: a pooled analysis of 1698 population-based measurement studies with 19.2 million participants. Lancet 2016;387:1377–96.

8. Ogden CL, Carroll MD, Fryar CD, et al. Prevalence of obesity among adults and youth: United States, 2011-2014. NCHS Data Brief; No. 219. Hyattsville (MD): National Center for Health Statistics; 2015.

9. Flegal KM, Knuszon-Moran D, Carroll MD, et al. Trends in obesity among adults in the United States, 2005-2014. J Am Med Assoc 2016;315(20):2284–91.

10. Ogden CL, Carroll MD, Kit BK, et al. Prevalence of childhood and adult obesity in the United States, 2011-2012. JAMA 2014;311(8):806–14.

11. Prospective Studies Collaborative. Body-mass index and cause-specific mortality in 900,000 adults: collaborative analysis of 57 prospective studies. Lancet 2009; 373:1083–96.

12. Berrington de Gonzalez A, Hartge P, Cerhan JR, et al. Body-mass index and mortality among 1.6 million white adults. N Engl J Med 2010;363:2211–21.

13. Nichols GA, Horberg M, Koebnick C, et al. Cardiometabolic risk factors among 1.3 million adults with overweight or obesity, but not diabetes, in 10 geographic diverse regions of the United States, 2012-2013. Prev Chronic Dis 2017;14: 160438.

14. The Global BMI Mortality Collaboration. Body-mass index and all-cause mortality: individual-participant-data meta-analysis of 239 prospective studies in four continents. Lancet 2016;388:776–86.

15. Aune D, Sen A, Prasad M, et al. BMI and all cause mortality: systematic review and non-linear dose-response meta-analysis of 230 cohort studies with 3.74 million deaths among 30.3 million participants. BMJ 2016;353:i2156.

16. Yu E, Ley SH, Manson JE, et al. Weight history and all-cause and cause-specific mortality in three prospective cohort studies. Ann Intern Med 2017;166(9): 613–20.

17. Petrick JL, Kelly SP, Liso LM, et al. Body weight trajectories and risk of oesophageal and gastric cardia adenocarcinomas: a pooled analysis of NIH-AARP and PLCO studies. Br J Cancer 2017;116:951–9.

18. Vistisen D, Witte DR, Tabak AG, et al. Patterns of obesity development before diagnosis of type 2 diabetes: the Whitehall II Cohort Study. PLoS Med 2014; 11(2):e1001602.

19. Wanigatunga AA, Sourdet SS, LaMonte MJ, et al, for the Women's Health Initiative Investigators. Physical impairment and body weight history in postmenopausal women: the Women's Health Initiative. Public Health Nutr 2016;19:3169–77.

20. Yuen MM, Kahan S, Kaplan LM, et al. Poster T-P-3166: a systematic review and evaluation of current evidence reveals 195 obesity-associated disorders. The Obesity Society. New Orleans, LA, October 31 - November 4, 2016.

21. Bray GA, Kim KK, Wilding JPH. Obesity: a chronic relapsing progressive disease process. A Position Statement of the World Obesity Federation. Obes Rev 2017; 18:715–23.
22. Ligibel JA, Alfano CM, Courneya KS, et al. American Society of Clinical Oncology Position Statement on Obesity and Cancer. J Clin Oncol 2014;32(31):3568–74.
23. Lauby-Secretan B, Scocdianti C, Loomis D, et al, for the International Agency for Research on Cancer Handbook Working Group. Body fatness and cancer–viewpoint of the IARC Working Group. N Engl J Med 2016;375:794–8.
24. Kygiou M, Kalliala I, Markozannes G, et al. Adiposity and cancer at major anatomical sites: umbrella review of the literature. BMJ 2017;356:477.
25. Acosta A, Street S, Kroh MD, et al. White paper AGA: POWER–practice guide on obesity and weight management, education, and resources. Clin Gastroenterol Hepatol 2017;15(5):631–49.
26. Sullivan S, Edmundowicz SA, Thompson CC. Endoscopic bariatric and metabolic therapies: new and emerging technologies. Gastroenterology 2017;152: 1791–801.
27. Jensen MD, Ryan DH, Apovian CM, American College of Cardiology/American Heart Association Task Force on Practice Guidelines, Obesity Society. 2013 AHA/ACC/TOS guidelines for the management of overweight and obesity is adults: a report of the American College of Cardiology/American Heart Association task force on practice guidelines and The Obesity Society. Circulation 2014; 129(25 Suppl 2):S102–38.
28. Garvey WT, Mechanick JI, Brett EM, et al. American Association of Clinical Endocrinologists and American College of Endocrinology Comprehensive clinical practice guidelines for medical care of patients with obesity. Endocr Pract 2016;22(7):842–84.
29. Obesity Algorithm: Clinical Guidelines for Obesity Treatment. Obesity Medical Association. Available at: https://obesitymedicine.org/obesity-algorithm/. Accessed September 21, 2017.
30. Apovian CM, Aronne LJ, Bessesen DH, et al. Pharmacological management of obesity: an Endocrine Society clinical practice guideline. J Clin Endocrinol Metab 2015;100(2):342–62.
31. Daniel S, Soleymani T, Garvey WT. A complications-based clinical staging of obesity to guide treatment modality and intensity. Curr Opin Endocrinol Diabetes Obes 2013;20:377–88.
32. Mechanick JI, Hurley DL, Garvey W. Adiposity-based chronic disease as a new diagnostic term: the American Association of Clinical Endocrinologists and American College of Endocrinology Position Statement. Endocr Pract 2017;23(3): 372–8.
33. Sharma AM, Kushner RF. A proposed clinical staging system for obesity. Int J Obes (Lond) 2009;33:289–95.
34. Kuk JL, Ardern CI, Church TS, et al. Edmonton obesity staging system: association with weight history and mortality risk. Appl Physiol Nutr Metab 2011;36: 570–6.
35. Padwal RS, Pajewski NM, Allison DB, et al. Using the Edmonton Obesity Staging System to predict mortality in a population-representative cohort of people with overweight and obesity. CMAJ 2011;183(14):E1059–66.
36. Klabuncde CN, Clauser SB, Liu B, et al. Organization of primary care practice for providing energy balance care. Am J Health Promot 2014;28(3):e67–80.
37. Steeves JA, Liu B, Willis G, et al. Physicians' personal beliefs about weight-related care and their associations with care delivery: the U.S. National

Survey of Energy Balance Related Care among Primary Care Physicians. Obes Res Clin Pract 2015;9:243–55.

38. Petrin C, Kahan S, Turner M, et al. Current attitudes and practices of obesity counselling by health care providers. Obes Res Pract 2017;11(3):352–9.

39. Talwalker A, McCarty F. Characteristics of physician office visits for obesity by adults aged 20 and over: United States, 2012. NCHS Data Brief; No. 237. Hyattsville (MD): National Center for Health Statistics; 2016.

40. Asselin J, Osuniana AM, Ogunieya AA, et al. Missing an opportunity: the embedded nature of weight management in primary care. Clin Obes 2015;5: 325–32.

41. NORC and ASMBS. New insights into Americans' perceptions and misperceptions of obesity treatments, and the struggles many face. Available at: http:// www.norc.org/PDFs/ASMBS%20Obesity/Issue%20Brief%20B_ASMBS%20NORC %20Obesity%20Poll.pdf. Accessed August 2, 2017.

42. Igel L, Kumar RB, Sanders KH, et al. Practical use of pharmacotherapy for obesity. Gastroenterology 2017;152:1765–79.

43. Samaranayake NR, Ong KL, Leung RYH, et al. Management of obesity in the National Health and Nutrition Examination Survey (NHANES), 2007-2008. Ann Epidemiol 2012;22(5):349–53.

44. Zhang S, Manne S, Lin J, et al. Characteristics of patients potentially eligible for pharmacotherapy for weight loss in primary car practice in the United States. Obes Sci Pract 2016;2(2):104–14.

45. Bodenheimer T, Wagner EH, Grumbach K. Improving primary care for patients with chronic illness. JAMA 2002;288(14):1775–9.

46. Dietz WH, Solomon LS, Pronk N, et al. An integrated framework for the prevention and treatment of obesity and its related chronic diseases. Health Aff 2015;34(9): 1456–63.

47. Deitz WH, Belay B, Bradley D, et al. A model framework that integrates community and clinical systems for the prevention and management of obesity and other chronic diseases. Washington, DC: National Academy of Medicine. Available at: https://nam.edu/wp-content/uploads/2017/01/A-Model-Frame-work-that-integrates-community-and-clinical-systems-for-the-prevention-and-management-of-obesity-and-other-chronic-diseases.pdf. Accessed July 30, 2017.

48. Campbell-Scherer DL, Asselin J, Osunlana AM, et al. Implementation and evaluation of the 5As framework of obesity management in primary care: design of the 5As Team (5AsT) randomized control trial. Implementation Sci 2014;9:78.

49. Ogunleye AA, Osunlana A, Asselin J, et al. The 5As team intervention: bridging the knowledge gap in obesity management among primary are practitioners. BMC Res Notes 2015;8:810.

50. Milani RV, Lavie CJ. Health Care 2020: reengineering health care delivery to combat chronic disease. Am J Med 2015;128(4):337–43.

51. Kushner RF, Brittan D, Cleek J, et al. The American Board of Obesity Medicine: five year report. Obesity 2017;25(6):982–3.

Obesity as a Disease

Jagriti Upadhyay, MD[a,b,c,]*, Olivia Farr, PhD[c],
Nikolaos Perakakis, MD, PhD[c], Wael Ghaly, MD[c], Christos Mantzoros, MD, PhD[a,c]

KEYWORDS

- Obesity • Metabolically healthy • Causes and mechanism
- Cardiovascular disease and metabolic syndrome

KEY POINTS

- Obesity is a complex disease with many causal factors.
- Obesity is associated with multiple comorbidities contributing to significant morbidity and mortality.
- Various peripheral and central mechanisms play a role in the development of obesity.

INTRODUCTION

Obesity is a complex, chronic medical condition with a major negative impact on human health.[1] Over the last 30 years, there has been an exponential growth in the prevalence of obesity worldwide with doubling rates for adult and childhood obesity (6–11 years) and tripling rates of adolescent obesity (12–19 years).[1,2] Obesity has become a public health burden with significant and profound impact on morbidity, mortality, and cost of health care.[1]

Obesity is often stigmatized and carries with it a false perception that it is caused mostly by lack of will leading to inappropriate dietary choices and physical inactivity. However, there is a rich evidence-based literature that presents obesity as a complicated chronic medical condition caused by the interplay of multiple genetic, environmental, metabolic, and behavioral factors. In 2008, an expert panel from the Obesity Society concluded "obesity is a complex condition with many causal contributors, including many factors that are largely beyond individuals' control; that obesity causes much suffering; that obesity causally contributes to ill health, functional impairment, reduced quality of life, serious disease, and greater mortality; that successful

Disclosure Statement: The authors have nothing to disclose.
[a] Section of Endocrinology, Diabetes and Metabolism, Boston VA Healthcare System, 150 South Huntington Avenue, Boston, MA 02130, USA; [b] Division of Endocrinology, Boston Medical Center, Boston University, 88 East Newton Street, Boston, MA 02118; [c] Division of Endocrinology, Diabetes and Metabolism, Department of Internal Medicine, Beth Israel Deaconess Medical Center, Harvard Medical School, 330 Brookline Avenue, Boston, MA 02215, USA
* Corresponding author. Beth Israel Deaconess Medical Center, 330 Brookline Avenue, Stoneman 820, Boston, MA 02215.
E-mail address: jupadhya@bidmc.harvard.edu

treatment, although difficult to achieve, produces many benefits." Obesity was thus recognized as a disease state. Acknowledging obesity as a serious public health threat, the American Medical Association also voted for obesity as a disease in June 2013. Several other societies have now recognized obesity as a disease (**Box 1**).[3,4] This recognition led the medical community and pharmaceutical companies to tackle this rising epidemic that affects 1 in 3 United States Americans.[5] Recently, the American Association of Clinical Endocrinologists and American College of Endocrinology concluded that a "more medically meaningful and actionable definition of obesity" was needed and hence published a position statement advocating for use of the word "adiposity based chronic disease or ABCD" for obesity to better describe the disease condition. Given such high prevalence of obesity and more than 30 medical conditions related to obesity, the disease has a significant impact on morbidity, mortality, and cost of health care. Obesity is a medical condition, a disease state, and should be treated as such.

Body mass index (BMI), calculated as kg/m^2, reflects body mass, in most but not all cases correlates well with the degree of obesity, and is a significant predictor of overall mortality with a reduction in median survival by approximately 2 to 4 years for persons with a BMI of 30 to 35 kg/m^2 and 8 to 10 years at a BMI of 40 to 45 kg/m^2,[6] even more with higher BMIs of longer duration. The increase in the prevalence of obesity has

---

Box 1
Associations or organizations that have declared obesity is a disease

- National Institutes of Health
- US Food and Drug Administration
- Federal Trade Commission
- American Medical Association
- World Health Organization
- American College of Physicians
- American Association of Clinical Endocrinologists
- American College of Cardiology
- The Endocrine Society
- American Academy of Family Physicians
- Institute of Medicine
- The Obesity Society
- World Obesity Federation
- American Heart Association
- American Diabetes Association
- American Academy of Family Physicians
- American Society for Reproductive Medicine
- American Urologic Association
- American College of Surgeons

Data from Kahan S, Zvenyach T. Obesity as a disease: current policies and implications for the future. Curr Obes Rep 2016;5(2):291–7; and Bray GA, Kim KK, Wilding JPH. Obesity: a chronic relapsing progressive disease process. A position statement of the World Obesity Federation. Obes Rev 2017;18(7):715–23.

occurred in parallel with the increase in prevalence of other medical conditions considered as comorbidities, including diabetes, stroke, cardiovascular disease, hyperlipidemia, cancers, nonalcoholic fatty liver disease, pulmonary disease, polycystic ovarian syndrome (PCOS), and osteoarthritis. As expected, the increase in morbidity and mortality from these diseases, mainly due to obesity, has led to an increasing financial burden. The cost of extra medications for a man or woman with obesity is estimated to be an additional US$1152 per year and US$3613 per year, respectively.[7] Extrapolation of these costs at the national level shows an estimated US$190 billion per year (21% of total US health care expenditure) in costs for the treatment of obesity and obesity-related morbidities.[7] In summary, obesity is a highly prevalent disease and poses an enormous health and economic burden to society. This article reviews the mechanisms of obesity and its related comorbidities.

CAUSES OR MECHANISMS OF OBESITY

Obesity is a disease that has rapidly escalated over the past several decades and is caused by environmental, humoral, and genetic factors, likely working in combination. The environmental factors contributing to the increase in obesity include but are not limited to decreased physical activity; increased television watching times and sedentary lifestyle[8]; increased food consumption, particularly of energy-dense, high-calorie, palatable food served in increasing portion sizes[9,10]; and the use of medications with weight gain as a side effect.[11] However, despite most individuals being exposed to these environmental factors, not all of people become obese, suggesting differing genetic mechanisms that predispose certain individuals to developing obesity.

Many genes have been identified as potentially contributing to obesity, possibly acting in combination; studies with twins have shown relatively high heritability for eating behaviors (53%–84%).[12,13] One of the most well-studied is the fat mass and obesity-associated (FTO) gene, which exerts modest effects on its own and seems to be modified by lifestyle.[14] Relatively few individuals have monogenic forms of obesity, although up to 200 types of single gene mutations have been found to cause obesity.[15] There are relatively few well-known monogenic mutations that explain no more than 10% of extreme obesity cases, such as mutations in leptin or the leptin receptor[16] and the melanocortin-4 receptor.[17] Syndromic forms of obesity also make up a relatively small amount of clinical cases and are related to genetic disorders that include a distinct set of clinical phenotypes and also demonstrate obesity. For instance, some of the most common forms include WAGR (Wilms tumor, aniridia, genitourinary anomalies, and mental retardation), Prader-Willi, Bardet Biedl, and Cohen syndromes.[18] Apart from genetics, certain other neuroendocrine causal factors for obesity include but are not limited to hypothyroidism, Cushing disease, pseudohypoparathyroidism, growth hormone deficiency, hypothalamic causes, and PCOS. Early referral to an endocrinologist and intervention is useful in patients suspected to have an underlying neuroendocrine or genetic cause for obesity.

More recently, studies have also implicated epigenetic factors, such as changes in DNA methylation, microRNA expression, and noncoding microRNAs, as contributing to obesity.[19–21] Unlike with genetics, epigenetics are susceptible to change throughout the lifespan and with lifestyle modifications through diet and physical activity. As research continues to grow in these areas, one begins to understand the complex gene-environment interactions that contribute to obesity and how these may be targeted as treatment.

To understand obesity further, one must examine the central nervous system (CNS) circuitry that controls appetite and how this may become dysregulated through the gene-environment changes previously discussed. Although the oldest research focuses on changes in the homeostatic CNS control of eating in the hypothalamus, more recent research points to other networks, such as reward, emotion or memory, attention, and cognitive control as playing a more potent role in the control of appetite in humans.[22] The hypothalamus regulates homeostatic energy intake and expenditure, integrating hormonal signals from the periphery and communicating them to the rest of the CNS. For instance, leptin is secreted by adipose tissue and circulates proportionally to the amount of body fat mass, also responding to acute changes in energy deprivation.[23–25] At low levels of body fat, leptin circulates at lower levels and communicates with neurons in the hypothalamus to increase energy intake and decrease energy expenditure.[24] In obesity, the opposite occurs and leptin circulates at high levels; however, leptin does not decrease energy intake and increase energy expenditure due to leptin resistance or tolerance, demonstrating a resistance to the homeostatic control of eating.[26–28] Thus, homeostatic control of energy intake is more critical in states of starvation. Increasing evidence demonstrates that other peripheral molecules may act on several areas in the brain, such as glucagon-like peptide 1 (GLP-1) and its analogues, which have been shown to act on the attention and reward networks.[29,30] Other molecules that are secreted by the periphery and may act in the brain have not yet been studied in humans, including amylin, pancreatic hormones, myokines such as irisin, and others. These may prove to be potential targets for therapy.

Aside from the homeostatic system, other neural systems may be more potent in terms of regulating appetite and obesity. The reward system, in particular, has been suggested to be at the root of obesity.[31–51] Food is naturally rewarding and this system may be altered in patients with obesity, leading to and/or exacerbating weight gain. The 2 primary theories are that either a hyporesponsivity to rewards leads individuals to seek highly rewarding, high-fat or high-calorie foods, or there is a hyperresponsivity to food cues that leads individuals to increasingly eat highly palatable foods. These theories are supported by the observed lower availability of rewarding dopamine D2 receptors in individuals with obesity[52–56] and the heightened activity of brain areas responding to reward, such as the orbitofrontal cortex and nucleus accumbens, to visual food cues.[57–61] Emotions are also potent regulators of appetite because depressed mood and anxiety are comorbidities of obesity and related to central obesity in particular.[62–66] Indeed, stress is also known to cause changes in appetite that can lead to the development of obesity.[67] Memory, regulated by the hippocampus, may also influence eating, and impaired functioning of the hippocampus leads to increased food intake and obesity, which in turn leads to further impairment of the hippocampus.[68,69] Thus, reward, emotion, and memory all may influence eating and the development of obesity.

Higher CNS centers, such as those controlling attention and cognitive control, are also altered in obesity. Individuals with obesity and even normal weight individuals who later gain weight show more attention to food cues and attentional bias toward eating when sated.[70–75] Attention, controlled primarily by the parietal and occipital visual cortices, is generally increased for items of salience and in obesity these areas demonstrate increased activation to highly palatable food cues.[76,77] Cognitive areas in the prefrontal cortex exert control inappropriate behaviors, such as eating when full or eating unhealthy foods.[78] Individuals with obesity and normal weight individuals who later gain weight have shown impaired inhibitory control toward food cues[79–92] and even when performing tasks not related to food.[85,92] Cognitive control may also suppress reward-related responses and, in the case of obesity in which cognitive control is impaired, this may enhance the activation of the reward system.[93,94] Altogether, the control of eating in the human brain is complex and involves several cortical and subcortical networks.

Inflammatory links between obesity and insulin resistance (IR) or metabolic syndrome were suggested when increased tumor necrosis factor (TNF)-α expression was found in the adipose tissue of obese humans and rodents almost 20 years ago.[95] Further research demonstrated involvement of multiple inflammatory pathways and increased cytokine levels in the mechanism of obesity and obesity-related IR.[96,97] Along the same lines, De Souza and colleagues[98] found that rats subjected to long-term high-fat diet (HFD) had increased activation of Jun N-terminal kinase (JnK) and Nuclear factor kappa B (NF-κB) inflammatory pathways resulting in increased cytokines (interleukin [IL]-6, TNFα, and IL-1β) in the mediobasal hypothalamic region. They further demonstrated that this inflammation led to significant impairment in insulin and leptin signaling pathways.[98] These results have since been replicated by other investigators with consistent finds in mice and also other nonhuman primates.[99,100] At the cellular level, HFD-induced inflammation involves reactive gliosis of the hypothalamus in rats.[100,101] Reactive gliosis, which involves recruitment, proliferation, and morphologic transformation of astrocytes and microglia, is observed as early as 24 hours after starting an HFD diet in rats and resolves after 4 weeks of returning to a normal chow diet.[100,101] However, prolonged HFD diet has shown to result in more significant and irreversible changes in hypothalamus, including gliosis, loss of synapsis in proopiomelanocortin (POMC) neurons, and reduction of neurogenesis in the hypothalamic region, leading to structural changes in the blood brain barrier.[102]Although studies in rodents have provided some critical insights, they may not fully capture the complexity of the human CNS and obesity.

METABOLICALLY HEALTHY VERSUS UNHEALTHY

BMI is most frequently used for the classification of obesity. Mortality, morbidity, and complications increase with the grade of obesity. Grade II and III obesity (BMI equal to or greater than 35 kg/m^2 and equal to or greater than 40 kg/m^2, respectively) have been associated with increased risk of cardiovascular disease and comorbidities compared with grade I obesity (BMI 30–35 kg/m^2).[103–106] However, there is a known subset of the obese population devoid, in the short-term, of cardiometabolic complications such as diabetes mellitus, hyperlipidemia, IR, and cardiovascular disease, and hence are known as metabolically healthy obese (MHO), which has gained much interest. Although several studies have better characterized this phenotype using cutoffs for blood pressure, IR measures (eg, fasting plasma glucose, hemoglobin [Hb]A1c, homeostatic model assessment [HOMA]- insulin resistance [IR]), and cholesterol (high-density lipoprotein [HDL], low-density lipoprotein [LDL], Total cholesterol (TC), Triglyceride (TG), or TG/HDL ratios), there are no set criteria that distinguish metabolically healthy from metabolically unhealthy obese (MUO) persons.[107,108] Importantly, none of the current guidelines distinguish between these 2 phenotypes and, therefore, recommend lifestyle interventions as the first-line treatment of all patients with obesity. As opposed to the MHO phenotype, another phenotype that has gained interest is the metabolically unhealthy normal weight (MUHNW) phenotype. These patients are not obese per BMI criteria but have a dysfunctional metabolic profile as would be typically found with obesity. This is more commonly observed with patients of Asian origin, particularly the Asian Indian and Chinese subgroups, who tend to have a normal BMI but increased visceral adiposity. Data from the Korean National Health and Nutrition Examination Survey showed a 12.7% prevalence of MUHNW phenotype among normal-weight individuals (BMI <25 kg/m^2) and 47.9% prevalence of the MHO phenotype among obese population (BMI >30 mg/m^2).[109] Several studies have examined all possible transitions among MHO, MUO, and MUHNW and many have suggested that MHO is a state in time and that the natural progression would eventually be to the MUO state.[110,111] A recent study followed more than 3500 women for 6 years to study the progression of different metabolic phenotypes. The study concluded that highest rate of metabolic improvement was noted in MUHNW women, whereas the highest rates of metabolic deterioration was seen in MHO women.[112] A third of women with the MHO phenotype transitioned to a MUO state at the end of 6 years,[112] suggesting that, given enough time, many patients who appear to be MHO would convert to MUO. A recent study involving 15,000 participants in the third National Health and Nutrition Examination Survey (NHANES) showed that patients with normal BMI but higher waist or hip ratio (>0.85 in women and >0.90 in men) had higher mortality compared with patients with normal fat distribution irrespective of BMI.[113] A combination of central adiposity along with metabolic status seems to be the most consistent and significant predictor of morbidity and mortality. Hence, weight loss and lifestyle changes should be recommended even for MHO patients.

Obesity is associated with an increased risk of more than 20 medical conditions, such as diabetes mellitus type 2, hypertension, dyslipidemia, Cardiovascular disease (CVD), stroke, sleep apnea, urogenital issues, gall bladder disease, and multiple cancers (**Fig. 1**). Not only does obesity have significant impact on physical health but also tremendously affects patients psychologically and is associated with very poor self-esteem, increased rates of depression, and poor quality of life. Obese patients often suffer from discrimination and social stigmatization. There are multiple pathophysiological mechanisms that interplay in development of comorbidities in relation to obesity (**Fig. 2**). Next a few of the major obesity-related comorbidities and their mechanisms are discussed.

METABOLIC SYNDROME, DIABETES, AND CARDIOVASCULAR DISEASE IN RELATION TO OBESITY

Obesity is associated with increased mortality.[6] Each 5 kg/m^2 increase in BMI above 25 kg/m^2 increases overall mortality by approximately 30%; vascular mortality by

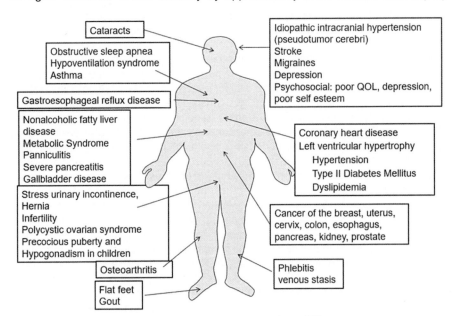

Fig. 1. Comorbidities associated with obesity. QOL, quality of life.

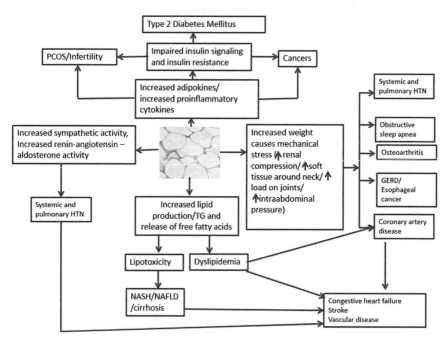

Fig. 2. Pathways through which obesity leads to comorbidities. GERD, Gastroesophageal reflux disease; HTN, Hypertension; NAFLD, Nonalcoholic fatty liver disease; NASH, Nonalcoholic steatohepatitis.

40%; and diabetic, renal, and hepatic mortality by 60% to 120%.[6] At 30 to 35 kg/m^2, median survival is reduced by 2 to 4 years and at 40 to 45 kg/m^2 by 8 to 10 years.[6] The main causes of death include ischemic heart disease,[114] stroke[115] and diabetes-related complications.[6] The vicious cycle resulting in increased mortality in obesity involves IR, as well as all the components of metabolic syndrome (ie, hyperglycemia, dyslipidemia, and hypertension).

Obesity is associated with an increased risk for IR.[116] HOMA-IR correlates strongly with visceral fat mass [correlation factor (r) r = 0.570], total fat mass (r = 0.492), BMI (r = 0.482), and waist circumference (r = 0.466).[116] In contrast, lower extremity fat is not associated with HOMA-IR.[116] Adipose tissue controls metabolism by regulating the levels of nonesterified fatty acids (NEFAs), glycerol, proinflammatory cytokines, cells of immune system (macrophages, lymphocytes), and hormones such as leptin and adiponectin.[117] In obesity, the production of most of these molecules is increased and can affect insulin sensitivity through multiple pathways. Much is known about the biochemical and physiologic effects of obesity on IR. First, increased NEFA delivery and consequently elevated intracellular levels compete with glucose for substrate oxidation, resulting in inhibition of important enzymes (ie, phosphofructokinase, pyruvate dehydrogenase, hexokinase II) participating in glycolysis.[117] Additionally, fatty acid metabolites (ie, ceramides, diacylglycerol [DAG], fatty acyl-coenzyme A [acyl-CoA]) are increased, resulting in serine or threonine phosphorylation of insulin receptor substrate (IRS)-1 and IRS-2, reduced activation of phosphatidylinositol (PI)-3-kinases, and inhibition downstream of insulin-receptor signaling.[117,118] Second, increased secretion of TNFα, IL-6, and monocyte chemoattractant protein-1 activate proinflammatory signaling pathways in adipose tissue, liver, and muscle.[119] The proinflammatory signaling pathways involve activation of JNK and inhibitor of nuclear factor kappa-B kinase, leading both to phosphorylation of IRS-1 and IRS-2, as well as to increased transcription of inflammatory genes.[119] Finally, increased levels of proteins, such as retinol-binding protein-4 and leptin, and reduced levels of adiponectin affect insulin sensitivity, by impairing PI (3) kinase signaling in muscle, inducing the expression of the gluconeogenic enzyme phosphoenolpyruvate carboxykinase in the liver and stimulating fatty acid oxidation. The net outcome of all the pathophysiological changes in obesity is the development of liver and muscle IR, depicted by impaired suppression of glucose output from the liver and reduced glucose uptake from the muscle.[119–121]

Obesity is strongly associated with the development of type 2 diabetes. IR in the liver, muscle, and adipose tissue demands an increase in insulin supplied by the pancreatic β cells to maintain normoglycemia.[117] Healthy pancreatic β cells can improve their function and mass to satisfy the increasing demands.[122] However, genetic and environmental factors may lead to a β cell dysfunction.[117,119] Certain mutations or single nucleotide polymorphisms in genes involved in critical β cell-pathways can directly affect beta cell function and survival.[123] Genetically susceptible β-cells will fail to satisfy the high insulin demands deriving from chronic increased caloric intake and reduced physical activity, resulting in hyperglycemia.[124] The combination of hyperglycemia and hyperlipidemia (glucolipotoxicity) will accelerate β cell death, reduce insulin secretion, and aggravate hyperglycemia.[125] The relative risk for incident diabetes is 1.87, 1.87, and 1.88 per standard deviation of body mass index, waist circumference, and waist or hip ratio, respectively.[126] The adjusted relative risk for incident type 2 diabetes is 8.93 in MUHO and 4.03 in MHO adults compared with healthy normal-weight individuals.[127] This shows that even healthy obesity is not a harmless condition. Additionally, the age of obesity onset is important. Individuals with childhood onset of obesity have approximately 24-fold risk of HbA1c greater than 7% after 45 years. This risk is lower for young (16-fold) and middle (2.99-fold) adulthood obesity onset.[128]

Obesity is associated with dyslipidemia. This is characterized by increased plasma triglycerides and apolipoprotein B (apoB), as well as by decreased HDL-cholesterol (HDL-C).[129] Accumulation of the lipolytically active visceral fat in combination with the development of IR lead to a prominent increase in the flux of free fatty acids in the portal vein and, subsequently, in the liver, resulting in high triglyceride synthesis.[129] In addition, hepatic secretion of very low density lipoprotein (VLDL)-apoB is increased and the catabolism of HDL-apoA-I is induced. A BMI greater than 30 kg/m^2 is associated with an odds ratio of approximately 6 for low HDL-C and approximately 3 for increased total cholesterol.[130] Given the high relevance between dyslipidemia and atherogenesis, the obesity-mediated changes in lipid profile significantly contribute to the increased cardiovascular mortality.

Obesity promotes hypertension.[131] Individuals with BMI greater than 30 kg/m^2 have a 9-fold increased risk for high blood pressure.[130] Several mechanisms are implicated in the pathophysiology of obesity-related hypertension. First, obesity is characterized by altered hemodynamics due to volume overload.[132] This results in high cardiac output, increased peripheral resistance, and pressure overload. Second, high salt intake due to increased food consumption impairs sodium homeostasis promoting hypertension.[131] In addition, higher sodium reabsorption combined with elevated renal blood flow and glomerular hyperfiltration lead to renal structural changes and dysfunction, contributing to elevated blood pressure.[133,134] Furthermore, hormonal changes (hyperaldosteronism, hyperinsulinemia, and hyperleptinemia) result in activation of the renin-aldosterone-angiotensin system, stimulation of sympathetic nervous system, and decrease of parasympathetic activity.[131,135] Finally, endothelial dysfunction combined with vascular stiffness, increased oxidative stress, and chronic low-grade inflammation lead to vascular injury.[131,136–138] All these hormonal and vascular changes increase blood pressure and lead to hypertension.

Altogether, obesity is associated in a causal way with IR, dyslipidemia, hypertension, hyperglycemia, and diabetes. This explains the high risk of cardiovascular events in obesity and specifically of myocardial infarction, heart failure, and stroke.[139–141] The metabolic consequences of obesity (ie, hypertension, dyslipidemia, diabetes), mediate 44% of the excess risk of obesity for coronary heart disease and 69% of stroke. Among them, hypertension seems to have the most important role, accounting for 31% of the excess risk for coronary heart disease and 65% for stroke.[140] However, even MHO individuals have a 2-fold relative risk of CVD events compared with healthy normal-weight people.[142] In addition, the risk seems to be much higher in adults with obesity who were overweight or obese as children.[143] In summary, early onset, long-duration, and excessive obesity aggravate the CVD risk and, consequently, cardiovascular-related mortality.

OTHER COMPLICATIONS AND COMORBIDITIES ASSOCIATED WITH OBESITY
Polycystic Ovarian Syndrome

There is a confirmed relationship between obesity and PCOS. The prevalence of obesity in women diagnosed with PCOS is as high as 80% in the United States.[144] PCOS is characterized by increased production of androgens, which affects the hypothalamus-hypophysis-ovarian axis (HHOA) and may affect fertility.[145] Obesity is considered a factor in the pathophysiological cascade of PCOS through 2 major pathways: IR and hyperandrogenism.[145] However, obesity can also be considered a complication of PCOS, considering the presence of increased visceral fat in PCOS.[146] Hyperinsulinemia and IR have shown to decrease sex hormone-binding globulin, leading to higher levels of free androgens in PCOS. This is indirectly conducted through downregulation of hepatic nuclear factor–4α.[145] Increased insulin levels is a key factor in the development of the disease and has shown to increase pulsatility of the HHOA, resulting in increased ovarian synthesis of androgens.[147] This correlation is further evidenced by use of metformin in the treatment of PCOS. Metformin improves IR, and at the same time improves the hyperandrogenemia in PCOS.[148] High insulin levels also stimulate the hypothalamus-hypophysis-adrenal axis (HHAA), resulting in enhanced secretion of adrenal androgens.[149]It was reported that 45% of girls with premature pubarche developed PCOS later in their lives.[150] Obesity in adolescence has been associated with hyperandrogenism due to the stimulatory effect of insulin and Insulin-like growth factor 1 (IGF-1) on steroidogenic enzymes in the adrenal glands.[151] Baptiste and colleagues[152] demonstrated another feedback mechanism in which hyperandrogenemia leads to increased free fatty acid levels and IR through serine phosphorylation of IRS-1. The third mechanism that explains the hyperandrogenism in patients with PCOS and obesity is hyperleptinemia, which leads to decreased production of the soluble leptin receptor with subsequent elevation in androgen levels.[151] Effective weight-loss measures have been reported to improve the regularity in menstruation.[153] More than 35% of women who lost greater than 5% of their body weight were reported to regain either their fertility or normal menstrual cycles in a study by Kiddy and colleagues.[154] Importantly, although much less common, PCOS is also reported in a subset of lean women, suggesting a different mechanism, such as increased androgen receptors sensitivity or the increased activity of HHAA.[149,155] However, a strong relationship exists between PCOS, hyperinsulinemia, and hyperandrogenism in relation to obesity that needs to be further explored.[156]

Obstructive Sleep Apnea

Obstructive sleep apnea (OSA) prevalence has been demonstrated to be high in patients with obesity[157] and coincides with several comorbidities, such as hypertension, type 2 diabetes mellitus, dyslipidemia, nonalcoholic fatty liver disease, congestive heart failure, and atrial fibrillation.[158,159] The prevalence of OSA is almost double in obese compared with lean individuals.[160] With the rising rates of obesity, the prevalence of OSA is expected to increase in the next few years.[161] Obesity is thought to be a predisposing factor of OSA due to fat deposition around the upper respiratory airways, chest wall, and truncal fat, which leads to a decrease in the functional residual capacity.[162] This is further evidenced by the direct correlation that exists between the apnea hypoxia index and adiposity measures.[160] Furthermore, treatment of OSA with continuous positive airway pressure has shown to improve visceral obesity, suggesting a role of OSA in the pathogenesis of obesity.[163] In physiologic conditions, the collapsibility of the upper airway tract is determined by the critical closing pressure inside the pharynx.[164] This pressure in maintained by a balance between the mechanical and neurologic factors, which keeps it toward the positive side.[165] This means that when the pressure inside the lumen decreases in rapid eye movement sleep, a neuromuscular impulse, also called negative pressure reflex, is elicited to dilate the muscles and restore its patency.[166] In OSA, this balance seems to be disturbed, either by the increased mechanical effect of anatomic alteration due to adiposity of the neck region or a defect of the neuromuscular signaling in these cases, or the combined effect of both factors.[167] The reflex dilatation is not sufficient because it requires higher level of activity to overcome the higher tissue mass in obesity.[165] In addition, obesity increases the soft palate length, which was found to be correlated with the severity of OSA.[168] Another proposed mechanism for the pathophysiology of OSA related to obesity is snoring.[169] The inflammatory process resulting from the vibration related to snoring leads to peripheral nerve damage, especially those responsible for the negative pressure reflex.[170] Studies have shown that decrease in body weight through lifestyle modification could improve all the symptoms related to OSA.[171]

Cancer

Obesity is a known risk factor for many cancers including pancreatic, liver, colorectal, postmenopausal breast cancer, esophageal adenocarcinoma, endometrial, and kidney cancers.[172,173] One in 5 of all cancers are thought to be related to obesity.[174] There is growing evidence that increasing BMI is associated with a parallel increase in risk of cancer with rates as high as 70% in BMI greater than 40 kg/m^2.[175] Mortality rates are 52% higher in obese men and 62% higher in obese women compared with the normal-weight population.[174] Furthermore, weight loss after bariatric surgery is associated with a decrease in the cancer risk, suggesting importance of healthy weight in cancer prevention.[176] Several mechanisms linking cancer and adiposity have been proposed. Etiologic factors include increase in IR, elevated IGF-1 levels, low-grade chronic inflammation due to obesity, dysregulation of adipocyte-derived factors, and alteration in sex hormones.[177,178] Although hypoadiponectinemia is associated with IR, in type 2 diabetes, cancer, and atherosclerosis, adiponectin has been shown to increase insulin sensitivity and has demonstrated antiproliferative effects, making it a potential diagnostic tool and therapeutic option in cancer.[179,180] Research is underway to decipher the various other unknown mechanisms and pathways involved in obesity and cancer.[181] Similarly, in humans, high levels of cytokines, such as IL-6 and TNF, have been shown to cause hepatic inflammation, which further activates the Janus kinase–Signal Transducer and Activator of Transcription pathway that includes oncogenic transcription factor STAT3.[182,183] Mechanisms linking obesity and cancer, however, still remain unclear and much research is needed to establish these links. All in all, healthy weight has multiple health benefits and thus the obesity pandemic needs to be addressed rather urgently.

SUMMARY

Obesity has emerged as an epidemic that poses an unprecedented public health challenge. Historically known to be a rare disease of the affluent, this disease has now flipped the coin and is more prevalent among the lower socioeconomic and less-educated classes. Although multiple risk factors have been identified for obesity, a deeper understanding of how these factors interact is yet to be determined. Major determinants and contributors of the obesity epidemic are the highly processed, high-calorie food available in large portions and at a cheaper rate, along with physical inactivity and increased screen time. These environmental changes overlay genetic and epigenetic mechanisms to regulate adiposity and lead to the development of obesity in many individuals. With increasing trends, this disease is also associated with a wide variety of complications and comorbidities, adding to the socioeconomic burden. Increasing trends of diabetes, hypertension, cardiometabolic disease, cancers, and mortality are just a few of the major comorbidities associated with obesity that lead to significant economic burdens.

Significant reductions in the cost of health care could occur if the progress of the rising trends of obesity could be slowed. Although various guidelines recommend a combined approach to treatment and pharmacotherapy as only an adjunct to diet and exercise, antiobesity medications are still underused in health care. Clearly, there is a need to generate awareness, not only among the general public but also among the medical community, for proper utilization of currently available therapies. Although there is good evidence that obesity is a daunting public health challenge, there are few effective programs and strategies to combat this epidemic. Although multiple interventions at many levels and for a long period of time would be required to achieve reversal of obesity epidemic, the declaration of obesity as a disease by AMA and multiple other organizations is the first step. Using similar to criteria for other disease states, obesity has been determined to be a disease state for several reasons, including

1. It is associated with impaired body function.
2. Although precipitated by environmental factors acting on a specific genetic predisposition, the final common pathways leading to obesity (or, obesities) signifies abnormal physiology.
3. It exacerbates or accelerates hundreds of comorbid disease states.
4. It is associated with substantial morbidity and mortality or premature death.

The determination that obesity is a disease state ultimately dictates and energizes practitioners toward an appropriate approach to obesity and allows a more effective strategy to marshal resources and tools, define clinical strategies, and structure payment policies to effectively combat this twenty-first century epidemic. Ultimately, this is expected to lead to a better understanding, prevention, and treatment in the not so distant future. Consequently, recognition of the problem would certainly help to allocate more resources and increase more awareness to decelerate the epidemic of obesity. There is an urgent need to draw public and government interest to allocate more resources, awareness, education, and research to curb the obesity epidemic in large populations worldwide. Recent study of obesity and better understanding of underlying mechanisms is expected to lead to pharmacologic treatments reaching the therapeutic armamentarium in the near future. Obesity is now considered a chronic disease state that needs a chronic treatment.

REFERENCES

1. Hu FB. Obesity and mortality: watch your waist, not just your weight. Arch Intern Med 2007;167(9):875–6.

2. Hedley AA, Ogden CL, Johnson CL, et al. Prevalence of overweight and obesity among US children, adolescents, and adults, 1999-2002. JAMA 2004;291(23): 2847–50.

3. Kahan S, Zvenyach T. Obesity as a disease: current policies and implications for the future. Curr Obes Rep 2016;5(2):291–7.

4. Bray GA, Kim KK, Wilding JPH. Obesity: a chronic relapsing progressive disease process. A position statement of the World Obesity Federation. Obes Rev 2017;18(7):715–23.

5. Baskin ML, Ard J, Franklin F, et al. Prevalence of obesity in the United States. Obes Rev 2005;6(1):5–7.

6. Whitlock G, Lewington S, Sherliker P, et al. Body-mass index and cause-specific mortality in 900 000 adults: collaborative analyses of 57 prospective studies. Lancet 2009;373(9669):1083–96.

7. Cawley J, Meyerhoefer C. The medical care costs of obesity: an instrumental variables approach. J Health Econ 2012;31(1):219–30.

8. Church TS, Thomas DM, Tudor-Locke C, et al. Trends over 5 decades in U.S. occupation-related physical activity and their associations with obesity. PLoS One 2011;6(5):e19657.

9. Popkin BM, Hawkes C. Sweetening of the global diet, particularly beverages: patterns, trends, and policy responses. Lancet Diabetes Endocrinol 2016; 4(2):174–86.

10. Njike VY, Smith TM, Shuval O, et al. Snack food, satiety, and weight. Adv Nutr 2016;7(5):866–78.

11. Medici V, McClave SA, Miller KR. Common medications which lead to unintended alterations in weight gain or organ lipotoxicity. Curr Gastroenterol Rep 2016;18(1):2.

12. Cooke L, Llewellyn C. Nature and nurture in early feeding behavior. Nestle Nutr Inst Workshop Ser 2016;85:155–65.

13. Bray MS, Loos RJ, McCaffery JM, et al. NIH working group report-using genomic information to guide weight management: From universal to precision treatment. Obesity (Silver Spring) 2016;24(1):14–22.

14. Bjornland T, Langaas M, Grill V, et al. Assessing gene-environment interaction effects of FTO, MC4R and lifestyle factors on obesity using an extreme phenotype sampling design: results from the HUNT study. PLoS One 2017;12(4): e0175071.

15. Albuquerque D, Stice E, Rodriguez-Lopez R, et al. Current review of genetics of human obesity: from molecular mechanisms to an evolutionary perspective. Mol Genet Genomics 2015;290(4):1191–221.

16. Farooqi IS, Matarese G, Lord GM, et al. Beneficial effects of leptin on obesity, T cell hyporesponsiveness, and neuroendocrine/metabolic dysfunction of human congenital leptin deficiency. J Clin Invest 2002;110(8):1093–103.

17. Ho G, MacKenzie RG. Functional characterization of mutations in melanocortin-4 receptor associated with human obesity. J Biol Chem 1999;274(50):35816–22.

18. Farooqi IS, O'Rahilly S. Monogenic obesity in humans. Annu Rev Med 2005;56: 443–58.

19. Ronn T, Volkov P, Davegardh C, et al. A six months exercise intervention influences the genome-wide DNA methylation pattern in human adipose tissue. PLoS Genet 2013;9(6):e1003572.

20. Widiker S, Karst S, Wagener A, et al. High-fat diet leads to a decreased methylation of the Mc4r gene in the obese BFMI and the lean B6 mouse lines. J Appl Genet 2010;51(2):193–7.

21. Almen MS, Jacobsson JA, Moschonis G, et al. Genome wide analysis reveals association of a FTO gene variant with epigenetic changes. Genomics 2012; 99(3):132–7.
22. Farr OM, Li CS, Mantzoros CS. Central nervous system regulation of eating: insights from human brain imaging. Metabolism 2016;65(5):699–713.
23. Farr OM, Gavrieli A, Mantzoros CS. Leptin applications in 2015: what have we learned about leptin and obesity? Curr Opin Endocrinol Diabetes Obes 2015; 22(5):353–9.
24. Farr OM, Tsoukas MA, Mantzoros CS. Leptin and the brain: influences on brain development, cognitive functioning and psychiatric disorders. Metabolism 2015;64(1):114–30.
25. Stieg MR, Sievers C, Farr O, et al. Leptin: a hormone linking activation of neuroendocrine axes with neuropathology. Psychoneuroendocrinology 2015;51: 47–57.
26. Balland E, Cowley MA. New insights in leptin resistance mechanisms in mice. Front Neuroendocrinol 2015;39:59–65.
27. Crujeiras AB, Carreira MC, Cabia B, et al. Leptin resistance in obesity: an epigenetic landscape. Life Sci 2015;140:57–63.
28. Sainz N, Barrenetxe J, Moreno-Aliaga MJ, et al. Leptin resistance and diet-induced obesity: central and peripheral actions of leptin. Metabolism 2015; 64(1):35–46.
29. Farr OM, Sofopoulos M, Tsoukas MA, et al. GLP-1 receptors exist in the parietal cortex, hypothalamus and medulla of human brains and the GLP-1 analogue liraglutide alters brain activity related to highly desirable food cues in individuals with diabetes: a crossover, randomised, placebo-controlled trial. Diabetologia 2016;65(10):2943–53.
30. Farr OM, Tsoukas MA, Triantafyllou G, et al. Short-term administration of the GLP-1 analog liraglutide decreases circulating leptin and increases GIP levels and these changes are associated with alterations in CNS responses to food cues: a randomized, placebo-controlled, crossover study. Metabolism 2016; 65(7):945–53.
31. Baik JH. Dopamine signaling in food addiction: role of dopamine D2 receptors. BMB Rep 2013;46(11):519–26.
32. Blum K, Thanos PK, Gold MS. Dopamine and glucose, obesity, and reward deficiency syndrome. Front Psychol 2014;5:919.
33. Burger KS, Stice E. Variability in reward responsivity and obesity: evidence from brain imaging studies. Curr Drug Abuse Rev 2011;4(3):182–9.
34. DiLeone RJ, Taylor JR, Picciotto MR. The drive to eat: comparisons and distinctions between mechanisms of food reward and drug addiction. Nat Neurosci 2012;15(10):1330–5.
35. Figlewicz DP. Adiposity signals and food reward: expanding the CNS roles of insulin and leptin. Am J Physiol Regul Integr Comp Physiol 2003;284(4): R882–92.
36. Garcia-Garcia I, Horstmann A, Jurado MA, et al. Reward processing in obesity, substance addiction and non-substance addiction. Obes Rev 2014;15(11): 853–69.
37. Gosnell BA, Levine AS. Reward systems and food intake: role of opioids. Int J Obes (Lond) 2009;33(Suppl 2):S54–8.
38. Kelley M, Khan NA, Rolls ET. Taste, olfactory, and food reward value processing in the brain. Adv Nutr 2015;127-128:64–90.

39. King BM. The modern obesity epidemic, ancestral hunter-gatherers, and the sensory/reward control of food intake. Am Psychol 2013;68(2):88–96.

40. Michaelides M, Thanos PK, Volkow ND, et al. Translational neuroimaging in drug addiction and obesity. ILAR J 2012;53(1):59–68.

41. Murray S, Tulloch A, Gold MS, et al. Hormonal and neural mechanisms of food reward, eating behaviour and obesity. Nat Rev Endocrinol 2014;10(9):540–52.

42. Small DM. Individual differences in the neurophysiology of reward and the obesity epidemic. Int J Obes (Lond) 2009;33(Suppl 2):S44–8.

43. Smith DG, Robbins TW. The neurobiological underpinnings of obesity and binge eating: a rationale for adopting the food addiction model. Biol Psychiatry 2013; 73(9):804–10.

44. Stice E, Figlewicz DP, Gosnell BA, et al. The contribution of brain reward circuits to the obesity epidemic. Neurosci Biobehav Rev 2013;37(9 Pt A):2047–58.

45. Volkow ND, Wang GJ, Fowler JS, et al. Food and drug reward: overlapping circuits in human obesity and addiction. Curr Top Behav Neurosci 2012;11:1–24.

46. Volkow ND, Wang GJ, Tomasi D, et al. The addictive dimensionality of obesity. Biol Psychiatry 2013;73(9):811–8.

47. Volkow ND, Wang GJ, Tomasi D, et al. Obesity and addiction: neurobiological overlaps. Obes Rev 2013;14(1):2–18.

48. Wang GJ, Volkow ND, Fowler JS. The role of dopamine in motivation for food in humans: implications for obesity. Expert Opin Ther Targets 2002;6(5):601–9.

49. Wang GJ, Volkow ND, Thanos PK, et al. Similarity between obesity and drug addiction as assessed by neurofunctional imaging: a concept review. J Addict Dis 2004;23(3):39–53.

50. Wise RA. Dual roles of dopamine in food and drug seeking: the drive-reward paradox. Biol Psychiatry 2013;73(9):819–26.

51. Ziauddeen H, Alonso-Alonso M, Hill JO. Obesity and the neurocognitive basis of food reward and the control of intake. Adv Nutr 2015;6(4):474–86.

52. Dunn JP, Kessler RM, Feurer ID, et al. Relationship of dopamine type 2 receptor binding potential with fasting neuroendocrine hormones and insulin sensitivity in human obesity. Diabetes Care 2012;35(5):1105–11.

53. Thanos PK, Michaelides M, Piyis YK, et al. Food restriction markedly increases dopamine D2 receptor (D2R) in a rat model of obesity as assessed with in-vivo muPET imaging ([11C] raclopride) and in-vitro ([3H] spiperone) autoradiography. Synapse 2008;62(1):50–61.

54. Dunn JP, Cowan RL, Volkow ND, et al. Decreased dopamine type 2 receptor availability after bariatric surgery: preliminary findings. Brain Res 2010;1350: 123–30.

55. Volkow ND, Wang GJ, Telang F, et al. Low dopamine striatal D2 receptors are associated with prefrontal metabolism in obese subjects: possible contributing factors. Neuroimage 2008;42(4):1537–43.

56. Wang GJ, Volkow ND, Logan J, et al. Brain dopamine and obesity. Lancet 2001; 357(9253):354–7.

57. Rothemund Y, Preuschhof C, Bohner G, et al. Differential activation of the dorsal striatum by high-calorie visual food stimuli in obese individuals. Neuroimage 2007;37(2):410–21.

58. Stice E, Yokum S, Bohon C, et al. Reward circuitry responsivity to food predicts future increases in body mass: moderating effects of DRD2 and DRD4. Neuroimage 2010;50(4):1618–25.

59. Beaver JD, Lawrence AD, van Ditzhuijzen J, et al. Individual differences in reward drive predict neural responses to images of food. J Neurosci 2006; 26(19):5160–6.
60. Pelchat ML, Johnson A, Chan R, et al. Images of desire: food-craving activation during fMRI. Neuroimage 2004;23(4):1486–93.
61. Yokum S, Ng J, Stice E. Attentional bias to food images associated with elevated weight and future weight gain: an fMRI study. Obesity (Silver Spring) 2011;19(9): 1775–83.
62. Dong C, Sanchez LE, Price RA. Relationship of obesity to depression: a family-based study. Int J Obes Relat Metab Disord 2004;28(6):790–5.
63. Novick JS, Stewart JW, Wisniewski SR, et al. Clinical and demographic features of atypical depression in outpatients with major depressive disorder: preliminary findings from STAR*D. J Clin Psychiatry 2005;66(8):1002–11.
64. Potenza MN. Obesity, food, and addiction: emerging neuroscience and clinical and public health implications. Neuropsychopharmacology 2014;39(1):249–50.
65. Roberts RE, Deleger S, Strawbridge WJ, et al. Prospective association between obesity and depression: evidence from the Alameda County Study. Int J Obes Relat Metab Disord 2003;27(4):514–21.
66. Simon GE, Von Korff M, Saunders K, et al. Association between obesity and psychiatric disorders in the US adult population. Arch Gen Psychiatry 2006;63(7): 824–30.
67. Farr OM, Sloan DM, Keane TM, et al. Stress- and PTSD-associated obesity and metabolic dysfunction: a growing problem requiring further research and novel treatments. Metabolism 2014;63(12):1463–8.
68. Martin AA, Davidson TL. Human cognitive function and the obesogenic environment. Physiol Behav 2014;136:185–93.
69. Parent MB, Darling JN, Henderson YO. Remembering to eat: hippocampal regulation of meal onset. Am J Physiol Regul Integr Comp Physiol 2014; 306(10):R701–13.
70. Doolan KJ, Breslin G, Hanna D, et al. Attentional bias to food-related visual cues: is there a role in obesity? Proc Nutr Soc 2015;74(1):37–45.
71. Leland DS, Pineda JA. Effects of food-related stimuli on visual spatial attention in fasting and nonfasting normal subjects: Behavior and electrophysiology. Clin Neurophysiol 2006;117(1):67–84.
72. Placanica JL, Faunce GJ, Soames Job RF. The effect of fasting on attentional biases for food and body shape/weight words in high and low Eating Disorder Inventory scorers. Int J Eat Disord 2002;32(1):79–90.
73. Ahern AL, Field M, Yokum S, et al. Relation of dietary restraint scores to cognitive biases and reward sensitivity. Appetite 2010;55(1):61–8.
74. Brignell C, Griffiths T, Bradley BP, et al. Attentional and approach biases for pictorial food cues. Influence of external eating. Appetite 2009;52(2):299–306.
75. Van Strien T, Schippers GM, Cox WM. On the relationship between emotional and external eating behavior. Addict Behav 1995;20(5):585–94.
76. Fuhrer D, Zysset S, Stumvoll M. Brain activity in hunger and satiety: an exploratory visually stimulated FMRI study. Obesity (Silver Spring) 2008;16(5):945–50.
77. Schur EA, Kleinhans NM, Goldberg J, et al. Activation in brain energy regulation and reward centers by food cues varies with choice of visual stimulus. Int J Obes 2009;33(6):653–61.
78. Aron AR. From reactive to proactive and selective control: developing a richer model for stopping inappropriate responses. Biol Psychiatry 2011;69(12): e55–68.

79. Anzman-Frasca S, Francis LA, Birch LL. Inhibitory control is associated with psychosocial, cognitive, and weight outcomes in a longitudinal sample of girls. Transl Issues Psychol Sci 2015;1(3):203–16.

80. Blanco-Gomez A, Ferre N, Luque V, et al. Being overweight or obese is associated with inhibition control in children from six to ten years of age. Acta Paediatr 2015;104(6):619–25.

81. Chamberlain SR, Derbyshire KL, Leppink E, et al. Obesity and dissociable forms of impulsivity in young adults. CNS Spectr 2015;20(5):500–7.

82. He Q, Xiao L, Xue G, et al. Poor ability to resist tempting calorie rich food is linked to altered balance between neural systems involved in urge and self-control. Nutr J 2014;13:92.

83. Khan NA, Raine LB, Drollette ES, et al. The relationship between total water intake and cognitive control among prepubertal children. Ann Nutr Metab 2015;66(Suppl 3):38–41.

84. Kullmann S, Heni M, Veit R, et al. Selective insulin resistance in homeostatic and cognitive control brain areas in overweight and obese adults. Diabetes Care 2015;38(6):1044–50.

85. Levitan RD, Rivera J, Silveira PP, et al. Gender differences in the association between stop-signal reaction times, body mass indices and/or spontaneous food intake in pre-school children: an early model of compromised inhibitory control and obesity. Int J Obes (Lond) 2015;39(4):614–9.

86. Reyes S, Peirano P, Peigneux P, et al. Inhibitory control in otherwise healthy overweight 10-year-old children. Int J Obes (Lond) 2015;39(8):1230–5.

87. Svaldi J, Naumann E, Trentowska M, et al. General and food-specific inhibitory deficits in binge eating disorder. Int J Eat Disord 2014;47(5):534–42.

88. Tuulari JJ, Karlsson HK, Hirvonen J, et al. Neural circuits for cognitive appetite control in healthy and obese individuals: an fMRI study. PLoS One 2015;10(2): e0116640.

89. Wirt T, Hundsdorfer V, Schreiber A, et al. Associations between inhibitory control and body weight in German primary school children. Eat Behav 2014;15(1): 9–12.

90. Wirt T, Schreiber A, Kesztyus D, et al. Early life cognitive abilities and body weight: cross-sectional study of the association of inhibitory control, cognitive flexibility, and sustained attention with BMI percentiles in primary school children. J Obes 2015;2015:534651.

91. Hendrick OM, Luo X, Zhang S, et al. Saliency processing and obesity: a preliminary imaging study of the stop signal task. Obesity (Silver Spring) 2012;20(9): 1796–802.

92. Nederkoorn C, Jansen E, Mulkens S, et al. Impulsivity predicts treatment outcome in obese children. Behav Res Ther 2007;45(5):1071–5.

93. Chapman CD, Benedict C, Brooks SJ, et al. Lifestyle determinants of the drive to eat: a meta-analysis. Am J Clin Nutr 2012;96(3):492–7.

94. Volkow ND, Wang GJ, Fowler JS, et al. Overlapping neuronal circuits in addiction and obesity: evidence of systems pathology. Philos Trans R Soc Lond B Biol Sci 2008;363(1507):3191–200.

95. Hotamisligil GS, Arner P, Caro JF, et al. Increased adipose tissue expression of tumor necrosis factor-alpha in human obesity and insulin resistance. J Clin Invest 1995;95(5):2409–15.

96. Lumeng CN, Saltiel AR. Inflammatory links between obesity and metabolic disease. J Clin Invest 2011;121(6):2111–7.

97. Brestoff JR, Artis D. Immune regulation of metabolic homeostasis in health and disease. Cell 2015;161(1):146–60.

98. De Souza CT, Araujo EP, Bordin S, et al. Consumption of a fat-rich diet activates a proinflammatory response and induces insulin resistance in the hypothalamus. Endocrinology 2005;146(10):4192–9.

99. Grayson BE, Levasseur PR, Williams SM, et al. Changes in melanocortin expression and inflammatory pathways in fetal offspring of nonhuman primates fed a high-fat diet. Endocrinology 2010;151(4):1622–32.

100. Thaler JP, Yi CX, Schur EA, et al. Obesity is associated with hypothalamic injury in rodents and humans. J Clin Invest 2012;122(1):153–62.

101. Valdearcos M, Robblee MM, Benjamin DI, et al. Microglia dictate the impact of saturated fat consumption on hypothalamic inflammation and neuronal function. Cell Rep 2014;9(6):2124–38.

102. Horvath TL, Sarman B, Garcia-Caceres C, et al. Synaptic input organization of the melanocortin system predicts diet-induced hypothalamic reactive gliosis and obesity. Proc Natl Acad Sci U S A 2010;107(33):14875–80.

103. Phillips CM, Dillon C, Harrington JM, et al. Defining metabolically healthy obesity: role of dietary and lifestyle factors. PLoS One 2013;8(10):e76188.

104. Wildman RP, Muntner P, Reynolds K, et al. The obese without cardiometabolic risk factor clustering and the normal weight with cardiometabolic risk factor clustering: prevalence and correlates of 2 phenotypes among the US population (NHANES 1999-2004). Arch Intern Med 2008;168(15):1617–24.

105. Van Gaal LF, Mertens IL, De Block CE. Mechanisms linking obesity with cardiovascular disease. Nature 2006;444(7121):875–80.

106. Mokdad AH, Ford ES, Bowman BA, et al. Prevalence of obesity, diabetes, and obesity-related health risk factors, 2001. JAMA 2003;289(1):76–9.

107. Achilike I, Hazuda HP, Fowler SP, et al. Predicting the development of the metabolically healthy obese phenotype. Int J Obes (Lond) 2015;39(2):228–34.

108. Velho S, Paccaud F, Waeber G, et al. Metabolically healthy obesity: different prevalences using different criteria. Eur J Clin Nutr 2010;64(10):1043–51.

109. Lee K. Metabolically obese but normal weight (MONW) and metabolically healthy but obese (MHO) phenotypes in Koreans: characteristics and health behaviors. Asia Pac J Clin Nutr 2009;18(2):280–4.

110. Bell JA, Hamer M, Sabia S, et al. The natural course of healthy obesity over 20 years. J Am Coll Cardiol 2015;65(1):101–2.

111. Appleton SL, Seaborn CJ, Visvanathan R, et al. Diabetes and cardiovascular disease outcomes in the metabolically healthy obese phenotype: a cohort study. Diabetes Care 2013;36(8):2388–94.

112. Kabat GC, Wu WY, Bea JW, et al. Metabolic phenotypes of obesity: frequency, correlates and change over time in a cohort of postmenopausal women. Int J Obes (Lond) 2017;41(1):170–7.

113. Sahakyan KR, Somers VK, Rodriguez-Escudero JP, et al. Normal-weight central obesity: implications for total and cardiovascular mortality. Ann Intern Med 2015;163(11):827–35.

114. Canoy D, Boekholdt SM, Wareham N, et al. Body fat distribution and risk of coronary heart disease in men and women in the European Prospective Investigation Into Cancer and Nutrition in Norfolk cohort: a population-based prospective study. Circulation 2007;116(25):2933–43.

115. Song YM, Sung J, Davey Smith G, et al. Body mass index and ischemic and hemorrhagic stroke: a prospective study in Korean men. Stroke 2004;35(4):831–6.

116. Zhang M, Hu T, Zhang S, et al. Associations of different adipose tissue depots with insulin resistance: a systematic review and meta-analysis of observational studies. Sci Rep 2015;5:18495.
117. Kahn SE, Hull RL, Utzschneider KM. Mechanisms linking obesity to insulin resistance and type 2 diabetes. Nature 2006;444(7121):840–6.
118. Shulman GI. Cellular mechanisms of insulin resistance. J Clin Invest 2000; 106(2):171–6.
119. Osborn O, Olefsky JM. The cellular and signaling networks linking the immune system and metabolism in disease. Nat Med 2012;18(3):363–74.
120. Kadowaki T, Yamauchi T, Kubota N, et al. Adiponectin and adiponectin receptors in insulin resistance, diabetes, and the metabolic syndrome. J Clin Invest 2006;116(7):1784–92.
121. Scherer PE. Adipose tissue: from lipid storage compartment to endocrine organ. Diabetes 2006;55(6):1537–45.
122. Kahn SE, Prigeon RL, McCulloch DK, et al. Quantification of the relationship between insulin sensitivity and beta-cell function in human subjects. Evidence for a hyperbolic function. Diabetes 1993;42(11):1663–72.
123. Hara K, Shojima N, Hosoe J, et al. Genetic architecture of type 2 diabetes. Biochem Biophys Res Commun 2014;452(2):213–20.
124. Kahn SE. Clinical review 135: The importance of beta-cell failure in the development and progression of type 2 diabetes. J Clin Endocrinol Metab 2001;86(9): 4047–58.
125. Butler AE, Janson J, Bonner-Weir S, et al. Beta-cell deficit and increased beta-cell apoptosis in humans with type 2 diabetes. Diabetes 2003;52(1):102–10.
126. Vazquez G, Duval S, Jacobs DR Jr, et al. Comparison of body mass index, waist circumference, and waist/hip ratio in predicting incident diabetes: a meta-analysis. Epidemiol Rev 2007;29:115–28.
127. Bell JA, Kivimaki M, Hamer M. Metabolically healthy obesity and risk of incident type 2 diabetes: a meta-analysis of prospective cohort studies. Obes Rev 2014; 15(6):504–15.
128. Power C, Thomas C. Changes in BMI, duration of overweight and obesity, and glucose metabolism: 45 years of follow-up of a birth cohort. Diabetes Care 2011; 34(9):1986–91.
129. Chan DC, Barrett HP, Watts GF. Dyslipidemia in visceral obesity: mechanisms, implications, and therapy. Am J Cardiovasc Drugs 2004;4(4):227–46.
130. Brown CD, Higgins M, Donato KA, et al. Body mass index and the prevalence of hypertension and dyslipidemia. Obes Res 2000;8(9):605–19.
131. Susic D, Varagic J. Obesity: a perspective from hypertension. Med Clin North Am 2017;101(1):139–57.
132. Messerli FH, Christie B, DeCarvalho JG, et al. Obesity and essential hypertension. Hemodynamics, intravascular volume, sodium excretion, and plasma renin activity. Arch Intern Med 1981;141(1):81–5.
133. Amann K, Benz K. Structural renal changes in obesity and diabetes. Semin Nephrol 2013;33(1):23–33.
134. Hall ME, do Carmo JM, da Silva AA, et al. Obesity, hypertension, and chronic kidney disease. Int J Nephrol Renovasc Dis 2014;7:75–88.
135. Kurukulasuriya LR, Stas S, Lastra G, et al. Hypertension in obesity. Med Clin North Am 2011;95(5):903–17.
136. Furukawa S, Fujita T, Shimabukuro M, et al. Increased oxidative stress in obesity and its impact on metabolic syndrome. J Clin Invest 2004;114(12):1752–61.

137. Kim JA, Montagnani M, Koh KK, et al. Reciprocal relationships between insulin resistance and endothelial dysfunction: molecular and pathophysiological mechanisms. Circulation 2006;113(15):1888–904.
138. Sprague AH, Khalil RA. Inflammatory cytokines in vascular dysfunction and vascular disease. Biochem Pharmacol 2009;78(6):539–52.
139. Kenchaiah S, Evans JC, Levy D, et al. Obesity and the risk of heart failure. N Engl J Med 2002;347(5):305–13.
140. Lu Y, Hajifathalian K, Ezzati M, et al. Metabolic mediators of the effects of body-mass index, overweight, and obesity on coronary heart disease and stroke: a pooled analysis of 97 prospective cohorts with 1.8 million participants. Lancet 2014;383(9921):970–83.
141. Wormser D, Kaptoge S, Di Angelantonio E, et al. Separate and combined associations of body-mass index and abdominal adiposity with cardiovascular disease: collaborative analysis of 58 prospective studies. Lancet 2011; 377(9771):1085–95.
142. Fan J, Song Y, Chen Y, et al. Combined effect of obesity and cardio-metabolic abnormality on the risk of cardiovascular disease: a meta-analysis of prospective cohort studies. Int J Cardiol 2013;168(5):4761–8.
143. Juonala M, Magnussen CG, Berenson GS, et al. Childhood adiposity, adult adiposity, and cardiovascular risk factors. N Engl J Med 2011;365(20):1876–85.
144. Gambineri A, Pelusi C, Vicennati V, et al. Obesity and the polycystic ovary syndrome. Int J Obes Relat Metab Disord 2002;26(7):883–96.
145. Rojas J, Chavez M, Olivar L, et al. Polycystic ovary syndrome, insulin resistance, and obesity: navigating the pathophysiologic labyrinth. Int J Reprod Med 2014; 2014:719050.
146. Baldani DP, Skrgatic L, Ougouag R. Polycystic ovary syndrome: important underrecognised cardiometabolic risk factor in reproductive-age women. Int J Endocrinol 2015;2015:786362.
147. Blank SK, McCartney CR, Chhabra S, et al. Modulation of gonadotropin-releasing hormone pulse generator sensitivity to progesterone inhibition in hyperandrogenic adolescent girls–implications for regulation of pubertal maturation. J Clin Endocrinol Metab 2009;94(7):2360–6.
148. Marshall JC, Dunaif A. Should all women with PCOS be treated for insulin resistance? Fertil Steril 2012;97(1):18–22.
149. Tock L, Carneiro G, Pereira AZ, et al. Adrenocortical production is associated with higher levels of luteinizing hormone in nonobese women with polycystic ovary syndrome. Int J Endocrinol 2014;2014:620605.
150. Ibanez L, Potau N, Virdis R, et al. Postpubertal outcome in girls diagnosed of premature pubarche during childhood: increased frequency of functional ovarian hyperandrogenism. J Clin Endocrinol Metab 1993;76(6):1599–603.
151. l'Allemand D, Schmidt S, Rousson V, et al. Associations between body mass, leptin, IGF-I and circulating adrenal androgens in children with obesity and premature adrenarche. Eur J Endocrinol 2002;146(4):537–43.
152. Baptiste CG, Battista MC, Trottier A, et al. Insulin and hyperandrogenism in women with polycystic ovary syndrome. J Steroid Biochem Mol Biol 2010; 122(1–3):42–52.
153. Norman RJ, Noakes M, Wu R, et al. Improving reproductive performance in overweight/obese women with effective weight management. Hum Reprod Update 2004;10(3):267–80.

154. Kiddy DS, Hamilton-Fairley D, Bush A, et al. Improvement in endocrine and ovarian function during dietary treatment of obese women with polycystic ovary syndrome. Clin Endocrinol 1992;36(1):105–11.

155. Yildiz BO, Bolour S, Woods K, et al. Visually scoring hirsutism. Hum Reprod Update 2010;16(1):51–64.

156. Sam S. Obesity and polycystic ovary syndrome. Obes Manag 2007;3(2):69–73.

157. Lee YH, Johan A, Wong KK, et al. Prevalence and risk factors for obstructive sleep apnea in a multiethnic population of patients presenting for bariatric surgery in Singapore. Sleep Med 2009;10(2):226–32.

158. Kositanurit W, Muntham D, Udomsawaengsup S, et al. Prevalence and associated factors of obstructive sleep apnea in morbidly obese patients undergoing bariatric surgery. Sleep Breath 2017. [Epub ahead of print].

159. Jean-Louis G, Zizi F, Clark LT, et al. Obstructive sleep apnea and cardiovascular disease: role of the metabolic syndrome and its components. J Clin Sleep Med 2008;4(3):261–72.

160. Romero-Corral A, Caples SM, Lopez-Jimenez F, et al. Interactions between obesity and obstructive sleep apnea: implications for treatment. Chest 2010; 137(3):711–9.

161. Hurt RT, Kulisek C, Buchanan LA, et al. The obesity epidemic: challenges, health initiatives, and implications for gastroenterologists. Gastroenterol Hepatol 2010;6(12):780–92.

162. Zammit C, Liddicoat H, Moonsie I, et al. Obesity and respiratory diseases. Int J Gen Med 2010;3:335–43.

163. Babu AR, Herdegen J, Fogelfeld L, et al. Type 2 diabetes, glycemic control, and continuous positive airway pressure in obstructive sleep apnea. Arch Intern Med 2005;165(4):447–52.

164. Strohl KP, Butler JP, Malhotra A. Mechanical properties of the upper airway. Compr Physiol 2012;2(3):1853–72.

165. Dempsey JA, Veasey SC, Morgan BJ, et al. Pathophysiology of sleep apnea. Physiol Rev 2010;90(1):47–112.

166. Schwartz AR, Smith PL, Oliven A. Electrical stimulation of the hypoglossal nerve: a potential therapy. J Appl Physiol (1985) 2014;116(3):337–44.

167. Schwartz AR, Patil SP, Laffan AM, et al. Obesity and obstructive sleep apnea: pathogenic mechanisms and therapeutic approaches. Proc Am Thorac Soc 2008;5(2):185–92.

168. Shigeta Y, Ogawa T, Tomoko I, et al. Soft palate length and upper airway relationship in OSA and non-OSA subjects. Sleep Breath 2010;14(4):353–8.

169. Zancanella E, Haddad FM, Oliveira LA, et al. Obstructive sleep apnea and primary snoring: diagnosis. Braz J Otorhinolaryngology 2014;80(1 Suppl 1):S1–16.

170. Daulatzai MA. Role of sensory stimulation in amelioration of obstructive sleep apnea. Sleep Disord 2011;2011:596879.

171. Tuomilehto HP, Seppa JM, Partinen MM, et al. Lifestyle intervention with weight reduction: first-line treatment in mild obstructive sleep apnea. Am J Respir Crit Care Med 2009;179(4):320–7.

172. Dobbins M, Decorby K, Choi BC. The association between obesity and cancer risk: a meta-analysis of observational studies from 1985 to 2011. ISRN Prev Med 2013;2013:680536.

173. Vainio H, Kaaks R, Bianchini F. Weight control and physical activity in cancer prevention: international evaluation of the evidence. Eur J Cancer Prev 2002; 11(Suppl 2):S94–100.

174. Calle EE, Rodriguez C, Walker-Thurmond K, et al. Overweight, obesity, and mortality from cancer in a prospectively studied cohort of U.S. adults. N Engl J Med 2003;348(17):1625–38.
175. Berrington de Gonzalez A, Hartge P, Cerhan JR, et al. Body-mass index and mortality among 1.46 million white adults. N Engl J Med 2010;363(23):2211–9.
176. Sjostrom L, Gummesson A, Sjostrom CD, et al. Effects of bariatric surgery on cancer incidence in obese patients in Sweden (Swedish Obese Subjects Study): a prospective, controlled intervention trial. Lancet Oncol 2009;10(7): 653–62.
177. Park J, Euhus DM, Scherer PE. Paracrine and endocrine effects of adipose tissue on cancer development and progression. Endocr Rev 2011;32(4):550–70.
178. Ziemke F, Mantzoros CS. Adiponectin in insulin resistance: lessons from translational research. Am J Clin Nutr 2010;91(1):258S–61S.
179. Kelesidis I, Kelesidis T, Mantzoros CS. Adiponectin and cancer: a systematic review. Br J Cancer 2006;94(9):1221–5.
180. Dalamaga M, Diakopoulos KN, Mantzoros CS. The role of adiponectin in cancer: a review of current evidence. Endocr Rev 2012;33(4):547–94.
181. Jain SS, Bird RP. Elevated expression of tumor necrosis factor-alpha signaling molecules in colonic tumors of Zucker obese (fa/fa) rats. Int J Cancer 2010; 127(9):2042–50.
182. Khandekar MJ, Cohen P, Spiegelman BM. Molecular mechanisms of cancer development in obesity. Nat Rev Cancer 2011;11(12):886–95.
183. Park EJ, Lee JH, Yu GY, et al. Dietary and genetic obesity promote liver inflammation and tumorigenesis by enhancing IL-6 and TNF expression. Cell 2010; 140(2):197–208.

Treatment of Obesity in Primary Care

Adam G. Tsai, MD, MSCE[a,b,*], Jocelyn E. Remmert, BA[c], Meghan L. Butryn, PhD[c], Thomas A. Wadden, PhD[d]

KEYWORDS

- Treatment • Obesity • Primary care • Interventions • Behavioral counseling
- Weight loss programs • Medication • Surgery

KEY POINTS

- The studies reviewed demonstrate that the interventions most likely to produce clinically important weight loss are those that provide high-intensity counseling. Primary care physicians (PCPs) can be effective in delivering weight loss counseling, particularly if they are able to individualize the message for a given patient.
- Given the behavioral and biological challenges involved in maintenance of weight loss, PCPs should be open to the idea of using medications and surgery to treat obesity. To the extent that PCPs themselves are open to these therapies, they will truly be treating obesity in the same way they treat other chronic medical illnesses.
- Whether or not a PCP becomes an expert in the treatment of obesity, she or he should show respect and empathy in discussing the topic with patients.
- Positive reinforcement of success with patients is very important, including redefining success (5%–10% loss of initial body weight), encouraging efforts at maintenance of weight loss, and refocusing on improvement in weight-related conditions, not body mass index alone.
- The physicians who will have the greatest success in managing obesity will be those individuals who are most adept at engaging patients in behavioral treatment, providing patient-centered counseling, and using biological tools when necessary to produce long-term weight loss.

In 2013, the American Medical Association declared obesity to be a chronic disease. Taking this view of obesity as a disease, obesity is the most prevalent chronic disease in the United States, with 37% of women and 35% of men having a body mass index

[a] Kaiser Permanente, Metabolic-Surgical Weight Management, 2045 Franklin Street, 3rd Floor, Denver, CO 80205, USA; [b] University of Colorado School of Medicine, Aurora, CO, USA; [c] Department of Psychology, Center for Weight, Eating, and Lifestyle Science, Drexel University, 3201 Chestnut Street, Philadelphia, PA 19104, USA; [d] Center for Weight and Eating Disorders, Perelman School of Medicine University of Pennsylvania, 3535 Market Street, Suite 3027, Philadelphia, PA 19104, USA
* Corresponding author. 1375 East 20th Avenue, 3rd Floor, Denver, CO 80205.
E-mail address: adam.tsai@kp.org

Med Clin N Am 102 (2018) 35–47
http://dx.doi.org/10.1016/j.mcna.2017.08.005
0025-7125/18/© 2017 Elsevier Inc. All rights reserved.
medical.theclinics.com

(BMI) of 30 kg/m^2 or greater. The prevalence of obesity has begun to stabilize but is still increasing, albeit more slowly.[1] Additionally, obesity itself is a risk factor for many other chronic diseases. These include diabetes, hypertension, and obstructive sleep apnea, all forms of cardiovascular disease (atherosclerotic, arrhythmias, and congestive heart failure), arthritis of weight-bearing joints, and depression.

Primary care physicians (PCPs) and other providers (nurse practitioners and physician assistants) are typically the first clinicians to evaluate and treat obesity and its related complications. If PCPs are able to address obesity in its own right, it has the potential to reduce the burden of chronic disease. The medical and health care policy communities have made some progress toward supporting PCPs in addressing obesity. For example, the Patient Protection and Affordable Care Act mandates that any service receiving an A or a B grade recommendation from the US Preventive Services Task Force be covered without patient copays.[2] The Task Force gave high-intensity weight loss counseling a B grade in its initial review in 2003 and again in 2012.[3,4] (A grade of B means that there is high certainty that the net benefit of providing a service is moderate, or that there is moderate certainty that the net benefit of providing a service is moderate to substantial.) Also, the Center for Medicare and Medicaid Services now reimburses up to 20, 15-minute weight loss counseling visits over 1 year,[5] when conducted in a primary setting. Updated guidelines for behavioral and surgical treatment of obesity[6] and for pharmacologic treatment of obesity[7] have provided PCPs with tools to better address obesity. There is now a board certification in obesity medicine (www.abom.org) and, although the specialty of obesity medicine is not yet recognized by the American Board of Medical Specialties, the number of internal medicine physicians taking the examination has now surpassed the number certifying in more traditional subspecialties, such as endocrinology and infectious disease.[8,9]

Despite this progress, the evidence continues to show that PCPs do not consistently address obesity in outpatient visits.[10–12] Although the treatment of obesity has become a higher priority from professional societies and policy makers, the frequency with which PCPs discuss weight has not improved.[13] The lack of improvement in obesity treatment may be a consequence of physicians not buying in to the model of obesity as a chronic disease, or it may be a consequence of PCP overwork and burnout in a time in which a career in outpatient internal medicine or family medicine is perceived as a low prestige choice.[14]

Regardless of why PCPs are not consistently addressing weight, this article outlines some of the behavioral, pharmacologic, and surgical interventions available to PCPs to help their patients with weight management. For systematic reviews on each of these topics, the reader is referred elsewhere.[7,15–19] Recognizing that interventions are not always feasible to implement (see later discussion), this article ends with several clinical suggestions on obesity management that PCPs can take back and use immediately in office practice.

LIFESTYLE MODIFICATION FOR TREATMENT OF OBESITY

The updated guidelines on behavioral and surgical treatment of obesity (American Heart Association [AHA]/American College of Cardiology [ACC]/The Obesity Society [TOS]) affirmed that the standard of care for behavioral treatment of obesity is a high-intensity, in-person intervention that is comprehensive in nature (ie, includes dietary and physical activity targets and the provision of behavioral counseling to achieve those targets).[6] The AHA/ACC/TOS guidelines defined high-intensity as at least 14 visits, delivered over 6 months, in either individual or group format. The guidelines also specified that visits must include personalized feedback from a trained interventionist. (For example, an individual weekly email from an employer with standardized weight loss advice sent out for 6 months does not qualify as a gold standard behavioral intervention. Conversely, an individual who attends a Weight Watchers group visit 14 times over 6 months has achieved the standard.) A systematic review of obesity treatment in primary care,[20] as well as a systematic review of primary care–relevant studies,[21] concluded that high-intensity interventions, delivered in primary care, can lead to clinically significant weight loss. The review by Wadden and colleagues[20] also found that low-intensity interventions and interventions using only alternative methods of counseling (eg, motivational interviewing, without specific goals for calorie intake or physical activity) did not lead to clinically significant weight loss. Rather than providing a systematic review, this article briefly reviews low-intensity and moderate-intensity interventions, and then focuses primarily on high-intensity interventions, defined as at least 2 visits per month for the first 6 months.[4]

Low-Intensity or Moderate-Intensity Interventions

Research consistently demonstrates that patients are more likely to attempt and to achieve weight loss when their physician discusses it.[22] However, when physician advice is delivered in a low-to-moderate intensity format ($\leq$1 visit per month), weight loss is minimal. For example, in a randomized trial, Martin and colleagues[23,24] assigned subjects to monthly counseling visits with their PCP or to usual care. Subjects in the treatment arm lost 1.4 kg at 12 months, compared with a weight gain of 0.3 kg in the control group (P = .01), but the difference at 18 months was not significant (-0.5 kg vs $+0.1$ kg; P = .39).[23,24] Christian and colleagues[25] tested an even lower intensity intervention in 2 randomized trials, both using PCPs to deliver counseling. One study provided quarterly counseling and the second trial provided just 2 visits over the 12 months of the trial.[26] In both studies, the intervention group also completed an interactive computer program that produced individualized recommendations for subjects to discuss with their PCPs. In both trials, however, differences between groups were small after 1 year (-0.1 kg intervention vs $+0.6$ control in the first study, P = .23; and -1.5 kg intervention vs $+0.2$ kg control in the second study; P = .002).

Physician time is costly and at least 1 trial has suggested that registered dietitians, when provided with the same tools, facilitate greater weight losses than physicians.[27] Thus, investigators have attempted to use other clinicians or staff in primary care offices to deliver weight loss counseling. In 1 trial, nurse practitioners delivered quarterly weight loss counseling visits; weight losses were 1.6% of initial body weight (intervention) and 0.3% (control) after 12 months (P = .08 for difference; estimated from a figure).[28] A separate trial used medical assistants to provide monthly counseling to subjects at their home primary care practices. The control group received brief counseling every 4 months from their PCP. Weight losses after 12 months were 1.6 kg in the intervention arm and 0.6 kg in the control arm (P = .15 for difference).[29] A third trial, also using medical assistants to deliver counseling, randomized primary care subjects to quarterly counseling visits with their PCPs, or to a series of 8 lifestyle counseling visits over 6 months (moderate intensity counseling), using a shortened version of the Diabetes Prevention Program (DPP) curriculum. Weight loss at 6 months was significantly greater in the treatment than control arm (4.4 kg vs 0.9 kg; P<.001), but at 12 months the difference was no longer significant (2.3 kg vs 1.1 kg; P = .31).[30]

The results of the trials previously described are all consistent, showing an additional weight loss of 1 to 2 kg after 12 months of low or moderate intensity counseling compared with standard medical care. The results are generally similar when the counseling is conducted by a physician or by another team member in the primary care office. It follows that PCPs should not expect most patients with obesity to lose a clinically significant amount of weight with infrequent visits (monthly or less often). Although the risk of offering low-intensity treatment is probably minimal for most individuals, some patients may feel frustrated if they do not lose weight and consequently have lower self-efficacy and motivation for persisting in behavior change.

High-Intensity Interventions

Most of the studies described next show that high-intensity counseling in primary care leads to clinically significant weight loss. The relatively small number of trials that have been able to achieve this standard speaks to the challenge of implementing intensive behavior change programs in busy primary care practices.

Two trials conducted as part of a collaborative funding effort by the National Institutes of Health found weight losses of 4 to 5 kg in primary care subjects provided with intensive or multimodality interventions. In the first study, subjects were randomized to standard care, to high-intensity counseling by telephone, or to high-intensity counseling in person. After 2 years, weight losses were 0.8 kg, 4.6 kg, and 5.1 kg in the 3 groups, respectively ($P<.0001$ for difference between standard care and both intensive groups).[31] In the second trial, subjects were randomly assigned to standard care, moderate-intensity counseling (monthly visits with a medical assistant), or moderate-intensity counseling with choice of an additional weight loss tool (meal replacements or weight loss medication). Weight losses after 2 years were 1.7 kg, 2.8 kg, and 4.6 kg in the 3 groups ($P = .003$ for comparison of standard care vs enhanced lifestyle counseling; $P = .08$ for moderate intensity counseling vs standard care).[32]

An additional randomized trial by Ma and colleagues recruited subjects with prediabetes or metabolic syndrome and randomized them to usual care versus in-person delivery of the DPP curriculum (weekly group meetings for 12 weeks, followed by monthly maintenance sessions) versus the DPP curriculum delivered at self-directed pace by DVD. After 2 years, weight losses in the 3 groups were 2.4, 5.4, and 4.5 kg, respectively ($P = .001$ for in-person vs control; $P = .03$ for self-directed vs control).[33,34]

High-intensity counseling during the period of weight-loss maintenance has also been shown to be beneficial. In a randomized trial, subjects who completed 6 months of high-intensity treatment (12 visits over 6 months) were randomized to standard maintenance (written materials delivered by e-mail or regular mail) versus intensive maintenance (monthly in-person visits, with telephone calls halfway between visits). All subjects had access to a subsidized regimen of portion-controlled foods (Nutrisystem) throughout the trial. Weight losses after 18 months were 6.1 kg with intensive maintenance versus 2.2 kg with standard maintenance ($P<.001$).[35]

The trial by Wadden and colleagues[32] previously described demonstrated the value of multimodality interventions, which was confirmed by another randomized trial with state employees in Louisiana conducted by Ryan and colleagues.[36] Participants were recruited from primary care practices and randomized to usual care or an intervention that incorporated intensive behavioral counseling, meal replacements, and weight loss medication over 24 months. Subjects received a 900 kcal per day medically supervised diet, followed by 4 months of high-intensity group counseling with continued partial meal replacement and optional weight loss medication, followed by 17 months of continued monthly group sessions, optional weight loss medication, and optional bursts of meal replacement. At the end of 24 months, average weight loss was 4.9% of initial body weight in the treatment arm versus 0.2% of initial body weight in the usual care arm ($P<.001$ for difference).[36] Of note, the dropout rate was 49% after

24 months. Subjects in the intervention group who completed the trial lost 8.3% of initial body weight.

Despite these promising results, not every study of high-intensity interventions led to clinically significant weight loss. In another trial, the 16-session DPP was shortened to 6 sessions and implemented by nurse practitioners in a primary office, with telephone visits delivered between the monthly office visits over a 6-month period. Weight loss was 2.5% of initial body weight in the intervention group compared with a weight gain of 0.8% in the control group. Although the intervention period in this trial lasted only 6 months, the intensity of contact is considered high, given the telephone calls conducted between the in-person contacts.[37]

Finally, another randomized trial demonstrated that frequent contact by telephone is effective and that group treatment is more effective than individual treatment.[38] In this study, primary care subjects with metabolic syndrome received the DPP curriculum, either by group conference call or by individual telephone calls. All subjects had 10 telephone calls in the first 6 months, and monthly calls for the rest of the first year. Optional monthly calls were offered during year 2. At the end of 2 years, the group conference call arm had a weight loss of 6.2 kg, and the individual telephone calls arm had a weight loss of 2.2 kg ($P<.001$ for difference).[39] As with the trial by Ryan and colleagues,[36] attrition was high (47.5% after 2 years).

As a group, the studies of high-intensity treatment in primary care show that frequent contact can lead to clinically significant weight loss. The intensity of treatment is the most important factor in producing weight loss. Both in-person and telephonic interventions achieved significant weight losses. The studies previously described also demonstrated that multimodality interventions (ie, counseling plus meal replacements plus weight loss medication) are effective at increasing weight losses.[32,36] High attrition was noted in 2 trials,[36,39] highlighting again the challenge of conducting intensive behavioral interventions in a largely unselected patient population. However, analyses accounted for high attrition, and clinically significant weight loss was still observed.

Studies Using Alternative Methods of Behavioral Counseling in Primary Care

As previously stated, the systematic review of obesity treatment in primary care[20] found that high-intensity interventions lead to consistently greater weight loss compared with low-intensity or moderate-intensity interventions. The second main finding of the systematic review was that so-called traditional behavioral counseling methods were associated with greater weight losses than other, less prescriptive methods of treatment. All the trials included in the systematic review were required to include counseling on diet, physical activity, and behavior modification. Traditional behavioral counseling was defined more specifically in the systematic review as including specific targets for calorie restriction and physical activity, and the use of behavioral strategies to facilitate achievement of those goals (eg, self-monitoring). The other studies were referred to as alternative treatment methods and used primarily motivational interviewing or stages of change.[40,41] Two studies published after this review also found similarly modest results for motivational interviewing-based interventions. One study[42] randomly assigned participants to either a no-intervention control group or to a program that included access to online-based lifestyle modification materials and 5 sessions of either motivational interviewing or psychoeducation. At 6 months, weight loss averaged 2.6 kg in the psychoeducation condition and 1.1 kg in the motivational interviewing condition; only the psychoeducation condition significantly outperformed the usual care group ($P = .004$). In the other study,[43] participants were randomly assigned to usual care or to a 3-month, biweekly, telephone-based intervention that combined motivational interviewing with training in several behavioral weight loss principles. Weight loss in the intervention group, which was 2.2 kg at 3 months and 2.6 kg at 6 months, was not superior to the usual care group at either time point (P = .09 and 0.22, respectively). The finding that alternative counseling methods generally do not lead to clinically significant weight loss, although disappointing, provides helpful guidance to clinicians and investigators seeking to evaluate weight loss interventions.

COMMERCIAL WEIGHT LOSS PROGRAMS

In the 2013 guidelines,[6] the AHA/ACC/TOS committee recommended that commercial weight loss programs can be used as an option for high-intensity behavioral treatment of obesity. Many PCPs, particularly those who work in small practices, may not have immediate access to or time for high-intensity interventions. In this situation, commercial programs are a reasonable alternative. The AHA/ACC/TOS guidelines specified that programs should provide published, peer-reviewed evidence of their safety and efficacy.

Several of the largest commercial weight loss providers have sponsored randomized controlled trials to test the efficacy of their programs, spurred by the publication of a systematic review in 2005 noting the paucity of evidence.[44] Gudzune and colleagues[45] conducted an updated systematic review of the literature on commercial weight loss programs. They found that Weight Watchers and Jenny Craig had long-term data (1 year or longer) to support their programs, and that Nutrisystem, Optifast, Health Management Resources, and Medifast had reported shorter-term randomized trials of their efficacy. Gudzune and colleagues[45] also found that Atkins and Slim-Fast, 2 companies producing meal replacement products for self-directed use, had reported evidence of safety and efficacy. Of note, the cost of many commercial programs is high, particularly those programs that require the purchase of food, and therefore may not be an option for all patients. A nonprofit alternative to commercial weight loss programs is Take Off Pounds Sensibly (TOPS). TOPS is a low-cost (approximately $32 a year), peer-led group intervention. No randomized trial data have been published to support it, but available published research suggests that it may be effective among individuals who continue treatment.[46,47]

MEDICAL AND SURGICAL OPTIONS FOR PRIMARY CARE PHYSICIANS TO CONSIDER
Adding Medications to Behavioral Treatment

As noted in the AHA/ACC/TOS guidelines, medications for the treatment of obesity are an option for patients who have not reached weight loss goals with behavioral treatment. In 2015, the Endocrine Society, together with TOS, published the definitive national guideline on using medications to treat obesity. This guideline is helpful for PCPs seeking to add pharmacotherapy for obesity to their practices. Several randomized trials[48–51] have demonstrated that the combination of intensive behavioral treatment and medication achieves nearly double the weight loss of either treatment delivered alone. However, the challenge remains of engaging patients in high-intensity behavioral treatment. Thus, the reality is that most patients will take medications for treatment of obesity in the context of self-directed efforts at lifestyle modification. The existing randomized trials of weight loss medications are likely a reasonable reflection of the weight losses that could be expected with use of these drugs by PCPs. Three published trials have used weight loss medications in primary care.[50,52,53] All 3 studies showed significantly greater weight loss among subjects randomly assigned to take medication. However, of these 3 trials, 2 used orlistat, a medication that is no longer commonly prescribed,[52,53] and 1 used sibutramine,[50] a medication that is now off the market.

Surgical Treatment of Obesity

Bariatric surgery has long been the most effective tool for the treatment of severe obesity, inducing weight losses of 20% to 30% of initial body weight. PCPs should consider referring their patients for evaluation for weight loss surgery if weight loss goals have not been met with the combination of high-intensity behavioral treatment and medication (and if the patient desires the evaluation for surgery). Surgery induces multiple changes in the body that make it easier for patients to adhere to healthy eating and ultimately to increased physical activity. Weight loss achieved through surgery has been shown to be maintained out to 20 years in the Swedish Obese Subjects study. Weight loss after surgery has been shown to be variable but also durable out to 7 years in the United States (B. Wolfe, MD, personal communication, 2017). The safety of weight loss surgery has increased greatly from 20 to 30 years ago, when most gastric bypass was done by open incision and the mortality rate was 1% to 2%.[54] Currently, most bariatric procedures are laparoscopic and the mortality rate in accredited centers is approximately 0.1%. Not all patients referred for weight loss surgery are offered an operation; patients must first undergo a multidisciplinary medical and behavioral evaluation. Thus, PCPs should be reassured about the safety of referring their patients for a surgical evaluation.

KEY MESSAGES FOR PRIMARY CARE PHYSICIANS CONCERNING OBESITY

As previously described, medical professional societies and health care policy makers are making efforts to improve the treatment of obesity. However, rates of weight loss counseling by PCPs have not improved. This is likely a combination of 2 factors: (1) the high workload in primary care practice and (2) the many physicians who believe that obesity is a lifestyle problem rather than a chronic metabolic disease. Most of the behavioral interventions in the studies previously outlined are not practical for primary care practitioners who are already stretched with their current workload. PCPs can prescribe medications; however, without concurrent intensive lifestyle interventions, the weight loss achieved is likely to be well below patient goals.[55,56] Weight loss surgery is the most effective intervention for severe obesity, but access to this treatment is limited and many patients do not want to undergo surgery. Where does this leave the PCP in terms of treating obesity? PCPs obviously cannot tackle the obesity epidemic alone. However, the authors believe that PCPs do have an important role to play in treating obesity because they have the most contact with patients, sometimes over many years. The following is an attempt to provide practitioners with several clinical pearls that they can use in office practice. Several of these points were also reviewed in a paper by Rutledge and colleagues.[57] Stress is an issue frequently raised by patients as a barrier to successful weight management. However, the addition of mindfulness training or forms of stress management has not been shown to improve weight loss or health-related quality of life beyond conventional behavioral treatment for obesity (which does address stress management).

The first take-home message for PCPs is the importance of getting their patients to engage in high-intensity behavioral treatment. The studies previously described show that low-intensity or moderate-intensity treatment does not usually produce clinically significant weight loss. Thus, the patient who says, "I already met with a dietitian" can still benefit from more intensive work. Whether the patient participates in a program within the health care system versus outside (eg, commercial programs) is less important than the intensity of treatment. If a patient engages in treatment and self-monitoring of diet, there is a good likelihood of achieving a 5% to 10% weight loss. This is not an easy sell for the busy PCP, given the time commitment required by the patient. However, as previously noted, intensive interventions delivered by telephone seem to hold promise.[31,39] Additionally, even a provider referral to intensive behavioral treatment increases weight loss.[58] Participants in a recent study were randomly assigned to either a referral condition or a control intervention in which the physician simply advised the subject that weight loss would be helpful to their health.[58] In the first condition, referral was made to a weight management group and, if referral was accepted, the physician followed up to ensure attendance. Weight loss at 12 months averaged 2.4 kg in the referral condition compared with 1.0 kg in the control group ($P<.001$). This demonstrates that even a very brief referral for services and follow-up contributes to greater uptake of weight loss treatment (40% in the referral condition vs 9% in the control) and greater weight loss at 12 months. Also of note, a recent study (nonrandomized) demonstrated the value of an intensive behavioral program delivered as a live webinar.[59] The PCP should remind patients that the definition of high-intensity treatment includes a live person on the other end providing feedback and recommendations,[6] regardless of the mode of treatment delivery (in-person, telephone, Internet).

A second take-home message for PCPs to start using in their practices concerns weight loss goals. At least 2 studies have reported that patients' weight loss goals are often very unrealistic relative to average weight losses achieved with behavioral, pharmacologic, and surgical treatment.[55,56] Thus, part of the PCPs job is to counsel the patients on the benefits of moderate weight loss.[60–62] Rather than always targeting a normal weight on BMI charts, patients and their PCPs should target a weight loss that produces a clinically important improvement in comorbid conditions (diabetes, hypertension, sleep apnea) and improves health-related quality of life. A secondary message here relates to elderly patients, many of whom have sarcopenic obesity. In these individuals, who may be seeking treatment of obesity, increases in physical activity seem to be at least as effective as weight loss in improving overall functional status.[63]

The third message that PCPs must understand involves the challenge of keeping off lost weight (ie, weight loss maintenance). From the patient perspective, experiencing weight loss is highly motivating. Once the scale stops moving, however, many patients lose motivation and reduce their efforts at lifestyle change. It is in this weight-reduced state that the body experiences reductions in basal metabolic rate,[64] as well as increases in appetite.[65] Thus, again from the patient perspective, the hard work only continues when the plateau occurs. If PCPs can help their patients understand the biological predisposition to weight regain, it may help them to continue their efforts at behavior modification to maintain their weight loss. Efforts to maintain weight loss are particularly important given a recent study reporting that repeated cycles of weight loss and regain are associated with an increased risk of diabetes and of major cardiovascular events.[66]

A fourth message for PCPs to use with their patients includes the consideration of so-called biological treatments for obesity (ie, medications and bariatric surgery). Given the biological adaptations to weight loss previously mentioned (the third message), patients may be more open to the idea of taking a weight loss medication long term or undergoing weight loss surgery. These tools can counteract the automatic increases in appetite that occur with weight loss, perhaps in part by reducing the brain's reaction to stimulation from food.[67,68] The willingness of PCPs to use medications and surgery to treat obesity helps patients understand the chronic metabolic nature of obesity as a disease in its own right. When used appropriately, these tools may increase the long-term success rates of weight loss.

The fifth and last message that PCPs can use in practice is the importance of sleep in managing weight. This message was reviewed in the paper by Rutledge and colleagues[57] Sleep deprivation from any cause (eg, insomnia, untreated sleep apnea) has an adverse impact on weight.[69] Thus, for some patients, efforts at weight management start with efforts to improve sleep hygiene. Currently, only about two-thirds of Americans report getting 7 hours per night or more of sleep.[70] The average sleep requirement is thought to be 8 hours (range, 7–9 hours), indicating that the American public is sleep deprived and that this is contributing to weight gain at a population level.[71]

SUMMARY

As previously described, medical professional societies and policy makers are paying more attention to obesity and urging PCPs to treat it more consistently. However, this is occurring at a time when primary care medicine remains low on the totem pole of career choices for physicians. In addition, the pressure to treat obesity is also delivered with a mixed message from health payers, in the context of inconsistent reimbursement for treatment of obesity. The studies previously reviewed demonstrate that the interventions most likely to produce clinically important weight loss are those that provide high-intensity counseling. The modality of treatment (in-person or by telephone) is less important than the intensity of contact and the inclusion of personalized feedback from a trained interventionist.[6] Given that most primary care practices are ill-equipped to take on large-scale interventions in their practices, PCPs should refer patients to programs that meet the criteria previously outlined (high-intensity contact, personalized feedback). Such a program may be within the walls of the PCP's practice, a university-based program, or a commercial or nonprofit program.

PCPs can be effective in delivering weight loss counseling, particularly if they are able to individualize the message for a given patient. For example, some patients need help realigning weight loss goals, whereas other patients may not realize the interrelationship of sleep and weight. Given the behavioral and biological challenges involved in maintenance of lost weight, PCPs should be open to the idea of using medications and surgery to treat obesity. To the extent that PCPs themselves are open to these therapies, they will truly be treating obesity in the same way they treat other chronic medical illnesses.

Whether a PCP becomes an expert in the treatment of obesity, she or he should show respect and empathy in discussing the topic with patients. Weight is often a sensitive topic, and PCPs should broach it with appropriate terms (weight, rather than obesity).[72,73] People-first language (a patient with diabetes rather than a diabetic patient) has become a standard in health care and is appropriate to use with both patients and clinician colleagues. Positive reinforcement of success with patients is very important, including redefining success (5%–10% loss of initial body weight), encouraging efforts at maintenance of weight loss, and refocusing on improvement in weight-related conditions rather than BMI alone. This is especially true given that most patients will not reach the weight loss goals they initially set for themselves. The physicians that will have the greatest success in managing obesity will be those who are most adept at engaging patients in behavioral treatment, providing patient-centered counseling, and using biological tools when necessary to produce long-term weight loss.

REFERENCES

1. Flegal KM, Kruszon-Moran D, Carroll MD, et al. Trends in obesity among adults in the United States, 2005 to 2014. JAMA 2016;315(21):2284–91.

2. United States Congress. Patient Protection and Affordable Care Act (PPACA), section 2713. 2010. Available at: https://www.gpo.gov/fdsys/pkg/PLAW-111publ148/pdf/PLAW-111publ148.pdf.

3. Moyer VA, U.S. Preventive Services Task Force. Screening for and management of obesity in adults: U.S. Preventive Services Task Force recommendation statement. Ann Intern Med 2012;157(5):373–8.

4. US Preventive Services Task Force. Screening for obesity in adults: recommendations and rationale. 2003. Available at: http://annals.org/aim/article/716966/screening-obesity-adults-recommendations-rationale. Accessed June 29, 2017.

5. Centers for Medicare & Medicaid Services. Decision memo for intensive behavioral therapy for obesity (CAG-00423N). Available at: http://www.cms.gov/medicare-coverage-database/details/nca-decision-memo.aspx?&NcaName=Intensive%20Behavioral%20Therapy%20for%20Obesity&bc=ACAAAAAAIAAA&NCAId=253&. Accessed June 29, 2017.

6. Jensen MD, Ryan DH, Apovian CM, et al. 2013 AHA/ACC/TOS guideline for the management of overweight and obesity in adults: a report of the American College of Cardiology/American Heart Association task force on practice guidelines and The Obesity Society. J Am Coll Cardiol 2014;63(25 Pt B):2985–3023.

7. Apovian CM, Aronne LJ, Bessesen DH, et al. Pharmacological management of obesity: an Endocrine Society clinical practice guideline. J Clin Endocrinol Metab 2015;100(2):342–62.

8. Kushner RF, Brittan D, Cleek J, et al. The American Board of Obesity Medicine: five-year report. Obesity (Silver Spring) 2017;25(6):982–4.

9. American Board of Internal Medicine. Number of candidates certified annually by the American Board of Internal Medicine, 2011-2015. 2016. Available at: http://www.abim.org/~/media/ABIM%20Public/Files/pdf/statistics-data/candidates-certiified-annually.pdf. Accessed June 29, 2017.

10. Sciamanna CN, Tate DF, Lang W, et al. Who reports receiving advice to lose weight?: results from a multistate survey. Arch Intern Med 2000;160(15):2334–9.

11. Jackson JE, Doescher MP, Saver BG, et al. Trends in professional advice to lose weight among obese adults, 1994 to 2000. J Gen Intern Med 2005;20(9):814–8.

12. Ma J, Xiao L, Stafford RS. Adult obesity and office-based quality of care in the United States. Obesity (Silver Spring) 2009;17(5):1077–85.

13. Kraschnewski JL, Sciamanna CN, Stuckey HL, et al. A silent response to the obesity epidemic: decline in US physician weight counseling. Med Care 2013;51(2):186–92.

14. Roberts DL, Shanafelt TD, Dyrbye LN, et al. A national comparison of burnout and work-life balance among internal medicine hospitalists and outpatient general internists. J Hosp Med 2014;9(3):176–81.

15. Alamuddin N, Wadden TA. Behavioral treatment of the patient with obesity. Endocrinol Metab Clin North Am 2016;45(3):565–80.

16. Wadden TA, Webb VL, Moran CH, et al. Lifestyle modification for obesity. Circulation 2012;125(9):1157–70.

17. Khera R, Murad MH, Chandar AK, et al. Association of pharmacological treatments for obesity with weight loss and adverse events: a systematic review and meta-analysis. JAMA 2016;315(22):2424–34.

18. Arterburn DE, Fisher DP. The current state of the evidence for bariatric surgery. JAMA 2014;312(9):898–9.

19. Mechanick JI, Youdim A, Jones DB, et al. Clinical practice guidelines for the perioperative nutritional, metabolic, and nonsurgical support of the bariatric surgery patient—2013 update. Obesity 2013;21(S1):S1–27.

20. Wadden TA, Butryn ML, Hong PS, et al. Behavioral treatment of obesity in patients encountered in primary care settings: a systematic review. JAMA 2014;312(17): 1779–91.
21. Leblanc ES, O'Connor E, Whitlock EP, et al. Effectiveness of primary care-relevant treatments for obesity in adults: a systematic evidence review for the U.S. Preventive Services Task Force. Ann Intern Med 2011;155(7):434–47.
22. Rose SA, Poynter PS, Anderson JW, et al. Physician weight loss advice and patient weight loss behavior change: a literature review and meta-analysis of survey data. Int J Obes (Lond) 2013;37(1):118–28.
23. Davis Martin P, Rhode PC, Dutton GR, et al. A primary care weight management intervention for low-income African-American women. Obesity (Silver Spring) 2006;14(8):1412–20.
24. Martin PD, Dutton GR, Rhode PC, et al. Weight loss maintenance following a primary care intervention for low-income minority women. Obesity 2008;16(11): 2462–7.
25. Christian JG, Bessesen DH, Byers TE, et al. Clinic-based support to help overweight patients with type 2 diabetes increase physical activity and lose weight. Arch Intern Med 2008;168(2):141–6.
26. Christian JG, Byers TE, Christian KK, et al. A computer support program that helps clinicians provide patients with metabolic syndrome tailored counseling to promote weight loss. J Am Diet Assoc 2011;111(1):75–83.
27. Ashley JM, Jeor STS, Schrage JP, et al. Weight control in the physician's office. Arch Intern Med 2001;161(13):1599–604.
28. ter Bogt NCW, Bemelmans WJE, Beltman FW, et al. Preventing weight gain by lifestyle intervention in a general practice setting: three-year results of a randomized controlled trial. Arch Intern Med 2011;171(4):306–13.
29. Kumanyika SK, Fassbender JE, Sarwer DB, et al. One-year results of the Think Health! study of weight management in primary care practices. Obesity (Silver Spring) 2012;20(6):1249–57.
30. Tsai AG, Wadden TA, Rogers MA, et al. A primary care intervention for weight loss: results of a randomized controlled pilot study. Obesity (Silver Spring) 2010;18(8):1614–8.
31. Appel LJ, Clark JM, Yeh H-C, et al. Comparative effectiveness of weight-loss interventions in clinical practice. N Engl J Med 2011;365(21):1959–68.
32. Wadden TA, Volger S, Sarwer DB, et al. A two-year randomized trial of obesity treatment in primary care practice. N Engl J Med 2011;365(21):1969–79.
33. Ma J, Yank V, Xiao L, et al. Translating the Diabetes Prevention Program lifestyle intervention for weight loss into primary care: a randomized trial. JAMA Intern Med 2013;173(2):113–21.
34. Xiao L, Yank V, Wilson SR, et al. Two-year weight-loss maintenance in primary care-based diabetes prevention program lifestyle interventions. Nutr Diabetes 2013;3:e76.
35. Tsai AG, Felton S, Wadden TA, et al. A randomized clinical trial of a weight loss maintenance intervention in a primary care population. Obesity (Silver Spring) 2015;23(10):2015–21.
36. Ryan DH, Johnson WD, Myers VH, et al. Nonsurgical weight loss for extreme obesity in primary care settings: results of the Louisiana obese subjects study. Arch Intern Med 2010;170(2):146–54.
37. Whittemore R, Melkus G, Wagner J, et al. Translating the Diabetes Prevention Program to primary care: a pilot study. Nurs Res 2009;58(1):2–12.

38. Renjilian DA, Perri MG, Nezu AM, et al. Individual versus group therapy for obesity: effects of matching participants to their treatment preferences. J Consult Clin Psychol 2001;69(4):717–21.

39. Weinstock RS, Trief PM, Cibula D, et al. Weight loss success in metabolic syndrome by telephone interventions: results from the SHINE Study. J Gen Intern Med 2013;28(12):1620–8.

40. Prochaska JO, Velicer WF. The transtheoretical model of health behavior change. Am J Health Promot 1997;12(1):38–48.

41. Miller WR, Rollnick S. Motivational interviewing: helping people change. New York (NY): Guilford Press; 2012.

42. Barnes RD, White MA, Martino S, et al. A randomized controlled trial comparing scalable weight loss treatments in primary care. Obesity (Silver Spring) 2014; 22(12):2508–16.

43. Huber JM, Shapiro JS, Wieland ML, et al. Telecoaching plus a portion control plate for weight care management: a randomized trial. Trials 2015;16:323.

44. Tsai AG, Wadden TA. Systematic review: an evaluation of major commercial weight loss programs in the United States. Ann Intern Med 2005;142(1):56–66.

45. Gudzune KA, Doshi RS, Mehta AK, et al. Efficacy of commercial weight-loss programs: an updated systematic review. Ann Intern Med 2015;162(7):501–12.

46. Mitchell NS, Dickinson LM, Kempe A, et al. Determining the effectiveness of Take Off Pounds Sensibly (TOPS), a nationally available nonprofit weight loss program. Obesity (Silver Spring) 2011;19(3):568–73.

47. Mitchell NS, Polsky S, Catenacci VA, et al. Up to 7 years of sustained weight loss for weight-loss program completers. Am J Prev Med 2015;49(2):248–58.

48. Stunkard A, Wilcoxon Craighead L, O'Brien R. Controlled trial of behaviour therapy, pharmacotherapy, and their combination in the treatment of obesity. Lancet 1980;316(8203):1045–7.

49. Wadden TA, Berkowitz RI, Sarwer DB, et al. Benefits of lifestyle modification in the pharmacologic treatment of obesity: a randomized trial. Arch Intern Med 2001; 161(2):218–27.

50. Wadden TA, Berkowitz RI, Womble LG, et al. Randomized trial of lifestyle modification and pharmacotherapy for obesity. N Engl J Med 2005;353(20):2111–20.

51. Digenio AG, Mancuso JP, Gerber RA, et al. Comparison of methods for delivering a lifestyle modification program for obese patients: a randomized trial. Ann Intern Med 2009;150(4):255–62.

52. Hauptman J, Lucas C, Boldrin MN, et al. Orlistat in the long-term treatment of obesity in primary care settings. Arch Fam Med 2000;9(2):160–7.

53. Poston WSC, Haddock CK, Pinkston MM, et al. Evaluation of a primary care-oriented brief counselling intervention for obesity with and without orlistat. J Intern Med 2006;260(4):388–98.

54. Longitudinal Assessment of Bariatric Surgery (LABS) Consortium, Flum DR, Belle SH, King WC, et al. Perioperative safety in the longitudinal assessment of bariatric surgery. N Engl J Med 2009;361(5):445–54.

55. Foster GD, Wadden TA, Vogt RA, et al. What is a reasonable weight loss? Patients' expectations and evaluations of obesity treatment outcomes. J Consult Clin Psychol 1997;65(1):79–85.

56. Wadden TA, Womble LG, Sarwer DB, et al. Great expectations: "I'm losing 25% of my weight no matter what you say". J Consult Clin Psychol 2003;71(6):1084–9.

57. Rutledge T, Groesz LM, Linke SE, et al. Behavioural weight management for the primary careprovider. Obes Rev 2011;12(5):e290–7.

58. Aveyard P, Lewis A, Tearne S, et al. Screening and brief intervention for obesity in primary care: a parallel, two-arm, randomised trial. Lancet 2016;388(10059): 2492–500.

59. Sepah SC, Jiang L, Peters AL. Long-term outcomes of a web-based diabetes prevention program: 2-year results of a single-arm longitudinal study. J Med Internet Res 2015;17(4):e92.

60. Goldstein DJ. Beneficial health effects of modest weight loss. Int J Obes Relat Metab Disord 1992;16(6):397–415.

61. Wing RR, Lang W, Wadden TA, et al. Benefits of modest weight loss in improving cardiovascular risk factors in overweight and obese individuals with type 2 diabetes. Diabetes Care 2011;34(7):1481–6.

62. Jensen MD, Ryan DH. New obesity guidelines: promise and potential. JAMA 2014;311(1):23–4.

63. Villareal DT, Chode S, Parimi N, et al. Weight loss, exercise, or both and physical function in obese older adults. N Engl J Med 2011;364(13):1218–29.

64. Rosenbaum M, Hirsch J, Gallagher DA, et al. Long-term persistence of adaptive thermogenesis in subjects who have maintained a reduced body weight. Am J Clin Nutr 2008;88(4):906–12.

65. Polidori D, Sanghvi A, Seeley RJ, et al. How strongly does appetite counter weight loss? Quantification of the feedback control of human energy intake. Obesity (Silver Spring) 2016;24(11):2289–95.

66. Bangalore S, Fayyad R, Laskey R, et al. Body-weight fluctuations and outcomes in coronary disease. N Engl J Med 2017;376(14):1332–40.

67. Faulconbridge LF, Ruparel K, Loughead J, et al. Changes in neural responsivity to highly palatable foods following roux-en-Y gastric bypass, sleeve gastrectomy, or weight stability: an fMRI study. Obesity 2016;24(5):1054–60.

68. Wang GJ, Tomasi D, Volkow ND, et al. Effect of combined naltrexone and bupropion therapy on the brain's reactivity to food cues. Int J Obes (Lond) 2014;38(5): 682–8.

69. Nedeltcheva AV, Kilkus JM, Imperial J, et al. Insufficient sleep undermines dietary efforts to reduce adiposity. Ann Intern Med 2010;153(7):435–41.

70. Liu Y, Wheaton AG, Chapman DP, et al. Prevalence of healthy sleep duration among adults–United States, 2014. MMWR Morb Mortal Wkly Rep 2016;65(6): 137–41.

71. Ogilvie RP, Redline S, Bertoni AG, et al. Actigraphy measured sleep indices and adiposity: the multi-ethnic study of atherosclerosis (MESA). Sleep 2016;39(9): 1701–8.

72. Wadden TA, Didie E. What's in a name? Patients' preferred terms for describing obesity. Obes Res 2003;11(9):1140–6.

73. Volger S, Vetter ML, Dougherty M, et al. Patients' preferred terms for describing their excess weight: discussing obesity in clinical practice. Obesity 2012;20(1): 147–50.

Guideline Recommendations for Obesity Management

Donna H. Ryan, MD[a],*, Scott Kahan, MD, MPH[b]

KEYWORDS

- Obesity guidelines • Weight management • Lifestyle intervention
- Obesity pharmacotherapy • Diet • Bariatric surgery • Medication

KEY POINTS

Primary care practitioners should be aware of the following practice recommendations:

- Body mass index (BMI) is a valuable part of the electronic health record, but it is a screening measure, not a diagnostic measure. The diagnosis of obesity is the presence of abnormal excess body fat that impairs health. Consider the patient's genetics an ethnicity as part o BMI and waist circumference and do not treat on BMI alone. Consider comorbidities and health risk when determining the intensity of treatment approach.

- Modest or moderate weight loss can produce health benefits. For more serious complications, more weight loss may be needed. For patients with severe obesity and complications, bariatric surgery should be considered.

- There are multiple pathways to dietary success. Prescribe a diet the patient can adhere to and that has health benefits. Successful lifestyle change requires skills training. Patients should have access to counseling sessins with at least 14 sessions over 6 months and followup for one year.

- Medications approved for chronic weight management can help patients better adhere to the diet plan and can help sustain hard-won weight loss. Medications should be prescribed and success evaluated at 12-16 weeks. If patients are successful, medications should be continued.

- Obesity is a complex, chronic disease and life-long management is indicated.

[a] Pennington Biomedical Research Center, 6400 Perkins Road, Baton Rouge, LA 70130, USA;
[b] Johns Hopkins Bloomberg School of Public Health, National Center for Weight and Wellness, Washington, DC, USA
* Corresponding author.
E-mail address: ryandh@pbrc.edu

Med Clin N Am 102 (2018) 49–63
http://dx.doi.org/10.1016/j.mcna.2017.08.006
0025-7125/18/© 2017 Elsevier Inc. All rights reserved.
medical.theclinics.com

INTRODUCTION

Responding to the growing epidemic of obesity and obesity-related chronic diseases, over the last 4 years numerous guidelines and position statements have been published to assist practitioners in addressing obesity in their patients. In particular, 3 major guidelines published by United States governmental health agencies and professional societies offer valuable, and mostly consistent, recommendations for primary care providers. Related to the problem of increasing obesity prevalence are increasing rates, observed globally, of type 2 diabetes and other obesity-associated disease, creating an enormous global health burden. Thus far, no country has been successful in reversing obesity prevalence.[1]

Primary care practitioners acknowledge that obesity is a major driver of the chronic disease burden, but managing weight effectively can be challenging, especially in primary care settings. The pathophysiology that drives weight gain in susceptible individuals and makes weight loss and weight loss maintenance difficult is a barrier to primary care physicians in a busy office practice.[2,3] The public health challenge has also stimulated drug discovery and approval, with 4 new medications approved by the US Food and Drug Administration (FDA) for chronic weight management since 2012. Primary care providers need knowledge and skills in the following areas:

- Diagnosis of obesity and overweight, and staging of disease
- Recognition and treatment of obesity-related comorbidities
- Determining which therapy or therapies is or are appropriate for an individual patient
- Management of weight loss, including:
  - Effective delivery of lifestyle intervention (diet, physical activity, and behavior modification)
  - Consideration of obesity pharmacotherapy, in appropriate patients
    - Weight-centric prescribing: avoiding medications that promote weight gain in favor of weight-neutral or medications that produce some weight loss
  - Appropriate prescription of medications approved for chronic weight management
  - Referral to specialty care (eg, obesity medicine specialists and/or bariatric surgical procedures) and
- Prevention of weight regain in patients who are successful with weight loss.

Three obesity guidelines are discussed in this article. Targeting primary care providers, the US National Institutes of Health and the American Heart Association, American College of Cardiology, and The Obesity Society (AHA/ACC/TOS) sponsored systematic evidence review and guidelines around 5 critical questions on assessment and management of obesity.[4] The Endocrine Society (ENDO) sponsored systematic evidence review and guidelines targeting pharmacotherapy, reviewing medications that promote weight gain and medications approved for obesity management.[5] The American Association of Clinical Endocrinologists (AACE) also published obesity guidelines in 2016,[6,7] which are particularly relevant for endocrinologists and for guidance on patients with more severe obesity and metabolic complications of obesity, such as diabetes (**Table 1**). This article reviews and compares findings and recommendations across these guidelines, identifies areas of controversy and concordance, and suggests how primary care practices may make use of the most appropriate recommendations for their circumstances. **Table 1** describes, in abbreviated language, the methodology, focus, key recommendations, whether those recommendations are broad or targeted, and areas of controversy for each of the documents.

Table 1
Comparison of recent clinical treatment guidelines for diagnosis and management of obesity in adults

2013 AHA/ACC/TOS[4] (Based on Systematic Evidence Review Sponsored by National Heart Lung and Blood Institute	2015 ENDO Obesity Pharmacotherapy[5]	AACE 2016[6]
Methodology: stringent; systematic evidence review; graded recommendations	Methodology: stringent; systematic evidence review; graded recommendations	Methodology: literature review and consensus of expert endocrinologists; targets treatment recommendations
Focus, narrow: 5 critical questions • Benefits of weight loss • Risks of excess weight • Best diet for weight loss • Efficacy of lifestyle intervention approaches • Efficacy and safety of bariatric surgery	Focus, narrow: 2 topical areas • Medications approved for weight loss • Weight effects of medications used for chronic disease management	Focus, broad 9 broad clinical questions and 126 recommendations • Complication-centric approach to management • Emphasis on identifying comorbidities with more detailed screening recommendations • Grading system identifies severity of disease and severity of comorbidity profile directs intensity of treatment
Recommendations: both broad and narrow; Narrow around 5 questions; Broad around, the treatment algorithm, "Chronic Disease Management Model for Primary Care of Patients With Overweight and Obesity" based on evidence statements and expert opinion	Recommendations: broad; target an overall approach to medicating the patient with obesity, both to augment weight loss efforts and to minimize weight gain effects of medications for chronic disease prescription	Recommendations: broad and comprehensive, with focus on staging severity of disease as a guide to treatment planning; more severe disease warrants more aggressive approach

(continued on next page)

Table 1
(continued)

2013 AHA/ACC/TOS[4] (Based on Systematic Evidence Review Sponsored by National Heart Lung and Blood Institute	2015 ENDO Obesity Pharmacotherapy[5]	AACE 2016[6]
Key points: • BMI is screening tool; waist circumference is a risk factor • It is not necessary to achieve normal weight; health improvements begin with modest weight loss • There is no magic diet • Lifestyle-intervention counseling conducted face-to-face in 14 or more sessions over 6 mo is the gold standard for weight loss intervention • Bariatric surgery should be discussed with patients who meet criteria and would benefit from it, and referrals should be made	Key points: • Weight-centric prescribing should be done for chronic diseases; in prescribing for chronic diseases, avoid medications that promote weight gain in favor of those that are weight neutral or are associated with weight loss • Medications are useful adjuncts to diet and exercise, when prescribed appropriately • Choosing which medication to use is a shared decision of prescriber and patient	Key points: • Complications of excess body weight should direct intensity of treatment and urgency of treatment • Medications for chronic weight management may be used initially (without lifestyle-alone attempt) for patients with more severe disease manifestations as an adjunct to lifestyle (multicomponent) measures • Individuals without comorbidities or risk factors are stage 0 and no medical intervention is required
Areas of controversy: • Does not include race-specific BMI cutpoints to assess risk • BMI 30 indicates medical intervention regardless of health status	Areas of controversy: • Does not indicate stepped approaches to medicating for chronic weight management; eg, all medications given equal consideration for first-line therapy	Areas of controversy: • Specialist focus; no recommendations for screening and early intervention in context of care across the lifespan • Confusion caused by BMI 25 <30 and risk factors being designated as obesity

BMI 25 <30 means BMI at least 25 and up to 30 kg/m2. This is usually classified as overweight, but in this guideline, it can be "obesity".

Guidelines Methodology Determines Scope

To understand the differences among guidelines, one must understand the methodology used to generate recommendations. There is a movement to make the development process for all guidelines more rigorous.[8,9] Guidelines that use more rigorous methodology take longer to develop, require painstaking steps and costs to assemble, and are presumably more trustworthy; however, they are necessarily limited in that they can only address a small number of critical questions. Guidelines that use this more rigorous methodology, such as those from AHA/ACC/TOS[4] and ENDO,[5] are by necessity more narrow but are more authoritative. Those that skip the step of formulating critical questions use less formal literature review and rely more on expert opinion of specialists (AACE[6]) are not held to the same strict constraints of evidence review methodology and can give broader recommendations and be more timely in an attempt to be more relevant to practitioners. The methodological approach informs the range of recommendation and strength of recommendation possible, as indicated in **Table 1**.

This discussion emphasizes discrepancies across the guidelines and explains how both approaches may be relevant in primary care and specialty offices.

Diagnosis of Obesity and Staging of Disease: Selecting Appropriate Candidates for Medical Intervention

All guidelines[4–6] use body mass index (BMI) as a screening measure. What is new, compared with guidelines of the past, is that the BMI-centric approach is fading in influence in all guidelines and BMI is not the sole director of treatment choice.

It is important that primary care providers understand that the diagnosis of obesity should not be made based on BMI alone.[10,11] BMI is a measure of body size. Obesity should be defined as a condition in which excess abnormal body fat impairs health.[10] BMI correlates well with total body fat on a population basis and has utility in tracking populations.[12] In the United States, BMI is a core measure available through the electronic health record at every visit; therefore, the BMI is here to stay. But BMI is only the first step in evaluating risk associated with excess weight. The second step in determining need for and intensity of medical management is to screen for other risk factors related to excess weight and to make a decision to offer medical treatment based on a combination of body size (BMI) and other risk factor assessment.

The AHA/ACC/TOS guidelines[4] emphasize the importance of including waist circumference as a risk factor to determine need for weight loss. In those guidelines, the cutpoints for waist circumference are 35 inches (89 cm) for women and 40 inches (101 cm) for men. Those guidelines also use the standard cutpoints for BMI (overweight is BMI ≥ 25 <30 kg/m^2 and obesity is BMI ≥ 30 kg/m^2). However, different populations have more propensity for visceral fat accumulation, which is associated with greater metabolic risk than subcutaneous fat and, therefore, are at increased risk for comorbidities. In Asians, the cutpoint for overweight is BMI greater than or equal to 23 kg/m^2 and for obesity it is BMI greater than or equal to 25 kg/m^2 and the waist circumference cutpoint is 31.5 inches (80 cm) for women and 35 inches (89 cm) for men.[12] In general, it is recommended that slightly lower waist circumference cutoffs are used for Asian, ethnic Central and South American, Sub-Saharan African, and Middle East populations.[6]

All guidelines agree that patients with excess weight and associated health risks should be treated for obesity. However, there is a discrepancy in guidelines for patients with BMI greater than 30 but without clear metabolic health risks. The AHA/ACC/TOS guidelines endorse medically directed, intensive weight loss intervention to improve health risk in all patients with BMI greater than 30, even if no comorbid risks are present, based on the rationale that there is likely to be progression over time to develop risk factors and comorbid conditions. In contrast, the AACE guidelines[6] highlight that individuals with BMI greater than 30 kg/m^2 but without metabolic risk factors, which is often referred to as metabolically healthy obesity, would not necessitate intensive weight reduction therapies. Given that the AACE guidelines are written primarily for endocrinologists, this discrepancy makes sense because patients are not seeking treatment from endocrinologists for a well patient visit. Most importantly, this is likely to be an area in which clinical judgment should play a central role in determining the intensity of intervention. Certainly, specialist care is not appropriate for medically directed weight loss in individuals without any associated health risks; but lifestyle intervention may be appropriately prescribed by primary care providers for individuals with BMI greater than 30 kg/m^2, even without associated health risk, to prevent further weight gain.

Controversy concerning the guidelines can arise when individuals have comorbidities or risk factors related to excess body fat and have BMI less than 25 kg/m^2. This can be the case in certain racial groups, especially Asians, and all guidelines acknowledge this fact. Although no formal evidence review supports such a recommendation among US immigrants from South Asia and China, the AHA/ACC/TOS guidelines[4] do support such an approach for Asians.

Choice of Initial Treatment Approach

The AHA/ACC/TOS guidelines[4] emphasize that comprehensive lifestyle intervention is the cornerstone for treating obesity and adjunctive therapies are reserved for individuals with more health risk who do not succeed with weight loss and maintenance. In clinical practice, most individuals have already tried self-help approaches before medical intervention is contemplated. The AACE guidelines[6] introduce staging (obesity stages 0, 1, and 2) that links severity of disease at presentation to degree of intensity of intervention. If comorbidities or risk factors are mild, AACE terms this obesity stage 1. If the associated comorbidities are moderate or severe, the term is obesity stage 2. This approach promotes the concept that the intensity of treatment needs to match the severity of disease, rather than the patient's size or BMI. However, AACE uses the term obesity for individuals with weight-related comorbidities and BMI greater than 25 kg/m^2, which is somewhat confusing. Still, the principle is sound: for individuals at higher risk, more intensive approaches are justified; for individuals with low health risks, overly aggressive intervention may not be warranted.

Primary care practitioners should take away several important principles from these somewhat different approaches. First, there is more urgency to intervene when patients have health risks or comorbidities associated with excess body weight; the greater the health risk, the greater the urgency, and the more justification for higher intensity approaches. Additionally, the patient's weight management history can be used to determine choice of treatment plan. Patients do not need to fail at behavioral management under the observation of the health care provider; a history of struggle should be enough justification to add adjunctive treatment, such as pharmacotherapy. Finally, because the goal of weight loss is improvement in health and quality of life, the targeted health goal should be the rationale for determining intensity of approach and for judging success of intervention.

Comprehensive Lifestyle Intervention

It is clear that medical advice to "just eat less and exercise more" is not effective for most patients to succeed at weight loss. Comprehensive lifestyle intervention includes building a skill set of behavioral knowledge and strategies to achieve and maintain sustainable improvements in food intake and physical activity. The AHA/ACC/TOS guidelines systematic evidence review[4] of lifestyle intervention was conducted to support inclusion of intensive behavioral therapy for weight management as a part of medical practice. It demonstrated that when these components are delivered in face-to-face (group or individual) sessions, with at least 14 sessions over 6 months and continued monthly follow-up thereafter, then average weight loss of 8% of baseline weight at 1 year is expected.[4] This degree of weight loss is clinically meaningful because it translates into clinically significant improvements in blood pressure, lipids, glycemic control, and reduction in risk for progression to type 2 diabetes.[4] Based on these and other findings, the US Preventive Services Task Force[13] has recommended that individuals with obesity and cardiovascular disease risk factors should be referred for intensive behavioral therapy and the Centers for Medicare and Medicaid Services now covers intensive counseling in primary care for Medicare patients.[14–16]

When in-person interaction is challenging, telephone-based or Web-based counseling and commercial programs can be used as alternatives, although less average weight loss should be expected.[4]

Diets for Weight Loss

The entrenched belief that there is a magic diet has stimulated studies that have focused on various macronutrients compositions, including low-fat diets, low-carbohydrate or high-protein diets, low glycemic-index diets, balanced deficit diets, vegetarian, vegan, and various diets based on dietary patterns and eliminating 1 or more major food groups. To address this issue, the creators of the AHA/ACC/TOS guidelines performed a systematic evidence review of 17 dietary patterns and showed that no diet type was superior in terms of ability to produce and sustain weight loss[4] (**Box 1**). Thus, there are many pathways to successful weight loss regardless of which diet is chosen. In all of the diets that were studied, the best predictor of success was dietary adherence. Thus, providers are advised to recommend diets according to patient preference to improve adherence to achieve reduced caloric intake and weight loss. This does not mean that diet composition is not important but merely that negative energy balance is the key factor in promoting weight loss. Referral to a registered dietitian is endorsed by the AHA/ACC/TOS guidelines[4] when the dietary recommendation has a specific health target.

Physical Activity

Increased physical activity is an essential component of a comprehensive lifestyle intervention. The AHA/ACC/TOS guidelines[4] typically prescribe increased aerobic physical activity (eg, brisk walking) for greater than 150 minutes per week (equal to >30 min/d, most days of the week). This echoes the 2001 and 2009 American College of Sports Medicine Position Stand,[17] which also supported 200 to 300 minutes per week for long-term weight loss and moderate-intensity physical activity between 150 and 250 minutes per week to be effective to prevent weight gain, although that intensity will provide only modest weight loss.[17] This Position Stand found that resistance training does not enhance weight loss but may increase fat-free mass, promote loss of fat mass, and is associated with reductions in health risk. Existing evidence indicates that endurance physical activity or resistance training, even without weight loss, improves health risk.[17]

Pharmacotherapy

The best source for authoritative recommendations on medications for obesity comes from the ENDO guidleines.[5] Foremost is the consideration of the role of medications in

---

Box 1
Dietary approaches with evidence of weight loss efficacy

- European Association for the Study of Diabetes guidelines–style diet targeting food groups, without formal prescribed energy restriction target but realized energy deficit

- Higher protein (25% of total calories from protein, 30% of total calories from fat, 45% of total calories from carbohydrate) with provision of foods that realized energy deficit

- Higher protein Zone diet (5 meals per day, each with 40% of total calories from carbohydrate, 30% of total calories from protein, 30% of total calories from fat) without formal prescribed energy restriction but realized energy deficit

- Lacto-ovo-vegetarian-style diet with prescribed energy restriction

- Low-calorie diet with prescribed energy restriction

- Low-carbohydrate diet (initially <20 g per day carbohydrate) without formal prescribed energy restriction but realized energy deficit

- Low-fat vegan style diet (10%–25% of total calories from fat) without formal prescribed energy restriction but realized energy deficit

- Low-fat diet (20% of total calories from fat) without formal prescribed energy restriction but realized energy deficit

- Low-glycemic-load diet, either with or without formal prescribed energy restriction

- Lower fat (≤30% fat), high dairy (4 servings/day) diets with or without increased fiber and/or low-glycemic index or load foods (low-glycemic load), with prescribed energy restriction

- Macronutrient-targeted diets (15% or 25% of total calories from protein; 20% or 40% of total calories from fat; 35%, 45%, 55%, or 65% of total calories from carbohydrate) with prescribed energy restriction

- Mediterranean-style diet with prescribed energy restriction

- Moderate protein (12% of total calories from protein, 58% of total calories from carbohydrate, 30% of total calories from fat) with provision of foods that realized energy deficit

- Provision of high-glycemic-load or low-glycemic-load meals with prescribed energy restriction

- The American Heart Association style Step 1 diet (with prescribed energy restriction of 1500–1800 kcal per day, <30% of total calories from fat, <10% of total calories from saturated fat)

Dietary approaches are listed in alphabetical order.
Adapted from Jensen MD, Ryan DH, Donato KA, et al. Guidelines (2013) for managing overweight and obesity in adults. Obesity 2014;22(S2):S75; with permission.

---

weight gain. An important part of evaluation of the patient with obesity is reviewing the medication list to ensure that the patient is not taking drugs that contribute to weight gain and to modify if possible, when medications associated with gain are found. Many medications in use for common chronic diseases may contribute to weight gain, and changing medications to weight-neutral alternatives, when possible, is advised. **Table 2** describes some of the medications commonly prescribed chronically and their weight effects.

All of these guidelines support pharmacotherapy as an adjunct to lifestyle changes to help patients who struggle with behavioral management alone. Across all guidelines,[4–6] the indications for adding pharmacotherapy to a weight loss effort are a history of failure to achieve clinically meaningful weight loss and/or to sustain lost weight,

Table 2
Medications associated with weight gain and alternatives

Indication or Class	Weight Gain Associated with Use	Weight Loss or Weight Neutrality Associated with Use (Weight Reduction in Parentheses)
Antidepressants, mood stabilizers, or tricyclic antidepressants	Amitriptyline Doxepin Imipramine Nortriptyline Trimipramine Mirtazapine	(Bupropion) Nefazodone Fluoxetine (short-term) Sertraline (<1 y)
Antidepressants, mood stabilizers, or SSRIs	Fluoxetine? Sertraline? Paroxetine Fluvoxamine	
Antidepressants, mood stabilizers, or MAO inhibitors	Phenelzine Tranylcypromine	
Mood stabilizer	Lithium	
Antidiabetic medications	Insulin (weight gain differs with type and regimen used) Sulfonylureas Thiazolidinediones Sitagliptin? Mitiglinide	(Metformin) (Acarbose) (Miglitol) (Pramlintide) (Exenatide) (Liraglutide) (SGLT 2 inhibitors)
Antihypertensive medications	α-blocker? β-blocker?	ACE inhibitors? Calcium channel blockers? Angiotensin-2 receptor antagonists

(continued on next page)

Table 2
(continued)

Indication or Class	Weight Gain Associated with Use	Weight Loss or Weight Neutrality Associated with Use (Weight Reduction in Parentheses)
Antipsychotics	Clozapine Risperidone Olanzapine Quetiapine Haloperidol Perphenazine Quetiapine	Ziprasidone Aripiprazole
Anticonvulsants	Carbamazepine Gabapentin Valproate	Lamotrigine? (Topiramate) (Zonisamide)
Contraceptives	Injectable progesterone Oral progesterone	Barrier methods Intrauterine devices Oral contraceptives preferable to injectable
Endometriosis treatment	Depot leuprolide acetate	Surgical treatment
Chronic inflammatory diseases	Glucocorticoids	Nonsteroidal antiinflammatory drugs Disease-modifying antirheumatic drugs
AIDS treatment	Antiretroviral therapies	Monitor body weight, body fat distribution, and cardiovascular risk factors

Abbreviations: ?, refers to uncertain or unknown effect on weight; SSRI, selective serotonin reuptake inhibtor.

From Apovian CM, Aronne LJ, Bessesen DH, et al. Pharmacologic management of obesity: an Endocrine Society clinical practice guideline. J Clin Endocrinol Metab 2015;100(2):342–62; with permission.

in patients who meet regulatory prescribing guidelines (BMI $\geq$27 kg/m^2 with 1 or more obesity comorbidities or a BMI >30 kg/m^2 with or without metabolic consequences).[4–6]

The ENDO guidelines on pharmacotherapy for obesity provide recommendations that serve as guiding principles.[5] First, effective behavioral support for weight loss should be provided in all patients. Obesity pharmacotherapy reinforces diets that result in an energy deficit, and combining medication and behavioral therapy leads to significantly greater weight loss than either alone. Second, the patient should be familiar with the drug and its potential side effects (**Table 3**). Third, if less than 5% weight occurs after 3 months, a new treatment plan should be considered because the patient is not likely responding to the medication. No single medication is effective in every patient, similar to treatment of other comorbidities that primary care providers treat on a daily basis. Finally, if medications result in improvement in health and weight, they should be continued long term. Medications approved for chronic weight management and their profiles are found in **Table 3**.

Bariatric Surgery

The AHA/ACC/TOS guidelines[4] offers the strongest recommendation yet that physicians should be proactive to identify and refer patients who would benefit from bariatric surgery. Adult patients with BMI greater than or equal to 40 or BMI greater than or equal to 35 with obesity-related comorbid conditions meet basic criteria for surgery. Bariatric surgery leads to substantial long-term weight loss, improves many obesity-related comorbid conditions, and reduces mortality. Safety of these procedures has been well-studied and is not significantly higher than routine abdominal surgeries. For patients with type 2 diabetes, bariatric surgery, especially Roux-en-Y gastric bypass surgery, is particularly effective. A recently published position statement offers additional guidance in using bariatric surgery for patients with obesity and poor control of type 2 diabetes.[18] These guidelines recommend that, for patients with type 2 diabetes, bariatric surgery should be recommended for those with BMI greater than or equal to 40 kg/m^2 and patients with BMI of 35.0 kg/m^2 to 39.9 kg/m^2 in the presence of poor glycemic control. This position statement goes even further, to suggest that patients with poor glycemic control could be considered for surgery even with BMI as low as 30 kg/m^2.

SUMMARY

The current menu of guidance around obesity management is revealing of progress in the field. The focus is on health risk assessment, not just body size. The various guidelines emphasize the importance of a multilayered approach to addressing the obesity epidemic. There is a need to intervene earlier, in primary care settings, with lifestyle intervention. Further, those interventions will only be effective if they are intensive behavioral therapy approaches. The guidelines emphasize the chronic nature of obesity and the need for long-term care. The guidelines debunk the notion of a magic diet and emphasize the importance of comprehensive approaches to lifestyle change: diet, physical activity, and behavioral changes. Further, the guidelines acknowledge the need for stepping up care when patients struggle and to add adjunctive approaches to lifestyle intervention when indicated. Practitioners now have the first guidelines based on a systematic evidence review of how and when to use medications in patients with obesity.[5] The growing evidence base for the role of bariatric surgery as a treatment approach for patients with severe obesity should lead health care providers to be more proactive in recommending these procedures. Future guidelines

Table 3
Medications approved in United States for chronic obesity management

Drug, Generic Name • Dose • Route of Administration	Mechanism of Action[5]	≥5% Weight Loss Efficacy at 1 y	≥10% Weight Loss Efficacy	Common Side Effects[5]	Contraindications and Warnings[5]
Orlistat • 120 mg tid, before meals Or • 60 mg tid before meals • Oral	Pancreatic lipase inhibitor; blocks absorption of dietary fat	In 5 studies, orlistat = 35.5%–54.8%; vs Placebo = 16%–27.4%	In 5 studies, orlistat = 16.4%–25.8%; vs Placebo = 3.8%–9.9%	• Steatorrhea • Oily spotting • Flatulence with discharge • Fecal urgency • Oily evacuation • Increased defecation • Fecal incontinence	• Contraindicated in pregnancy • Warning: ↑cyclosporine exposure • Liver failure (rare) • Requires coadministration of multiple vitamin • Increased risk of gall bladder disease • Increased urine oxalate; monitor renal function
Lorcaserin • 10 mg bid Or • 20 mg qd • Oral	5-HT$_{2C}$ serotonin agonist with little affinity for other serotonergic receptors; reduces food intake	In 2 studies combined, lorcaserin = 47.1%; vs Placebo = 22.6% Difference from placebo = 24.5%	In 2 studies combined, lorcaserin = 22.4%; vs Placebo = 8.7% Difference from placebo = 13.8%	• Headache • Dizziness • Nausea • Dry mouth • Fatigue • Constipation	• Contraindicated in pregnancy • Use with caution with SSRI, SNRI, MAOIs, St John's wort, triptans, bupropion, dextromethorphan
Phentermine or topiramate ER (Phen/TPM) • 7.5 mg/46 mg qd • 15 mg/92 mg qd, indicated as rescue • Oral, once daily dosing (requires titration)	Sympathomimetic Anticonvulsant (GABA receptor modulation, carbonic anhydrase inhibition, glutamate antagonism); reduces food intake	In 2 studies, Phen/TPM (3 doses) = 45%–70%; vs Placebo = 17%–21% Difference from placebo = 27.6%–49.4%	In 2 studies, Phen/TPM (3 doses) = 19%–48%; vs Placebo = 7% Difference from placebo = 11.4%–40.3%	• Insomnia • Dry mouth • Constipation • Paresthesias • Dizziness • Dysgeusia	• Contraindicated in pregnancy • Fetal toxicity; monthly pregnancy test suggested • Contraindicated with hyperthyroidism, glaucoma • Do not use with MAOIs or sympathomimetic amines • Acute myopia (rare)

Drug/Dosing	Mechanism of action	Efficacy (≥5%)	Efficacy (≥10%)	Common side effects	Safety issues
Naltrexone SR or bupropion SR (NB) • 32 mg/360 mg • Oral; bid dosing (requires titration)	Opioid receptor antagonist and dopamine and noradrenaline reuptake inhibitor; reduces food intake	In 3 studies, NB = 44.2%–62.3%; vs Placebo = 17%–43% Difference from placebo = 14%–25%	In 3 studies, NB = 15%–35%; vs Placebo = 5%–21% Difference from placebo = 10%–14%	• Nausea • Constipation • Headache • Vomiting • Dizziness	• Boxed warning: suicide risk in depression • Contraindicated in pregnancy • Contraindicated in seizure disorders, uncontrolled hypertension, glaucoma • Do not use with opioids, MAOIs • Hepatotoxicity (rare)
Liraglutide • 3.0 mg • Injection; once daily dosing (requires titration)	GLP-1 receptor agonist; reduces food intake	In 2 studies, liraglutide = 62% and 49%; vs Placebo = 34.4% and 16.4% Difference from placebo = 32.6% and 22.6%	In 2 studies, liraglutide = 22.4% and 33.9%; vs Placebo = 5.5% and 15.4% Difference from placebo = 16.9% and 18.5%	• Nausea • Vomiting • Diarrhea • Constipation • Headache • Dyspepsia • Fatigue • Dizziness • Abdominal pain	• Boxed warning: thyroid C-cell tumors in rodents • Contraindicated with personal or family history of medullary thyroid cancer or multiple endocrine neoplasia • Pancreatitis • Hypoglycemia in diabetes • Increased risk of gall bladder disease

Abbreviations: GABA, gaba amino benzoic acid; GLP, glucagon-like peptide; MAOI, monoamine oxidase reuptake inhibitor; NB, naltrexone/bupropion; SR, sustained release.

Mechanism of action, dosing, efficacy (range in proportion of treated individuals who achieve >5% and >10% during phase 3 clinical trials), common side effects and safety issues. Information from product labels, except where noted. The efficacy data are obtained from the US FDA product labels.

Data from Apovian CM, Aronne LJ, Bessesen DH, et al. Pharmacologic Management of obesity: An Endocrine Society clinical practice guideline. J Clin Endocrinol Metab 2015; 100(2):342–62.

should include a focus on obesity devices, for which 5 (ie, 3 types of gastric balloons, an electrical stimulating system, and a gastric aspiration device) have been approved by FDA since 2015.[19] There are guidelines for primary care and for specialist care, with specialist care targeting patients with obesity-related complications. The menu illustrates that one size does not fit all in terms of where to go for advice. Still, there is remarkable concordance in the overall direction of the guidelines, with all making an emphatic statement that it is an obligation for all health care providers to participate in obesity management. These guidelines are not mandates, and should be interpreted with clinical judgment.

REFERENCES

1. Ng M, Fleming T, Robinson M, et al. Global, regional, and national prevalence of overweight and obesity in children and adults during 1980–2013: a systematic analysis for the Global Burden of Disease Study 2013. Lancet 2014;384(9945): 766–81.
2. Heymsfield SB, Wadden TA. Mechanisms, pathophysiology, and management of obesity. N Engl J Med 2017;376:254–326.
3. Bray GA, Frühbeck G, Ryan DH, et al. Management of obesity. Lancet 2016; 387(10031):1947–56.
4. Jensen MD, Ryan DH, Donato KA, et al. Guidelines (2013) for managing overweight and obesity in adults. Obesity 2014;22(S2):S1–410.
5. Apovian CM, Aronne LJ, Bessesen DH, et al. Pharmacologic management of obesity: an Endocrine Society clinical practice guideline. J Clin Endocrinol Metab 2015;100(2):342–62.
6. Garvey WT, Mechanick JI, Brett EM, et al, Reviewers of the AACE/ACE Obesity Clinical Practice Guidelines. American Association of Clinical Endocrinologists and American College of Endocrinology Comprehensive Clinical Practice Guidelines for Medical Care of Patients with Obesity-Executive Summary. Endocr Pract 2016;22(7):842–84.
7. Flegal KM, Carroll RJ, Kuczmarski RJ, et al. Overweight and obesity in the United States: prevalence and trends, 1960-1994. Int J Obes 1998;22(1): 39–47.
8. Finding what works in health care standards for systematic reviews. Available at: http://www.iom.edu/Reports/2011/Finding-What-Works-in-Health-Care-Standards-for-Systematic-Reviews.aspx. Accessed January 15, 2015.
9. Clinical practice guidelines we can trust. Available at: http://www.iom.edu/Reports/2011/Clinical-Practice-Guidelines-We-Can-Trust.aspx. Accessed January 15, 2015.
10. Sharma AM, Campbell-Scherer DL. Redefining obesity: beyond the numbers. Obesity 2017;25:660–1.
11. Ryan DH, Ravussin E. Keeping the baby and throwing out the bathwater. Obesity 2017;25:659.
12. WHO Expert Consultation (Held in Singapore). Appropriate body-mass index for Asian populations and its implications for policy and intervention strategies. Lancet 2004;363:157–63.
13. LeFevre ML. Behavioral counseling to promote a healthful diet and physical activity for cardiovascular disease prevention in adults with cardiovascular risk factors: U.S. preventive services task force recommendation statement. Ann Intern Med 2014;161(8):587–93.

14. Decision Memo for Intensive Behavioral Therapy for Obesity (CAG-00423N). Available at: https://www.cms.gov/medicare-coverage-database/details/nca-decision-memo.aspx?&NcaName=Intensive%20Behavioral%20Therapy%20for%20Obesity&bc=ACAAAAAAIAAA&NCAId=253&. Accessed September 22, 2015.

15. Eckel RH, Jakicic JM, Ard JD, et al, American College of Cardiology/American Heart Association Task Force on Practice Guidelines. 2013 AHA/ACC guideline on lifestyle management to reduce cardiovascular risk: a report of the American College of Cardiology/American Heart Association Task Force on Practice Guidelines. J Am Coll Cardiol 2014;63(25 Pt B):2960–84.

16. The 2015 Dietary Guidelines Advisory Committee (February 2015). Scientific Report of the 2015 Dietary Guidelines Advisory Committee. Available at: http://www.health.gov/dietaryguidelines/2015-scientific-report. Accessed September 15, 2015.

17. Donnelly JE, Blair SN, Jakicic JM, et al, American College of Sports Medicine. American College of Sports Medicine Position Stand. Appropriate physical activity intervention strategies for weight loss and prevention of weight regain for adults. Med Sci Sports Exerc 2009;41(2):459–71.

18. Rubino F, Nathan DM, Eckel RH, et al. Metabolic surgery in the treatment algorithm for type 2 diabetes: a Joint Statement by International Diabetes Organizations. Diabetes Care 2016;39:861–77.

19. FDA Approved Obesity Treatment Devices. Available at: http://www.fda.gov/MedicalDevices/ProductsandMedicalProcedures/ObesityDevices/ucm350134.htm. Accessed September 15, 2015.

Addressing Obesity in Aging Patients

John A. Batsis, MD, AGSF*, Alexandra B. Zagaria, BA

KEYWORDS

- Obesity • Older adult • Weight loss • Physical function • Pharmacotherapy
- Bariatric surgery • Review

KEY POINTS

- Older adults with obesity will be an emerging demographic for which primary care practitioners will need to develop skills in managing.
- Intentional weight loss in this population can be successful and safe.
- Appropriate understanding of the dangers of weight loss for muscle and bone are required.
- Pharmacotherapies that are US Food and Drug Administration approved for adults have not been extensively studied in older adult populations.
- Bariatric surgery can be considered in selected candidates.

EPIDEMIOLOGY OF AGING AND OBESITY

By the year 2030 in the United States, more than 20% of the population will be more than 65 years of age[1] (**Fig. 1**), up from 15% of the population now.[2] The fastest growing demographic are the so-called oldest old: individuals aged more than 85 years. Much of the demographic shift is caused by the emergence of baby

Conflicts of Interest and Funding: Dr J.A. Batsis' research reported in this publication was supported in part by the National Institute on Aging of the National Institutes of Health under award number K23AG051681. The content is solely the responsibility of the authors and does not necessarily represent the official views of the National Institutes of Health. This work was also supported by the Dartmouth Health Promotion and Disease Prevention Research Center (cooperative agreement number U48DP005018) from the Centers for Disease Control and Prevention. The findings and conclusions in this article are those of the authors and do not necessarily represent the official position of the Centers for Disease Control and Prevention. Dr J.A. Batsis has received honoraria from the Royal College of Physicians of Ireland for policy statement review and an honorarium from the Endocrine Society for an educational CME presentation at its annual conference.

Section of General Internal Medicine, Geisel School of Medicine at Dartmouth, The Dartmouth Institute for Health Policy and Clinical Practice, Dartmouth-Hitchcock Medical Center, 1 Medical Center Drive, Lebanon, NH 03756, USA

* Corresponding author. Section of General Internal Medicine, Dartmouth-Hitchcock Medical Center, 1 Medical Center Drive, Lebanon, NH 03756

E-mail address: john.batsis@gmail.com

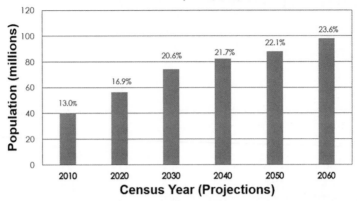

Fig. 1. Projected elderly population aged 65 years and older (represented as percentages) in the United States based on the 2010 census and future projections. (*Data from* United States Census Bureau. 2010 Census data. Available at: https://www.census.gov/2010census/data/. Accessed January 20, 2013.)

boomers, adults born mid-1946 to mid-1964, into older adulthood (aged ≥65 years). Improvements in medical care, chronic disease management, and infection control over the past century have also led to increases in life expectancy.[3,4] Based on recent census data, life expectancy at age 65 years is now 82.8 years in men and 85.3 years in women.[5] The demographic changes observed during the aging process lead to a trajectory of disability,[6] independent of other influencing comorbidities. For instance, individuals surviving into old age are at risk of functional impairments (inability to transfer, walk, dress, eat, toilet, and bathe[7]), which subsequently leads to a loss of independence, impairment in quality of life, and institutionalization.[8–10] Individuals are exposed to a longer period of time in which they may develop comorbidities and be at risk for developing incident disability.[11]

The obesity epidemic is not unique to a middle-aged or a pediatric population. The prevalence of obesity in older adults, classified using body mass index (BMI), continues to increase over time. Recent estimates from the National Health and Nutrition Examination Survey (NHANES) show that adults more than 60 years of age have obesity rates exceeding 37.5% in men and 39.4% in women[12] (**Fig. 2**). These estimates have been replicated and are increasing in other developed countries as well, including the United Kingdom[13] and Canada.[14]

DEFINING OBESITY IN OLDER ADULTS

Body composition changes with aging. Throughout adulthood, a natural increase in body fat develops up to the eighth decade of life, after which there is a reduction.[15] Redistribution of fat from peripheral and subcutaneous sources to a central location leads to increased waist circumference and waist/hip ratio in older adults. Importantly, there is a natural loss of muscle mass and strength with aging, termed sarcopenia.[16] Sarcopenia can also be accelerated in other processes, including deconditioning, immobility, or other acute illnesses.[17–19] Muscle mass and strength are thought to be vitally important in the preservation of physical function and independence in

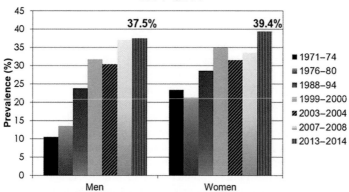

Prevalence of Obesity in Ages 60+
National Health & Nutrition Examination Surveys
1971–2014

Fig. 2. Prevalence of obesity in people aged 60 years and older using NHANESs over the past 4 decades based on body mass index. Current estimates indicate that obesity is present in 37.5% of men and 39.4% of women in the population. (*Data from* Flegal KM, Kruszon-Moran D, Carroll MD, et al. Trends in obesity among adults in the United States, 2005 to 2014. JAMA 2016;315(21):2284–91.)

this population.[20] Using standard adult classifications for weight status, such as BMI, may thus underestimate adiposity for a given individual.

Many epidemiologic and intervention-based studies have used BMI as a surrogate for adiposity. Standard BMI categories are used ubiquitously in clinical practice and are based on the World Health Organization cut points of underweight (BMI<18.5 kg/m^2), normal weight (18.5–24.9 kg/m^2), overweight (25–29.9 kg/m^2), and obese ($\geq$30 kg/m^2). BMI is easy to use, cheap, and can be measured using a simple stadiometer and a weight scale; however, BMI is a poor measure of adiposity in older adults. First, individuals lose height as they age. The Baltimore Longitudinal Study of Aging noted that both men and women lost height with age,[21] which affects the BMI's denominator, possibly leading to an overestimation of its overall value in this population. Second, although BMI is clearly valuable as a population-level measure, it has poor diagnostic accuracy for identifying older adults with obesity.[22–24] Using data from the 1999 to 2004 NHANES, the sensitivity of BMI in accurately identifying adiposity was 32.9% in men and 38.5% in women. Third, as previously described, older adults tend to gain weight in central regions of the body. BMI fails to distinguish between peripheral and visceral obesity, which is an important consideration in individuals who are classified as having normal-weight central obesity.[25] Based solely on BMI, this category of individuals is often not a target for obesity therapy because they are within the normal range (BMI of 18.5–24.9 kg/m^2). Individuals with central obesity presenting with a normal BMI may also be at risk for adverse cardiometabolic dysfunction, including dyslipidemia, coronary disease, hypertension, and early mortality.[26–28] One large-scale epidemiologic study using 15,184 adults aged 18 to 90 years with normal BMI and central adiposity based on waist/hip ratio[29] found that individuals with normal-weight central obesity had a higher risk of total and cardiovascular mortality (hazard ratio [HR] of 1.87 [95% CI (confidence interval): 1.53,2.29] in men and 1.48 [95% CI: 1.35,1.62] in women). These relationships have been observed in older adults as well, whereby women have higher short-term cardiovascular mortality than men, and men have higher long-term cardiovascular mortality than women.[27] Irrespective of sex, individuals with normal-weight central obesity (waist/hip ratio or waist circumference) are at higher risk of long-term disability.[28] Identifying and evaluating individuals in clinical practice who otherwise may not be identified as high risk is needed. Such misclassification can be problematic from a population-based management standpoint. In addition, BMI accounts for both fat-free mass (muscle) and fat mass, the former of which declines during the aging process, which can further lead to misclassification and potential underestimation of adiposity and risk.

However, gold-standard methods for identifying adiposity with accuracy, including MRI and computed tomography, are noncovered indications in clinical practice unless performed for other reasons. Dual-energy absorptiometry is more routinely available, but assessment of body composition is not covered by Medicare. Bioelectrical impedance can be a crude measure for body composition assessment in older adults and portable devices are available; however, the alterations in fluid balance in older adults,[30] along with a higher incidence of prosthetic implants[31] and implantable cardiovascular devices,[32] makes this modality less favorable. As such, BMI combined with a marker of central adiposity may provide a cost-effective approach to improved diagnostic accuracy within a clinical practice.

Established BMI cut points correspond with adverse disease processes, including mortality.[33] Multiple population-based cohort studies have examined the relationship between obesity and premature death. In one study, obesity led to an estimated 111,909 excess deaths.[34] Although obesity in midlife is associated with reduced life expectancy, the duration of obesity has a considerable effect on long-term mortality,[35] disability,[36] and nursing home placement,[37] as shown in numerous epidemiologic studies. The relationship between BMI and mortality in populations has been shown to be representative of a U-shaped curve[34]; individuals classified as underweight and obese are at the extremes with higher risks of mortality. With age, the curve flattens and shifts to the right, indicating that standard BMI cut points differ in older adults compared with younger populations. A meta-analysis that evaluated 32 studies between 1990 and 2013 (including 197,940 adults aged 65 years and older) also showed a U-shaped curve.[38] However, the lowest risk of mortality was observed in those with a BMI of $\sim$27.5 kg/m^2. The risk of death only increases at a BMI greater than 33.0 (HR, 1.08 [95% CI: 1.00, 1.15]).

In select older adult populations, not all participants with increased BMIs should be considered at high risk. An obesity paradox exists whereby increased body weight may be protective, mitigating death in select populations. For instance, a nursing home systematic review evaluated 19,538 subjects with a BMI greater than or equal to 30 kg/m^2 and found that the risk of death was significantly lower than for the referent (normal BMI) group (HR, 0.69 [95% CI: 0.60, 0.79]; $P<.001$).[39] Several factors are thought to explain this. First, issues related to the inability of BMI to discern between visceral and subcutaneous fat. Second, cardiovascular fitness likely moderates the relationship between obesity and death (individuals with high levels of cardiovascular fitness, irrespective of their obesity classification, portend to better outcomes[40]). Third, excess adiposity in high-risk populations at risk for frailty, itself a predictor of death, may be protective. Populations such as hemodialysis patients, patients with congestive heart failure, or nursing home residents all tend to lose weight (consisting of both fat and muscle) with aging, which promotes wasting, cachexia, and mortality.[41] Fourth, there may be self-selection; individuals with excess adiposity who have survived to old age may have a survival advantage compared with those who have died earlier in life. As such, practitioners should be made aware of these considerations in select populations, particularly when using BMI as a measure for adiposity in older adults with these specific comorbidities.

IMPACT OF OBESITY ON PHYSICAL FUNCTION/DISABILITY

Overweight and obesity predisposes to disability and decreased physical functioning. Using the Health, Aging, and Body Composition data, adults classified as overweight or with obesity using BMI at ages 25, 50, and 70 to 79 years had an HR of 2.38 for incident disability over a 7-year period.[35] Similar relationships have been observed using either waist circumference or body fat percentage, both in men and women. A systematic review by Schaap and colleagues[42] showed that adults with a BMI greater than or equal to 30 kg/m^2 aged 65 years and older had a 60% higher risk of incident disability [95% CI, 1.43, 1.80]. A U-shaped relationship is also observed between BMI and nursing home admission from community-dwelling adults.[43] Longitudinally, there seems to be a relationship. As the obesity epidemic has emerged in the past few decades, recent evidence suggests that its relationship with disability continues to be problematic, but may be leveling off.[44] A recent study evaluated 3 consecutive time periods using NHANES (1988–1994, 1999–2004, and 2005–2012) and evaluated the association between obesity and disability. The population attributable fraction for obesity having a functional impairment and severe impairment in activities of daily living was 23.2% [95% CI, 20.5, 25.7] and 24.6% [95% CI, 12.3, 35.2], respectively, in individuals aged 60 years and older. Individuals classified as having obesity were still at much higher risk of limitations, but limited wave-to-wave variability was observed. Other measures of adiposity, including body fat percentage and waist circumference, have also been associated with impaired physical function and disability and parallel these estimates. A study evaluating the cross-sectional association between obesity using body fat and disability showed significant odds of disability.[45,46] Although there are challenges in the diagnostic accuracy of obesity, irrespective of the body composition or anthropometric measure used, in community-dwelling adults, obesity is associated with a poorer prognosis of physical function.

Obesity is also associated with increased risk of falling in older adults. More than one-third of adults aged 65 years and older fall each year,[47] making it necessary to screen for fall risk in the primary care setting.[48,49] Two studies using Health and Retirement Study 1998 to 2006,[50] and the Behavioral Risk Factor Surveillance System 2014 data[51] showed that the degree of obesity (class I vs II vs III) was associated with a higher risk of falling. Using the Health and Retirement Study data, people with class III obesity (BMI>35 kg/m^2) have an odds ratio of 1.50 [95% CI: 1.21–1.86] for falling, whereas estimates from the Behavioral Risk Factor Surveillance System are slightly lower (OR, 1.23 [95% CI: 1.13,1.35] in women; OR, 1.18 [95% CI: 1.06,1.32] in men). Although fall risk is increased, risk of hip fractures from obesity is lower in this population.[52] Evaluating individuals who are at risk can prevent falls that may otherwise lead to restriction of social function, fractures, and death.[48,50]

SARCOPENIC OBESITY: A SUBSET OF HIGH-RISK INDIVIDUALS

Sarcopenia in individuals with obesity is a subgroup that deserves specific attention. Sarcopenia is derived from the Greek words sarcos, meaning flesh, and penia, meaning lack of. Infiltration of fat occurs within muscle tissue and can lead to impairments in muscle physiologic parameters.[53,54] The definition of sarcopenia and obesity (sarcopenic obesity) continues to be fraught with methodological challenges[55] and discrepancies in defining sarcopenia (muscle mass vs muscle strength) and obesity (body fat vs waist circumference vs BMI). Nonetheless, such individuals are at considerably higher risk than those with either of the two conditions independently. Although the medical definition has evolved over the past 3 decades,[55] based on the 2014

Foundations for the National Institutes of Health Conference,[20] sarcopenia is simply the loss of muscle mass and function with aging. Specific cut points have been developed for use. Although several earlier studies focused on loss of muscle mass as the key determinant of sarcopenia,[56] emerging evidence suggests that muscle strength may be a more powerful determinant of incident disability.[57]

The development of sarcopenia in old age is a natural phenomenon that can be partially mitigated with lifestyle interventions, altering the threshold at which disability ensues.[16,58] Short-term and long-term changes of both muscle mass and strength occur. However, changes in strength may occur without corresponding changes in muscle mass, as observed in an earlier study using Health, Aging and Body Composition data.[59] Earlier work using the New Mexico Aging Study showed that individuals with sarcopenic obesity had an HR of 2.63 [95% CI, 1.19–5.85] for developing an impairment of their instrumental activities of daily living over the course of an 8-year period.[60] This study defined sarcopenic obesity using appendicular skeletal muscle mass and body fat cut points.[61] Data from the InChianti study showed that individuals with low muscle strength and obesity (based on knee extensor strength and BMI) had lower walking speeds than their counterparts over a 6-year period of time.[62] Much of our own work has used dual x-ray absorptiometry–defined muscle mass with the Foundations for the National Institute of Health (FNIH) cut points with body fat–defined obesity (men, >25%; women, 35%), suggesting a significant relationship with limitations[63] and mortality.[64] Mortality is less clear, as shown using NHANES III data[65] (using bioelectrical impedance (BIA)-defined muscle mass) and NHANES 1999 to 2004 data (using dual x-ray absorptiometry–defined muscle mass).[64] Impaired muscle strength in conjunction with obesity, irrespective of its definition, is associated in cross-sectional and longitudinal studies with adverse and negative outcomes, more so than muscle mass.[42] Thus, identifying patients with both sarcopenia and obesity is of paramount importance.

EVIDENCE FOR WEIGHT LOSS IN OLDER ADULTS

Previous epidemiologic studies have provided conflicting findings on outcomes following weight loss in older adults; however, these studies failed to differentiate between intentional versus unintentional weight loss and do not account for important confounding variables and reverse causality.[66,67] A joint consensus statement, published in 2005 by members of The Obesity Society, American Society of Nutrition, and The National Association for the Study of Obesity, provided some evidence on managing this disease in older adults,[68] and several randomized controlled trials have since been published showing the benefits and the harms of weight loss in older adults[69] (note that this article defines weight loss as intentional in the following discussion).

A healthy lifestyle has been shown to compress the number of years of disability, according to data from the Cardiovascular Health Study 1989 to 2015.[70] Monitoring multiple lifestyle factors, including physical activity, diet, and BMI, 5248 community adults aged 65 years and older who were not wheelchair dependent were identified. Activities of daily living were assessed and the ratio of the number of years living without any disability to the total number of years lived was ascertained to indicate compression or expansion of the disabling period. Obesity was associated with a decrease of 7.3% [95% CI, 5.4–9.2] compared with normal-weight individuals. The lowest quintile of the Alternative Healthy Eating Index was associated with a 3.7% [95% CI, 1.6–5.9] lower score than the highest quintile. However, engaging in physical activity showed that for every 25 blocks walked in a week, a 0.5% [95% CI, 0.3–0.8] higher proportion of years was gained disability free. The article concluded that healthy lifestyles can compress the duration of disability in people's remaining lifetimes.

A recent qualitative systematic review evaluated 6 randomized controlled trials from 2005 to 2015 in adults aged 60 years and older (mean age >65 years).[69] Obesity was defined as BMI greater than or equal to 30 kg/m^2 or waist circumference greater than or equal to 88 cm/102 cm in women/men respectively. Of 5741 citations, 19 trials were identified, of which 6 were unique cohorts. Results suggested that a dietary weight reduction program combined with a physical activity program (aerobic and resistance) improved physical performance and quality of life and decreased the risk of reduced muscle mass, reduced strength, and bone loss. Weight loss ranged from 0.5 to 10.7 kg. A recently published randomized trial with 141 participants showed that weight loss inclusive of both aerobic and resistance exercises led to improvements in the physical performance test, peak oxygen consumption, and muscle strength, despite only marginal reductions in lean muscle mass.[71] In addition, there was no difference in exercise-related adverse events. In a separate review, weight loss in older adults with obesity was associated with reduced risk of death.[72] The investigators identified 15 randomized controlled trials including 17,186 participants with a mean age of 52 years at randomization. The mean BMI was 30 to 46 kg/m^2 with an average follow-up period of 27 months (ranging from 18 months to 12.6 years). The weight-loss group experienced a 15% lower all-cause mortality risk (relative risk, 0.85 [95% CI, 0.73, 1.00]). Although further evidence is needed to ascertain the impact on long-term mortality, weight loss seems to be safe and effective in older adults with obesity.

CAUTIONS OF LOSING WEIGHT IN OLDER ADULTS

There are important risks that often get overlooked in this population by practitioners. Loss of weight leads not only to loss of fat mass but also to loss of muscle mass, thereby promoting sarcopenia and its ensuing adverse outcomes.[73] The general principle that each kilogram lost equates to 75% fat and 25% muscle has been debated but is generally accepted.[74] Moreover, loss of weight affects bone metabolism and turnover, promoting osteoporosis.[75–77]

Although sarcopenia is a natural phenomenon of the aging process, its acceleration with weight-loss efforts is of considerable concern. Weight loss induced by diet or diet and exercise induces hormonal changes that negatively affect muscle mass and strength and this is exacerbated by moderate caloric restriction. A review of 33 interventions showed significant decreases from baseline in knee extensor strength (−7.5%) and handgrip strength (−4.6%) following diet-induced weight loss with moderate energy restriction.[76] Failure to engage patients in isokinetic resistance exercises is likely to led to loss of muscle mass and strength and to reduce the impact of the gains in function individuals may otherwise attain with weight loss.[78]

Several randomized controlled trials have shown that caloric restriction alone leads to loss of bone mineral density (BMD). Villareal and colleagues[58,71] showed that a loss of hip BMD was attenuated, in part, when resistance exercise was coupled with a weight-loss program, preventing an increase in bone turnover. In another study, a meta-analysis of 32 randomized controlled trials, weight loss had no significant effect on total BMD.[75] However, the pooled study data suggested that hip and lumbar spine BMD were significantly lower after 4 months, particularly in adults who were classified as having obesity. Lumbar spine BMD was also lower after calorie restriction in interventions longer than 13 months. Although these results were from adults aged 50 years and older, the sensitivity analysis stratified by age revealed that hip BMD loss was highest in adults aged 65 years and older. This finding has considerable implications for older adults who are at risk of falling. Approximately 30% of falls among older adults result in injury, 10% of which are fractures.[79] Hip fractures are especially serious in this population and portend considerable morbidity and mortality.[80]

In general, weight loss in the older adult population is safe and effective and can lead to considerable improvements in cardiometabolic risk and physical function. Although there are important known risks associated with weight loss in this population, they likely can be mitigated with appropriate health promotion interventions. As with all patients in a geriatrics practice, practitioners need to manage the benefits versus the risks of any interventions, and, in select individuals, weight loss should be encouraged.

OBESITY IN THE PRIMARY CARE SETTING

Obesity prevention efforts should be based in primary care settings, where front-line clinicians have longitudinal relationships to provide brief, motivational interviewing to engage patients in behavioral change. Intensive behavioral counseling can induce clinically meaningful weight loss of between 0.3 and 6.6 kg, but little research is available on primary care practitioners providing this care. A systematic review suggested that different interventionists can deliver counseling, both in person and by telephone, in this setting.[81] An additional review suggested that a multidisciplinary team approach consisting of collaborative care was much more effective.[82] This review conflicts with a recent 2-arm randomized trial of 2728 patients that showed that a behaviorally informed, very brief (30-second) physician-delivered opportunistic intervention was acceptable and effective in reducing population mean weight (1.43 kg [95% CI, 0.89, 1.97]).[83]

In 2011, in the United States, the Centers for Medicare and Medicaid Services began reimbursing obesity counseling (current procedural terminology code G0447) for clinicians in a primary care setting to provide 22 targeted, 15-minute intensive behavioral therapy counseling in a continuous 12-month period.[84] The goal was to achieve a mean weight loss of 3 kg in beneficiaries whose BMI was greater than or equal to 30 kg/m^2. Practice management barriers[85] exist in implementing this benefits, although novel technologies[86] may be helpful in addressing these issues. In 2012, the first full year of data, 27,338 (0.1%) of Medicare beneficiaries more than 65 years of age availed themselves of the benefit.[87] This number increased slightly in 2013 to 46,821 (0.17%). The estimated proportion of persons with obesity using the benefit increased from 0.35% to 0.60%, with a mean of 1.99 and 2.16 claims per user. These data suggest that its low uptake may not only be caused by poor implementation patterns but that other support staff, such as health coaches and dieticians, should be involved in delivering this important service. Novel delivery modalities to engage patients may be a strong consideration moving forward, including transition to value-based care models or increased reimbursements.

MEDICAL EVALUATION SPECIFIC TO OLDER ADULTS WITH OBESITY

The nutritional needs and caloric intake for healthy older adults is known to decrease with age in both sexes. The caloric difference between early adulthood and older adulthood ranges between 300 and 500 kCal/d. Much of this is caused by age-related phenomena related to basal metabolic rate, which decreases considerably with age.[88] Specific concerns are discussed here that primary care providers should consider using a geriatric-specific approach, compared with a middle-aged adult with obesity.[89]

Communication in clinical settings with older adults requires careful communication strategies that are often overlooked by clinicians. Behavioral techniques must be adapted to accommodate not only the sensory deficits that older adults face, such as hearing and vision, but need to be adapted to changes in cognition and executive function,[90] and older adults' preference for shared decision making.[91] Others have noted a gap between intentions and behavioral change,[92] which itself can be predicted by measures of executive function.[93] An inability to implement intentions leads to poor execution of the desired change.[94] Older adults may also be better focused on single-health-behavior change interventions compared with multiple,[95] focusing on a specific content. These approaches are less confusing and can be understood much more adequately. In contrast, complex conditions in older adults require multiple strategies to deliver health promotion efforts, which can be challenging to clinicians. Engaging individuals in strategies to improve self-efficacy through social support and change can be helpful to provide information to set goals, engage in change, and to promote self-monitoring.[96] Researchers continue to caution clinicians in applying behavioral change principles to older adults because they may require adaptation from a younger population.

Although primary care providers care for older adults, the lack of specific geriatric training can be problematic in delivering behavioral change interventions. First, motivational interviewing, a core tenet in eliciting change and in the Medicare Obesity Benefit, is heavily influenced by the contextual aspects of delivery and by clinicians,[97] and internists may approach elements differently than geriatricians. Second, geropsychological principles are often not integrated in routine interventions,[98] including social participation, which is strongly related to better health and can lead to forming new goals in people's lives.[99] This lack of integration allows a reframing of the discussion to engaging in change. Third, goals in seniors are different, in part because of multimorbidity[100] but also because of the changing perceptions on aging and health.[101–104] Fourth, aging individuals have limited lifespans and, hence, patients focus more on the present than on the future. These elements lead to significant challenges in busy primary care settings.

A thorough medical evaluation is needed in older patients who wish to improve their health and physical function through weight loss. Primary care clinicians (or obesity medicine specialists) should identify whether there are any recent changes in health status (medical or economic) or recent hospitalizations and changes in functional status (eg, joint replacement leading to physical inactivity) that may lead to weight gain.[105] Other standard questioning methods on weight history, previous strategies, and alcohol use parallel methods used in the general population. Notably, this article highlights 2 main concerns specific to older adults: medications and social support.

The number of medications prescribed increases with age and with the number of chronic conditions. Polypharmacy is a significant risk in older adults because it is associated with increased risk of cognitive impairment, urinary incontinence, falls, and declines in physical function.[106] The American Geriatric Society has developed the Beers Criteria,[107] which clearly identify potentially inappropriate medications in older adults and assists health care providers in improving medication safety for this population. The purpose of the criteria is to inform clinical decision making concerning the prescribing of medications for older adults in order to improve safety and quality of care. There are several medications that are considered obesogenic and that should be reevaluated as part of the evaluation. Because older adults have a high incidence of diabetes,[108] depression,[109] pain,[110] and hypertension,[111] medications treating these chronic diseases may increase the risk of a person gaining weight. In addition, several of these medications are listed in the Beers Criteria. The primary care practitioner, in concert with a clinical pharmacist on the multidisciplinary team, can assist in streamlining not only the number of medications but also the class of medications that promote weight gain. **Table 1** briefly highlights some of the common medications that predispose to weight gain.

Socioeconomic and ethnic disparities are two specific social determinants of health that increasingly are being recognized as important predictors in obesity management and adverse health. Elder on fixed incomes (often social security incomes) must make choices between food consumption and other care needs. Food insecurity is defined as the limited or uncertain availability of nutritionally adequate and safe foods, or the limited or uncertain ability to acquire acceptable foods in socially acceptable ways.[112] Food-insecure older individuals have poorer dietary intake, nutritional status, and health status than food-secure older adults.[113] Simple questions that should be asked include:

- Where is your food coming from?
- Who purchases your food?
- Do you have to pay for your medical bills and scrimp on food?

Such questions are helpful in that they lead to information on the affordability of food. A true multidisciplinary team led by the physician and including a dietician, social worker, and care manager can be helpful in intervening in this population. Dieticians are of utmost importance in that they are not only able to perform the usual functions of evaluation and counseling but can assist this population in engage in substituting choices that they can afford.

Most established trials have evaluated calorie-restricted diets ranging from 500 to 750 kCal/d under the guidance of a registered dietician.[69] In older adults, there is ample evidence that diets such as the Dietary Approaches to Stop Hypertension[114] or the Mediterranean diet[115] have shown improvements in metabolic parameters, weight loss, long-term disability, mortality, and cognition. Very-low-energy or protein-sparing diets should be avoided in older adults because of the risks of dramatic fluid and electrolyte shifts and proportionally can lead to augmented muscle mass loss. Villareal and colleagues[58,71] proposed a loss of ~10% of baseline weight at 6 months.[58,71] Supplemental vitamin D of ~800 to 1000 units and 1200 mg of calcium should be considered. The latter can be from dietary or supplement sources, although the authors emphasize the consumption from dietary calcium if possible considering the recent controversies. Protein intake should also be augmented in older adults. Recommended dietary allowance is 1.0 g/kg/d, but, because older adults produce less protein than younger persons, this should be revised to 1.0 to 1.2 g/kg/d.[116] Also, a

Table 1
Commonly prescribed medications in older adults predisposing to weight gain

Disease/Class of Medication	Examples
Diabetes	Insulin, TDZ[a], sulfonylureas[a]
Depression	Tricyclics[a], SSRIs[a]
Antipsychotics	First + second generation[a]
Neuropathic	Gabapentin
Antihistamines	Diphenhydramine[a]
Hypertension	β-Blockers

Abbreviations: SSRI, selective serotonin reuptake inhibitor; TDZ, thiazolidinedione.
[a] Medications that are listed in the 2015 Beers Criteria.[107]

larger amount of protein is required to produce an equal response.[116] Notably, a recent Cochrane Review showed that protein supplements did not lead to improved outcomes.[117] Early pilot studies during weight-loss interventions suggest improved short physical performance battery measures. The MeasureUP[118] in 67 subjects showed, at 6 months, a −8.7 ± 7.4 kg and −7.5 ± 6.2 kg weight loss in the protein and control groups, respectively. The investigators observed improvements in physical function based on the short physical performance battery of +2.4 ± 1.7 units and +0.9 ± 1.7 units, respectively ($P = .02$). Future studies should determine the amount of protein intake, the type of protein (meat vs plant), and whether advised supplements for the treatment of sarcopenia (whey, leucine, carnitine) can augment physical function and further mitigate sarcopenia.

Primary care providers have little training in counseling on physical activity.[119] However, they can provide targeted information on exercise prescriptions. Such prescriptions should be individually tailored based on the individual's functional status and capacity. The American College of Sports Medicine suggests at least 150 minutes of low to moderate intensity aerobic activity in all patients, including older adults.[120] Seniors who do not have sufficient cardiovascular fitness may subdivide this time period into smaller increments to not only build their endurance but assist in ongoing behavioral change. Practitioners and their teams can encourage patients to slowly increase their capacity to do so. During weight-loss efforts, resistance exercises are of paramount importance for the prevention of sarcopenia. All individuals should engage in flexibility, balance, and strengthening activities with resistance bands or weights, which can be free or can be attached to wrists or legs. In those with financial difficulties, the authors advise individuals to use common household items (ie, soup cans or jugs of milk). The weekly goals are 2 to 3 days, with at least 48 hours' rest between sessions. Each of these sessions should last between 30 and 40 minutes, rotating muscle groups and exercises, with 10 to 12 repetitions for each session. Fatigue normally occurs between 8 and 12 repetitions and some fatigue is advisable, but it is important to prevent injuries by starting low and going slow, starting with .5 to 1 kg (1–2 pounds) or with the lowest resistance color band. Physical therapists can assess a person's 1-repetition maximum and advise advancement. The authors advocate that current multidisciplinary physical activity programs should be based on the Life Study,[121] a multicenter randomized controlled study that showed reduced disability over a mean 2.6-year follow-up in 818 patients. Compared with a self-instructed exercise program, participants in this structured program showed a 28% reduction in incident major mobility disability [95% CI, 0.57, 0.91]. These materials are freely available at http://www.thelifestudy.org. In addition, the National Institute on Aging has a booklet of exercises that can be accessed and downloaded at http://www.nia.nih.gov/health/publication/exercise-physical-activity/introduction, free of charge for clinicians and patients to engage in at home.

Clinicians can play a paramount role in the monitoring of their older patients undergoing weight loss. Although there is no firm evidence pertaining to monitoring parameters, the authors recommend the following. First, consideration should be given to assessing baseline bone density during such efforts. Medicare indications for women are broad (ie, postmenopausal) but those for men may be slightly more challenging to find. The United States Preventive Services Task Force recommendations for osteoporosis screening in men do not provide a firm statement and conclude that the evidence is insufficient to assess the balance of benefits and harms of screening.[122] Some potential indications in men include radiograph evidence of possible osteopenia, osteoporosis, or vertebral fractures; a person taking steroids; hyperparathyroidism; and monitoring whether osteoporosis drug therapy is working. Examples of biomarkers of bone turnover that can be considered in the evaluative process include osteocalcin, type I procollagen, and urine collagen type-1 cross-linked N-telopeptide. These biomarkers may help direct the impact of weight loss on bone turnover. Baseline and longitudinal monitoring of grip strength is an office procedure that can easily be integrated in any busy practice. The recent approval of an ICD-10 (International Statistical Classification of Diseases and Related Health Problems, Tenth Revision) code for sarcopenia may allow further screening and routine integration in practice. In addition, monitoring of vitamin D levels may be helpful. Different societies have different views on monitoring of levels.[49] Our practice is to assess baseline vitamin D levels during routine weight-loss management. As with any intervention in older adults, assessment of the risks versus benefits of monitoring is needed, and further studies should best inform the appropriate indices that clinicians should considering during such efforts.

PHARMACOTHERAPY

With the emergence of newer medications that are effective in weight management, older adults are increasingly asking about the possibility of taking such medications. The American Association of Clinical Endocrinologists/American College of Endocrinology guidelines explicitly state that there is insufficient evidence to recommend weight-loss medications in older adults.[123] As is the case with most pharmaceutical-based clinical trials, to prove efficacy, older adults were excluded from most trials, biasing outcomes toward younger patients. However, the authors advise caution in extrapolating such results to older adults whose pharmacokinetic and pharmacodynamic properties differ from those in younger, robust populations of patients who often have fewer comorbid conditions and are on fewer medications.

Of the obesity medications available, 2 trials (using phentermine/topiramate and liraglutide) have documented efficacy analyses between older adults and their younger counterparts. These trials enrolled 7% (n = 254) and 6.9% (n = 232) older adults, respectively, among their study subjects.[123–128] There were no observed differences in efficacy, safety, and pharmacokinetics between subgroups. The other commercial medications had insufficient study sample sizes to make any statistical comparisons. Preliminary data suggest that pharmacokinetic data on phentermine/topiramate, liraglutide, lorcaserin, or naltrexone/bupropion were no different between younger and older patients. The propensity to add to an older adult's polypharmacy should approached with caution because polypharmacy leads to medication errors and subsequent adverse drug events, increased risk for falls, increased risk for delirium, and increased costs. **Table 2** highlights some of the absolute contraindications to these medications and some of the common side effects and major risks that older adults may face, irrespective of the lack of evidence. Given the need for obesity treatments and the limited data currently available, further research in older adult populations is important.

BARIATRIC SURGERY

An effective treatment approved by the National Institutes of Health in 1991 is bariatric surgery.[129] This procedure has gained considerable popularity and is increasingly being performed in persons with obesity who are at high risk of medical complications and/or have comorbidities. In the general population, there are considerable epidemiologic and trial data showing its safety, efficacy, and effectiveness.[130–135] The extent of the safety and efficacy in older adults continues to be debated in the surgical literature. Studies have used varying cut points for older adults (50– 65 years) and are

Table 2
Relative and absolute contraindications to weight-loss medications in older adults

Generic Name	Absolute Contraindications	Side Effects (>10%) and Major Risks in Older Adults
Lorcaserin	—	Renal insufficiency (tramadol), heart failure, serotonin excess, hypoglycemia
Phentermine/topiramate	Glaucoma, MAOI hyperthyroidism	Constipation, headache, xerostomia
Phentermine	Glaucoma, heart failure, CAD, hyperthyroidism, arrhythmias	Renal insufficiency, reduced exercise tolerance
Orlistat	Malabsorption, cholestasis	Fecal urgency, flatulence, steatorrhea
Bupropion/naltrexone	HTN, seizures, hepatic impairment	More sensitive to CNS effects, renal insufficiency, headache, constipation, NV
Liraglutide	Angioedema, MEN-2, MTC	Constipation, diarrhea, hypoglycemia, palpitations, NV

Abbreviations: CAD, coronary artery disease; CNS, central nervous system; HTN, hypertension; MAOI, monoamine oxidase inhibitor; MEN-2, multiple endocrine neoplasia type 2; MTC, medullary thyroid carcinoma; NV, nausea and vomiting.

fraught with considerable methodological problems, including reduced study power, study time period bias, and inconsistent definitions. In addition, the evolving surgical and medical care of this patient population, and the establishment of high-volume bariatric surgery centers of excellence, have led to considerably improved outcomes.[136,137] Several systematic reviews have been published discussing the short-term and long-term outcomes of bariatric surgery in older adult populations,[138] but these are outside the scope of this article.

European guidelines[139] have noted that the procedure should be considered in carefully selected patients. The authors previously developed an approach in older adults that highlights physiologic as opposed to chronologic age.[140] A laparoscopic approach is favored compared with an open approach. By applying the principles of a comprehensive geriatric assessment of patients evaluated for surgery, the hope is that those carefully selected individuals will have improved short-term and long-term outcomes. Highlighting the importance of future life expectancy, presence of undiagnosed cognitive impairment, medical comorbidity that could be affected by the surgical procedure, and important social support mechanisms for the immediate postoperative care are of utmost importance. Previous history of postoperative delirium and impairments in vision and hearing are also important factors in successful recovery. Understanding such limitations could sway a decision to consider surgical intervention or not in a given patient. Being classified as geriatric should not preclude evaluation of surgery in those motivated older adults who fulfill many of the elements noted earlier in the geriatric evaluation.

SUMMARY

The epidemic of geriatric obesity will continue to affect the role of primary care providers with time. The importance of lifespan prevention measures to delay the onset of disability and impairments in health-related quality of life cannot be overstated. Effective lifestyle modifications for weight loss can easily be implemented within a busy primary care setting to engage individuals. Community-based physical activity interventions are easy, cost-effective ways to delay disability and enhance physical function. Future studies should focus on disseminating and implementing practical ways to integrate established evidence-based practices into routine clinical care, without overburdening clinical staff. Emerging technologies may be helpful adjuncts. Evaluation of pharmacotherapy in this high-risk population remains a priority and including older, robust adults may be a reasonable first step in evaluating their safety and efficacy. The authors recommend that bariatric surgery be considered for older adults following a comprehensive geriatric assessment, and an interdisciplinary team–based approach is helpful in evaluating and engaging these patients in this process.

REFERENCES

1. Government US. Census bureau statistics. 2012. Available at: www.census.gov. Accessed January 20, 2013.
2. Mather M, Jacobsen LA, Pollard KM. Aging in the United States. Population Reference Bureau. 2015. Available at: http://www.prb.org/pdf16/aging-us-population-bulletin.pdf. Accessed September 19, 2017.
3. Lubitz J, Cai L, Kramarow E, et al. Health, life expectancy, and health care spending among the elderly. N Engl J Med 2003;349(11):1048–55.
4. Katz S, Branch LG, Branson MH, et al. Active life expectancy. N Engl J Med 1983;309(20):1218–24.
5. Arias E. United States life tables, 2011. Natl Vital Stat Rep 2015;64(11):1–63.
6. Dunlop DD, Hughes SL, Manheim LM. Disability in activities of daily living: patterns of change and a hierarchy of disability. Am J Public Health 1997;87(3): 378–83.
7. Katz S, Ford AB, Moskowitz RW, et al. Studies of illness in the aged. The index of ADL: a standardized measure of biological and psychosocial function. JAMA 1963;185:914–9.
8. Bish CL, Michels Blanck H, Maynard LM, et al. Health-related quality of life and weight loss among overweight and obese U.S. adults, 2001 to 2002. Obesity (Silver Spring) 2006;14(11):2042–53.
9. Cai Q, Salmon JW, Rodgers ME. Factors associated with long-stay nursing home admissions among the U.S. elderly population: comparison of logistic regression and the Cox proportional hazards model with policy implications for social work. Soc Work Health Care 2009;48(2):154–68.
10. Chambers BA, Guo SS, Siervogel R, et al. Cumulative effects of cardiovascular disease risk factors on quality of life. J Nutr Health Aging 2002;6(3):179–84.
11. Cigolle CT, Langa KM, Kabeto MU, et al. Geriatric conditions and disability: the health and retirement study. Ann Intern Med 2007;147(3):156–64.
12. Flegal KM, Kruszon-Moran D, Carroll MD, et al. Trends in obesity among adults in the United States, 2005 to 2014. JAMA 2016;315(21):2284–91.
13. Carl Baker. House of Commons Library, 20 January 2017. Obesity Statistics. Available at: www.parliament.uk/commons-library. Accessed September 19, 2017.
14. Twells LK, Gregory DM, Reddigan J, et al. Current and predicted prevalence of obesity in Canada: a trend analysis. CMAJ Open 2014;2(1):E18–26.
15. Baumgartner RN. Body composition in healthy aging. Ann N Y Acad Sci 2000; 904:437–48.

16. Sayer AA, Syddall H, Martin H, et al. The developmental origins of sarcopenia. J Nutr Health Aging 2008;12(7):427–32.
17. Fielding RA, Vellas B, Evans WJ, et al. Sarcopenia: an undiagnosed condition in older adults. Current consensus definition: prevalence, etiology, and consequences. International working group on sarcopenia. J Am Med Dir Assoc 2011;12(4):249–56.
18. Dutta C. Significance of sarcopenia in the elderly. J Nutr 1997;127(5 Suppl): 992S–3S.
19. Bales CW, Ritchie CS. Sarcopenia, weight loss, and nutritional frailty in the elderly. Annu Rev Nutr 2002;22:309–23.
20. Studenski SA, Peters KW, Alley DE, et al. The FNIH sarcopenia project: rationale, study description, conference recommendations, and final estimates. J Gerontol A Biol Sci Med Sci 2014;69(5):547–58.
21. Sorkin JD, Muller DC, Andres R. Longitudinal change in height of men and women: implications for interpretation of the body mass index: the Baltimore Longitudinal Study of Aging. Am J Epidemiol 1999;150(9):969–77.
22. Romero-Corral A, Somers VK, Sierra-Johnson J, et al. Accuracy of body mass index in diagnosing obesity in the adult general population. Int J Obes (Lond) 2008;32(6):959–66.
23. Okorodudu DO, Jumean MF, Montori VM, et al. Diagnostic performance of body mass index to identify obesity as defined by body adiposity: a systematic review and meta-analysis. Int J Obes (Lond) 2010;34(5):791–9.
24. Batsis JA, Mackenzie TA, Bartels SJ, et al. Diagnostic accuracy of body mass index to identify obesity in older adults: NHANES 1999-2004. Int J Obes (Lond) 2016;40(5):761–7.
25. Batsis JA, Zbehlik AJ, Scherer EA, et al. Normal weight with central obesity, physical activity, and functional decline: data from the osteoarthritis initiative. J Am Geriatr Soc 2015;63(8):1552–60.
26. Romero-Corral A, Somers VK, Sierra-Johnson J, et al. Normal weight obesity: a risk factor for cardiometabolic dysregulation and cardiovascular mortality. Eur Heart J 2010;31(6):737–46.
27. Batsis JA, Sahakyan KR, Rodriguez-Escudero JP, et al. Normal weight obesity and mortality in United States subjects ≥60 years of age (from the Third National Health and Nutrition Examination Survey). Am J Cardiol 2013;112(10):1592–8.
28. Batsis JA, Sahakyan KR, Rodriguez-Escudero JP, et al. Normal weight obesity and functional outcomes in older adults. Eur J Intern Med 2014;25(6):517–22.
29. Sahakyan KR, Somers VK, Rodriguez-Escudero JP, et al. Normal-weight central obesity: implications for total and cardiovascular mortality. Ann Intern Med 2015; 163(11):827–35.
30. Schlanger LE, Bailey JL, Sands JM. Electrolytes in the aging. Adv Chronic Kidney Dis 2010;17(4):308–19.
31. Maradit Kremers H, Larson DR, Crowson CS, et al. Prevalence of total hip and knee replacement in the United States. J Bone Joint Surg Am 2015;97(17): 1386–97.
32. Silverman BG, Gross TP, Kaczmarek RG, et al. The epidemiology of pacemaker implantation in the United States. Public Health Rep 1995;110(1):42–6.
33. Flegal KM, Kit BK, Orpana H, et al. Association of all-cause mortality with overweight and obesity using standard body mass index categories: a systematic review and meta-analysis. JAMA 2013;309(1):71–82.
34. Flegal KM, Graubard BI, Williamson DF, et al. Excess deaths associated with underweight, overweight, and obesity. JAMA 2005;293(15):1861–7.

35. Houston DK, Ding J, Nicklas BJ, et al. Overweight and obesity over the adult life course and incident mobility limitation in older adults: the Health, Aging and Body Composition Study. Am J Epidemiol 2009;169(8):927–36.

36. Strandberg TE, Sirola J, Pitkala KH, et al. Association of midlife obesity and cardiovascular risk with old age frailty: a 26-year follow-up of initially healthy men. Int J Obes (Lond) 2012;36(9):1153–7.

37. Elkins JS, Whitmer RA, Sidney S, et al. Midlife obesity and long-term risk of nursing home admission. Obesity (Silver Spring) 2006;14(8):1472–8.

38. Winter JE, MacInnis RJ, Wattanapenpaiboon N, et al. BMI and all-cause mortality in older adults: a meta-analysis. Am J Clin Nutr 2014;99(4):875–90.

39. Veronese N, Cereda E, Solmi M, et al. Inverse relationship between body mass index and mortality in older nursing home residents: a meta-analysis of 19,538 elderly subjects. Obes Rev 2015;16(11):1001–15.

40. Lee CD, Blair SN, Jackson AS. Cardiorespiratory fitness, body composition, and all-cause and cardiovascular disease mortality in men. Am J Clin Nutr 1999; 69(3):373–80.

41. McAuley PA, Artero EG, Sui X, et al. The obesity paradox, cardiorespiratory fitness, and coronary heart disease. Mayo Clin Proc 2012;87(5):443–51.

42. Schaap LA, Koster A, Visser M. Adiposity, muscle mass, and muscle strength in relation to functional decline in older persons. Epidemiol Rev 2013;35:51–65.

43. Zizza CA, Herring A, Stevens J, et al. Obesity affects nursing-care facility admission among whites but not blacks. Obes Res 2002;10(8):816–23.

44. Chang VW, Alley DE, Dowd JB. Trends in the relationship of obesity and disability, 1988-2012. Am J Epidemiol 2017. [Epub ahead of print].

45. Visser M, Langlois J, Guralnik JM, et al. High body fatness, but not low fat-free mass, predicts disability in older men and women: the Cardiovascular Health Study. Am J Clin Nutr 1998;68(3):584–90.

46. Visser M, Harris TB, Langlois J, et al. Body fat and skeletal muscle mass in relation to physical disability in very old men and women of the Framingham Heart Study. J Gerontol A Biol Sci Med Sci 1998;53(3):M214–21.

47. Masud T, Morris RO. Epidemiology of falls. Age Ageing 2001;30(Suppl 4):3–7.

48. Tinetti ME. Clinical practice. Preventing falls in elderly persons. N Engl J Med 2003;348(1):42–9.

49. American Geriatrics Society Workgroup on Vitamin D Supplementation for Older Adults. Recommendations abstracted from the American Geriatrics Society consensus statement on vitamin D for prevention of falls and their consequences. J Am Geriatr Soc 2014;62(1):147–52.

50. Himes CL, Reynolds SL. Effect of obesity on falls, injury, and disability. J Am Geriatr Soc 2012;60(1):124–9.

51. Ylitalo KR, Karvonen-Gutierrez CA. Body mass index, falls, and injurious falls among U.S. adults: findings from the 2014 Behavioral Risk Factor Surveillance System. Prev Med 2016;91:217–23.

52. Tang X, Liu G, Kang J, et al. Obesity and risk of hip fracture in adults: a meta-analysis of prospective cohort studies. PLoS One 2013;8(4):e55077.

53. Delmonico MJ, Harris TB, Visser M, et al. Longitudinal study of muscle strength, quality, and adipose tissue infiltration. Am J Clin Nutr 2009;90(6):1579–85.

54. Visser M, Kritchevsky SB, Goodpaster BH, et al. Leg muscle mass and composition in relation to lower extremity performance in men and women aged 70 to 79: the Health, Aging and Body Composition Study. J Am Geriatr Soc 2002; 50(5):897–904.

55. Batsis JA, Barre LK, Mackenzie TA, et al. Variation in the prevalence of sarcopenia and sarcopenic obesity in older adults associated with different research definitions: dual-energy X-ray absorptiometry data from the National Health and Nutrition Examination Survey 1999-2004. J Am Geriatr Soc 2013;61(6): 974–80.

56. Clark BC, Manini TM. Functional consequences of sarcopenia and dynapenia in the elderly. Curr Opin Clin Nutr Metab Care 2010;13(3):271–6.

57. Menant JC, Weber F, Lo J, et al. Strength measures are better than muscle mass measures in predicting health-related outcomes in older people: time to abandon the term sarcopenia? Osteoporos Int 2017;28(1):59–70.

58. Villareal DT, Chode S, Parimi N, et al. Weight loss, exercise, or both and physical function in obese older adults. N Engl J Med 2011;364(13):1218–29.

59. Goodpaster BH, Park SW, Harris TB, et al. The loss of skeletal muscle strength, mass, and quality in older adults: the Health, Aging and Body Composition Study. J Gerontol A Biol Sci Med Sci 2006;61(10):1059–64.

60. Baumgartner RN, Wayne SJ, Waters DL, et al. Sarcopenic obesity predicts instrumental activities of daily living disability in the elderly. Obes Res 2004; 12(12):1995–2004.

61. Baumgartner RN, Koehler KM, Gallagher D, et al. Epidemiology of sarcopenia among the elderly in New Mexico. Am J Epidemiol 1998;147(8):755–63.

62. Stenholm S, Alley D, Bandinelli S, et al. The effect of obesity combined with low muscle strength on decline in mobility in older persons: results from the InCHIANTI study. Int J Obes (Lond) 2009;33(6):635–44.

63. Batsis JA, Mackenzie TA, Lopez-Jimenez F, et al. Sarcopenia, sarcopenic obesity, and functional impairments in older adults: National Health and Nutrition Examination Surveys 1999-2004. Nutr Res 2015;35(12):1031–9.

64. Batsis JA, Mackenzie TA, Emeny RT, et al. Low lean mass with and without obesity, and mortality: results from the 1999-2004 National Health and Nutrition Examination Survey. J Gerontol A Biol Sci Med Sci 2017;72(10):1445–51.

65. Batsis JA, Mackenzie TA, Barre LK, et al. Sarcopenia, sarcopenic obesity and mortality in older adults: results from the National Health and Nutrition Examination Survey III. Eur J Clin Nutr 2014;68(9):1001–7.

66. Hardy R, Kuh D. Commentary: BMI and mortality in the elderly–a life course perspective. Int J Epidemiol 2006;35(1):179–80.

67. Richman EL, Stampfer MJ. Weight loss and mortality in the elderly: separating cause and effect. J Intern Med 2010;268(2):103–5.

68. Villareal DT, Apovian CM, Kushner RF, et al, American Society for Nutrition, NAASO, The Obesity Society. Obesity in older adults: technical review and position statement of the American Society for Nutrition and NAASO, The Obesity Society. Am J Clin Nutr 2005;82(5):923–34.

69. Batsis JA, Gill LE, Masutani RK, et al. Weight loss interventions in older adults with obesity: a systematic review of randomized controlled trials since 2005. J Am Geriatr Soc 2017;65(2):257–68.

70. Jacob ME, Yee LM, Diehr PH, et al. Can a healthy lifestyle compress the disabled period in older adults? J Am Geriatr Soc 2016;64(10):1952–61.

71. Villareal DT, Aguirre L, Gurney AB, et al. Aerobic or resistance exercise, or both in dieting obese older adults. N Engl J Med 2017;376:1943–55.

72. Kritchevsky SB, Beavers KM, Miller ME, et al. Intentional weight loss and all-cause mortality: a meta-analysis of randomized clinical trials. PLoS One 2015; 10(3):e0121993.

73. Gill LE, Bartels SJ, Batsis JA. Weight management in older adults. Curr Obes Rep 2015;4(3):379–88.

74. Heymsfield SB, Gonzalez MC, Shen W, et al. Weight loss composition is one-fourth fat-free mass: a critical review and critique of this widely cited rule. Obes Rev 2014;15(4):310–21.

75. Soltani S, Hunter GR, Kazemi A, et al. The effects of weight loss approaches on bone mineral density in adults: a systematic review and meta-analysis of randomized controlled trials. Osteoporos Int 2016;27(9):2655–71.

76. Zibellini J, Seimon RV, Lee CM, et al. Effect of diet-induced weight loss on muscle strength in adults with overweight or obesity - a systematic review and meta-analysis of clinical trials. Obes Rev 2016;17(8):647–63.

77. Zibellini J, Seimon RV, Lee CM, et al. Does diet-induced weight loss lead to bone loss in overweight or obese adults? A systematic review and meta-analysis of clinical trials. J Bone Miner Res 2015;30(12):2168–78.

78. Shah K, Armamento-Villareal R, Parimi N, et al. Exercise training in obese older adults prevents increase in bone turnover and attenuates decrease in hip bone mineral density induced by weight loss despite decline in bone-active hormones. J Bone Miner Res 2011;26(12):2851–9.

79. Tinetti ME, Doucette J, Claus E, et al. Risk factors for serious injury during falls by older persons in the community. J Am Geriatr Soc 1995;43(11):1214–21.

80. Batsis JA, Huddleston JM, Melton LJ, et al. Body mass index and risk of adverse cardiac events in elderly patients with hip fracture: a population-based study. J Am Geriatr Soc 2009;57(3):419–26.

81. Wadden TA, Butryn ML, Hong PS, et al. Behavioral treatment of obesity in patients encountered in primary care settings: a systematic review. JAMA 2014; 312(17):1779–91.

82. Tsai AG, Wadden TA. Treatment of obesity in primary care practice in the United States: a systematic review. J Gen Intern Med 2009;24(9):1073–9.

83. Aveyard P, Lewis A, Tearne S, et al. Screening and brief intervention for obesity in primary care: a parallel, two-arm, randomised trial. Lancet 2016;388(10059): 2492–500.

84. Decision memo for intensive behavioral therapy for obesity (CAG-00423N) Centers for Medicare & Medicaid Services 2011. Available at: http://www.cms.gov/medicare-coverage-database/details/nca-decision-memo.aspx?&NcaName=Intensive%20Behavioral%20Therapy%20for%20Obesity&bc=ACAAAAAAIAAA&NCAId=253. Accessed March 22, 2013.

85. Batsis JA, Huyck KL, Bartels SJ. Challenges with the Medicare obesity benefit: practical concerns & proposed solutions. J Gen Intern Med 2015;30(1):118–22.

86. Batsis JA, Pletcher SN, Stahl JE. Telemedicine and primary care obesity management in rural areas - innovative approach for older adults? BMC Geriatr 2017;17(1):6.

87. Batsis JA, Bynum JP. Uptake of the centers for Medicare and Medicaid obesity benefit: 2012-2013. Obesity (Silver Spring) 2016;24(9):1983–8.

88. Waters DL, Baumgartner RN, Garry PJ, et al. Advantages of dietary, exercise-related, and therapeutic interventions to prevent and treat sarcopenia in adult patients: an update. Clin Interv Aging 2010;5:259–70.

89. Jensen MD, Ryan DH, Apovian CM, et al. 2013 AHA/ACC/TOS guideline for the management of overweight and obesity in adults. Circulation 2014;129(25 suppl 2):S102–38.

90. De Luca CR, Leventer RJ. Developmental trajectories of executive functions across the lifespan. Washington, DC: Taylor & Francis; 2008.

91. Ende J, Kazis L, Ash A, et al. Measuring patients' desire for autonomy: decision making and information-seeking preferences among medical patients. J Gen Intern Med 1989;4(1):23–30.

92. Orbell S, Sheeran P. 'Inclined abstainers': a problem for predicting health-related behaviour. Br J Soc Psychol 1998;37(Pt 2):151–65.

93. Allan JL, Sniehotta FF, Johnston M. The best laid plans: planning skill determines the effectiveness of action plans and implementation intentions. Ann Behav Med 2013;46(1):114–20.

94. Allan JL, Johnston M, Campbell N. Missed by an inch or a mile? Predicting the size of intention-behaviour gap from measures of executive control. Psychol Health 2011;26(6):635–50.

95. Nigg CR, Long CR. A systematic review of single health behavior change interventions vs. multiple health behavior change interventions among older adults. Transl Behav Med 2012;2(2):163–79.

96. French DP, Olander EK, Chisholm A, et al. Which behaviour change techniques are most effective at increasing older adults' self-efficacy and physical activity behaviour? A systematic review. Ann Behav Med 2014;48(2):225–34.

97. Purath J, Keck A, Fitzgerald CE. Motivational interviewing for older adults in primary care: a systematic review. Geriatr Nurs 2014;35(3):219–24.

98. Ziegelmann JP, Knoll N. future directions in the study of health behavior among older adults. Gerontology 2015;61(5):469–76.

99. Lum TY, Lightfoot E. The effects of volunteering on the physical and mental health of older people. Res Aging 2005;27:31–55.

100. Guiding principles for the care of older adults with multimorbidity: an approach for clinicians. Guiding principles for the care of older adults with multimorbidity: an approach for clinicians: American Geriatrics Society Expert Panel on the Care of Older Adults with Multimorbidity. J Am Geriatr Soc 2012;60(10):E1–25.

101. Freund AM. Age-differential motivational consequences of optimization versus compensation focus in younger and older adults. Psychol Aging 2006;21(2):240–52.

102. Levy BR, Slade MD, Kasl SV. Longitudinal benefit of positive self-perceptions of aging on functional health. J Gerontol B Psychol Sci Soc Sci 2002;57(5):P409–17.

103. Lockenhoff CE, Carstensen LL. Socioemotional selectivity theory, aging, and health: the increasingly delicate balance between regulating emotions and making tough choices. J Pers 2004;72(6):1395–424.

104. Newsom JT, Huguet N, McCarthy MJ, et al. Health behavior change following chronic illness in middle and later life. J Gerontol B Psychol Sci Soc Sci 2012;67(3):279–88.

105. Keller H, Laporte M, Payette H, et al. Prevalence and predictors of weight change post discharge from hospital: a study of the Canadian Malnutrition Task Force. Eur J Clin Nutr 2017;71(6):766–72.

106. Fulton MM, Allen ER. Polypharmacy in the elderly: a literature review. J Am Acad Nurse Pract 2005;17(4):123–32.

107. By the American Geriatrics Society 2015 Beers Criteria Update Expert Panel. American Geriatrics Society 2015 updated Beers Criteria for potentially inappropriate medication use in older adults. J Am Geriatr Soc 2015;63(11):2227–46.

108. Kirkman MS, Briscoe VJ, Clark N, et al. Diabetes in older adults: a consensus report. J Am Geriatr Soc 2012;60(12):2342–56.

109. Soysal P, Veronese N, Thompson T, et al. Relationship between depression and frailty in older adults: a systematic review and meta-analysis. Ageing Res Rev 2017;36:78–87.

110. Sibille KT, McBeth J, Smith D, et al. Allostatic load and pain severity in older adults: results from the English Longitudinal Study of Ageing. Exp Gerontol 2017;88:51–8.

111. Mendelson G, Ness J, Aronow WS. Drug treatment of hypertension in older persons in an academic hospital-based geriatrics practice. J Am Geriatr Soc 1999; 47(5):597–9.

112. Castillo DC, Ramsey NLM, Yu SSK, et al. Inconsistent access to food and cardiometabolic disease: the effect of food insecurity. Curr Cardiovasc Risk Rep 2012;6(3):245–50.

113. Lee JS, Frongillo EA. Nutritional and health consequences are associated with food insecurity among U.S. elderly persons. J Nutr 2001;131:1503–9.

114. Appel LJ, Moore TJ, Obarzanek E, et al. A clinical trial of the effects of dietary patterns on blood pressure. DASH Collaborative Research Group. N Engl J Med 1997;336(16):1117–24.

115. Esposito K, Kastorini CM, Panagiotakos DB, et al. Mediterranean diet and weight loss: meta-analysis of randomized controlled trials. Metab Syndr Relat Disord 2011;9(1):1–12.

116. Bauer J, Biolo G, Cederholm T, et al. Evidence-based recommendations for optimal dietary protein intake in older people: a position paper from the PROT-AGE Study Group. J Am Med Dir Assoc 2013;14(8):542–59.

117. Colonetti T, Grande AJ, Milton K, et al. Effects of whey protein supplement in the elderly submitted to resistance training: systematic review and meta-analysis. Int J Food Sci Nutr 2017;68(3):257–64.

118. Porter Starr KN, Pieper CF, Orenduff MC, et al. Improved function with enhanced protein intake per meal: a pilot study of weight reduction in frail, obese older adults. J Gerontol A Biol Sci Med Sci 2016;71(10):1369–75.

119. Carroll JK, Antognoli E, Flocke SA. Evaluation of physical activity counseling in primary care using direct observation of the 5As. Ann Fam Med 2011;9(5): 416–22.

120. Garber CE, Blissmer B, Deschenes MR, et al. American College of Sports Medicine position stand. Quantity and quality of exercise for developing and maintaining cardiorespiratory, musculoskeletal, and neuromotor fitness in apparently healthy adults: guidance for prescribing exercise. Med Sci Sports Exerc 2011;43(7):1334–59.

121. Pahor M, Guralnik JM, Ambrosius WT, et al. Effect of structured physical activity on prevention of major mobility disability in older adults: the LIFE study randomized clinical trial. JAMA 2014;311(23):2387–96.

122. Screening for osteoporosis. U.S. preventive services task force recommendation statement. Ann Intern Med 2011;154(5):356–64.

123. Garvey WT, Mechanick JI, Brett EM, et al. American Association of Clinical Endocrinologists and American College of Endocrinology comprehensive clinical practice guidelines for medical care of patients with obesity. Endocr Pract 2016;22(Suppl 3):1–203.

124. Davies MJ, Bergenstal R, Bode B, et al. Efficacy of liraglutide for weight loss among patients with type 2 diabetes: the SCALE diabetes randomized clinical trial. JAMA 2015;314(7):687–99.

125. Gadde KM, Allison DB, Ryan DH, et al. Effects of low-dose, controlled-release, phentermine plus topiramate combination on weight and associated

comorbidities in overweight and obese adults (CONQUER): a randomised, placebo-controlled, phase 3 trial. Lancet 2011;377(9774):1341–52.

126. Perna S, Guido D, Bologna C, et al. Liraglutide and obesity in elderly: efficacy in fat loss and safety in order to prevent sarcopenia. A perspective case series study. Aging Clin Exp Res 2016;28(6):1251–7.

127. Pi-Sunyer X, Astrup A, Fujioka K, et al. A randomized, controlled trial of 3.0 mg of liraglutide in weight management. N Engl J Med 2015;373(1):11–22.

128. Wadden TA, Hollander P, Klein S, et al. Weight maintenance and additional weight loss with liraglutide after low-calorie-diet-induced weight loss: the SCALE Maintenance randomized study. Int J Obes (Lond) 2013;37(11):1443–51.

129. Gastrointestinal surgery for severe obesity. Proceedings of a National Institutes of Health consensus development conference. March 25-27, 1991, Bethesda, MD. Am J Clin Nutr 1992;55(2 Suppl):487s–619s.

130. Meron Eldar S, Henegahn H, Kroh M, et al. Bariatric surgery in the elderly - Comparing the 3 major bariatric procedures. Obes Surg 2011;21(8):1134–5.

131. Batsis JA, Miranda WR, Prasad C, et al. Effect of bariatric surgery on cardiometabolic risk in elderly patients: a population-based study. Geriatr Gerontol Int 2016;16(5):618–24.

132. Flum DR, Kwon S, MacLeod K, et al. The use, safety and cost of bariatric surgery before and after Medicare's national coverage decision. Ann Surg 2011; 254(6):860–5.

133. O'Keefe KL, Kemmeter PR, Kemmeter KD. Bariatric surgery outcomes in patients aged 65 years and older at an American Society for Metabolic and Bariatric Surgery center of excellence. Obes Surg 2010;20(9):1199–205.

134. Quebbemann B, Engstrom D, Siegfried T, et al. Bariatric surgery in patients older than 65 years is safe and effective. Surg Obes Relat Dis 2005;1(4): 389–92 [discussion: 392–3].

135. Ramirez A, Roy M, Hidalgo JE, et al. Outcomes of bariatric surgery in patients >70 years old. Surg Obes Relat Dis 2012;8(4):458–62.

136. Ibrahim AM, Ghaferi AA, Thumma JR, et al. Variation in outcomes at bariatric surgery centers of excellence. JAMA Surg 2017;152(7):629–36.

137. Livingston EH. Bariatric surgery outcomes at designated centers of excellence vs nondesignated programs. Arch Surg 2009;144(4):319–25 [discussion: 325].

138. Giordano S, Victorzon M. Bariatric surgery in elderly patients: a systematic review. Clin Interv Aging 2015;10:1627–35.

139. Mathus-Vliegen EM, Obesity Management Task Force of the European Association for the Study of Obesity. Prevalence, pathophysiology, health consequences and treatment options of obesity in the elderly: a guideline. Obes Facts 2012;5(3):460–83.

140. Batsis JA, Dolkart KM. Evaluation of older adults with obesity for bariatric surgery: geriatricians' perspective. J Clin Gerontol Geriatr 2015;6(2):45–53.

Obesity in Pregnancy

Optimizing Outcomes for Mom and Baby

Heidi Dutton, MD[a], Sarah Jean Borengasser, PhD[b], Laura Marie Gaudet, MD, MSc[c], Linda A. Barbour, MD, MSPH[d], Erin Joanne Keely, MD[a],*

KEYWORDS

• Obesity • Pregnancy • Preconception • Intergenerational obesity

KEY POINTS

• Weight and obesity-related comorbidities should be optimized in women with obesity before conception.
• Special considerations in pregnant women with obesity include optimization of gestational weight gain, prevention and management of gestational diabetes and hypertensive disorders of pregnancy, and being aware of risks to fetal health.
• Labor and delivery in women with obesity carries an increased risk of surgical and anesthetic complications.
• Postpartum considerations in women with obesity include prevention of complications, reduction of postpartum weight retention, and breastfeeding promotion.
• There is emerging evidence of adverse metabolic effects on the offspring of women with obesity.

INTRODUCTION

The high rates of obesity in women of childbearing age has made obesity the most common medical problem in pregnancy. According to the 2013 to 2014 Nutrition Examination Survey data, 37% of women between 20 and 39 years of age have obesity and rates continue to increase.[1] The rates vary dramatically by ethnic group, from 10% of Asian women, 33% of non-Hispanic white women, 43% of Hispanic women, and 57% of non-Hispanic black women.[1] Women with obesity are at a much higher rate of poor obstetric outcomes across the continuum of reduced fertility, pregnancy complications, and postpartum adverse events, of which some, but not all, are preventable

Conflict of interest: The authors have no relevant conflicts of interest to disclose.
[a] University of Ottawa, 1967 Riverside Drive, Ottawa, ON K1h7W9, Canada; [b] University of Colorado–Anschutz, 12631 East 17th Avenue, Mailstop F561, Aurora, CO 80045, USA; [c] University of Ottawa, 1053 Carling Avenue, Ottawa, ON K1Y 4E9, Canada; [d] University of Colorado School of Medicine, 12801 East 17th Avenue, RC1 South Room 7103, Aurora, CO 80405, USA
* Corresponding author.
E-mail address: ekeely@toh.ca

Med Clin N Am 102 (2018) 87–106
https://doi.org/10.1016/j.mcna.2017.08.008
0025-7125/18/© 2017 Elsevier Inc. All rights reserved.

through targeted medical care. The lack of good evidence for intervention has resulted in differences across national clinical practice guidelines.[2]

In addition to being more at risk, women with obesity may experience discrimination and humiliation at a time that should be joyful. In a study of obstetrics providers, 31% identified that they had made derogatory comments about obese women to colleagues and 66% thought more derogatory comments are made about women with obesity than those without obesity.[3] Providers who care for women with obesity who are of childbearing age need to identify strategies and tools that promote open, nonjudgmental communication about the risks in pregnancy and provide safer care through adequate resources, specialized equipment, and structured protocols.[4–7]

GOALS AND STRATEGIES
Preconception

Improve fertility
Obesity in women is associated with subfertility and with a longer time to achieve pregnancy.[8–10] Although partially explained by the higher prevalence of the polycystic ovarian syndrome (PCOS),[11] which is characterized by anovulation and hyperandrogenism,[12] the association between infertility and obesity exists even in women with ovulatory menstrual cycles.[8–10] In addition, women with obesity have higher miscarriage rates[13]; those using assisted reproductive technologies (ART), such as in vitro fertilization, seem to have decreased pregnancy and live birth rates compared with those with a normal body mass index (BMI).[14] Thus, obesity is associated with numerous factors that decrease the likelihood of achieving and maintaining a pregnancy.

There is a paucity of rigorous studies evaluating interventions to improve fertility in women with obesity. Observational evidence suggests that lifestyle interventions may improve pregnancy and live birth rates before undergoing ART.[15] One multicenter randomized controlled trial (RCT) evaluated the effect of a 6-month lifestyle intervention followed by 18 months of infertility treatment in infertile women with a BMI greater than 29, compared with a control group receiving 24 months of prompt infertility treatment.[16] The control group had a higher frequency of the primary outcome, a vaginal term birth of a healthy singleton, than the intervention group (35.2% vs 27.1%), although women in the intervention group were more likely to achieve conception without infertility treatments. In contrast, in women with obesity and PCOS, post hoc data aggregation from 2 separate RCTs suggest that lifestyle intervention for weight loss before ovulation induction with clomiphene citrate increases live birth rates compared with immediate ovulation induction.[17] Observational studies suggest that bariatric surgery improves fertility in women with obesity[18]; however, infertility is not considered an indication for bariatric surgery.[19,20] Thus, infertility treatments are most effective at achieving a live birth in women with obesity; however, in younger women in whom there is less urgency to conceive, weight loss via lifestyle interventions is a reasonable first step for infertility management, as it is likely associated with other benefits.

Preconception weight loss
Guidelines advise weight loss before conception for women with obesity.[21,22] Most evidence supporting this recommendation comes from studies of women who have undergone bariatric surgery. Pregnant women who have previously undergone bariatric surgery are less likely to develop gestational diabetes mellitus (GDM), hypertensive disorders of pregnancy (HDP), postpartum hemorrhage, and fetal macrosomia,

compared with controls who have not undergone bariatric surgery.[23] However, the risks of preterm birth and having a small for gestational age (SGA) newborn are increased.[23–25] Given that interventions during pregnancy have been found to be relatively ineffective in preventing comorbidities, such as GDM,[26] studies are currently underway to evaluate whether prepregnancy lifestyle interventions will be more effective in reducing adverse pregnancy outcomes in women with obesity.[27]

The current guidelines recommend a waiting period of 12 to 24 months following bariatric surgery before conceiving.[19,22,28] Reduced absorption of oral hormonal contraception may occur following bariatric surgery,[20] and alternate forms of contraception should be prescribed.[19] Women who have previously undergone bariatric surgery require careful monitoring during pregnancy, as there is a risk of nutrient deficiencies[21] and anatomic surgical complications in this population.[22] The benefits of postponing pregnancy to undertake bariatric surgery must also be weighed against the risk of declining fertility as maternal age increases.[22]

Congenital anomaly reduction

There is a dose-dependent increase in the rate of congenital anomalies among offspring of women with obesity. There are more neutral tube defects (odds ratio [OR] 1.87; 95% confidence interval [CI] 1.62–2.15), heart defects (OR 1.15; 1.07–1.23; including left and right ventricular outflow defects and hypoplastic left heart syndrome but not conotruncal defects), cleft lip and/or palate (OR 1.20; 95% CI 1.09–1.31), anorectal atresia (OR 1.48; 95% CI 1.12–1.97), hydrocephaly (OR 1.68; 95% CI 1.19–2.36), and limb reduction anomalies (OR 1.34; 95% CI 1.03–1.73).[29–31] The exact cause for this increased risk remains debatable but includes abnormal glucose metabolism and nutrient deficiencies.[32]

Targeted management strategies are needed, but evidence for these remains elusive. Human organogenesis is largely complete by 9 weeks' gestational age. Although most women do access prenatal care in the first trimester, true prevention must begin preconceptually. Most importantly, abnormal glucose metabolism must be identified and glycemic control optimized before conception. Folic acid supplementation has been shown to reduce congenital anomalies. Women with obesity are less likely to take preconception supplementation, which may be related to other health behaviors or unplanned pregnancies.[33] Also, BMI may affect the distribution of folate, with obese women having lower serum levels relative to red blood cell folate levels.[34] Although further study into optimal nutritional supplementation is needed for women with obesity, current guidelines differ in recommendations, with some suggesting 5.0 mg and others recommending 0.4 mg of folate.[2,35] Consideration should be given to recommending additional folic acid compared with normal weight for 3 months prenatally and until 12 weeks' gestation and vitamin D (10 μg daily during pregnancy).[35,36]

Detect and optimize comorbidities

Women with obesity are more likely to have other comorbidities, including type 2 diabetes mellitus (T2DM), hypertension, hyperlipidemia, sleep apnea, and nonalcoholic steatohepatitis (NASH), which may or may not have been previously identified and treated. Each of these conditions can contribute to poor obstetric outcomes and may worsen as part of the normal physiologic changes in pregnancy. It is essential that women be screened for these before pregnancy allowing for investigations to be completed and treatment adjusted for an upcoming planned pregnancy. Although a detailed discussion is out of scope for this article, key points for optimizing outcomes for each of these conditions are listed in **Box 1.**

Box 1
Key points for screening for and optimizing preexisting comorbidities

- Hyperglycemia
  - Screen: using HgA1c and/or fasting glucose before pregnancy
  - Before pregnancy
    - Target A1c of less than 7% to reduce congenital anomalies
    - Discontinue medications without known safety profile, including SGLT2 inhibitors, DPP4 inhibitors, GLP-1 analogues
    - Consider discontinuing sulfonylureas and metformin (unless metformin is being used for ovulation induction)
    - Optimize insulin and self-management skills
    - Assess for microvascular complications

- Hypertension[58]
  - Screen: if indicated, screen for secondary causes of hypertension
  - Before pregnancy
    - Discontinue medications without known safety profile, including ACE inhibitors, angiotensin receptor blockers, aldosterone antagonists
    - Consider using labetalol, methyldopa, nifedipine

- Hyperlipidemia
  - Screen: reevaluate indication for treatment as safety during pregnancy not established
  - Before pregnancy
    - Optimize nutritional management, especially for cases of severe hypertriglyceridemia
    - Consider discontinuing lipid-lowering agents unless there is a clear indication

- Sleep apnea[146–148]
  - Screen: use validated screening tools and perform sleep studies as indicated
  - Before pregnancy
    - Optimize sleep treatments, such as CPAP and mandibular repositioning devices

- Nonalcoholic steatohepatitis[149,150]
  - Screen: screen for other causes of liver dysfunction, consider ultrasound/transient elastography

- Optimize lifestyle modifications; if treated medically with pioglitazone or other agents, consider discontinuation if there are no safety data in pregnancy

Abbreviations: ACE, angiotensin-converting enzymes; CPAP, continuous positive airway pressure; DPP4, dipeptidyl-peptidase 4; GLP-1, glucagonlike peptide 1; HgA1c, hemoglobin A1c; SGLT2, sodium-glucose cotransporter 2.

Pregnancy

Limit gestational weight gain

Excess gestational weight gain (GWG) is associated with adverse outcomes, including an increased risk of developing GDM, T2DM, and HDP[37]; elevated infant birth weight and adiposity; and increased risk of metabolic syndrome and childhood obesity in offspring.[38] Women with prepregnancy overweight and obesity are more likely to gain excess weight during pregnancy.[39,40] One Canadian study found that 47% of normal-weight women compared with 78% of overweight and 72% of women with obesity exceeded the recommended GWG.[40]

The Institute of Medicine (IOM) recommends GWG ranges based on maternal prepregnancy BMI (**Table 1**), with less weight gain recommended for higher BMI categories.[41] A systematic review found that in women with obesity, less GWG than that recommended by the IOM is associated with an increased risk of preterm birth and having an SGA infant but also with reduced risk of macrosomia, HDP, and cesarean delivery.[42] Some studies have even suggested that weight loss in women with obesity during pregnancy may be associated with some reduced adverse outcomes.[43,44]

Table 1
Recommended gestational weight gain by prepregnancy body mass index

Prepregnancy BMI	BMI (kg/m²)	Total Weight Gain Range (lb)	Rates of Weight Gain Second and Third Trimester (Mean Range in lb/wk)
Underweight	<18.5	28–40	1 (1.0–1.3)
Normal weight	18.5–24.9	25–35	1 (0.8–1.0)
Overweight	25.0–29.9	15–25	0.6 (0.5–0.7)
Obese (includes all classes)	≥30.0	11–20	0.5 (0.4–0.6)

From Committee to Reexamine IOM Pregnancy Weight Guidelines. Institute of Medicine and National Research Council. Rasmussen KM, Yaktine AL, editors. Weight gain during pregnancy: reexamining the guidelines. Washington, DC: The National Academies Press; 2009; with permission.

Professional guidelines state that although recommendations must be individualized, women with obesity who are gaining less weight than recommended by the IOM need not increase their weight gain if fetal growth is adequate.[45]

GWG targets should be calculated and discussed with women early in pregnancy.[21,46] A recent systematic review and meta-analysis evaluated RCTs of antenatal interventions for preventing excess GWG and found that diet, exercise, or diet plus exercise interventions reduced the risk of excess GWG by an average of 20% (relative risk [RR] 0.80, 95% CI 0.73–0.87).[47] The results also suggested a lower risk of cesarean delivery, maternal hypertension, macrosomia, and newborn respiratory distress syndrome in mothers who received the interventions. Pregnant women with obesity should receive diet and exercise counseling to assist with managing GWG.[21] After the treating clinician has ruled out any contraindications to exercise,[48] an eventual goal of moderate-intensity exercises for 20 to 30 minutes per day on most days of the week can be advised.[48] An RCT evaluating the use of metformin versus placebo starting at 12 to 18 weeks' gestation in pregnant women with obesity but without diabetes resulted in reduced median GWG in the metformin group (4.6 kg vs 6.3 kg) but no difference in the primary outcome of neonatal birth-weight z score. However, there was no significant difference in neonatal or obstetric outcomes; thus, the use of metformin to reduce GWG in women with obesity cannot be routinely recommended.

Screen early for hyperglycemia
Women with obesity who are not known to have T2DM should be screened at the first antenatal visit for hyperglycemia. There are 2 strategies for testing glucose levels in early pregnancy: using the nonpregnancy recommended screening tests (fasting plasma glucose [FPG] or HbA1c) or using the typical 24- to 28-week GDM screening criteria.[49] There has been no rigorous validation that criteria accepted for the diagnosis of GDM in the second or third trimester are appropriate for use in the first trimester. A fasting glucose greater than 7.0 mmol/L or A1c of 6.5% or greater should be diagnosed as likely overt diabetes and treatment implemented. However, both FPG and A1c decrease early in pregnancy and may lead to underdiagnosis of preexisting diabetes. One study screened 16,122 women at a median of 47 days' gestation and found higher rates of major congenital anomalies (RR 2.67, 1.28–5.53), preeclampsia (RR 2.42, 1.28–5.53), shoulder dystocia (RR 2.47, 1.05–5.85), and perinatal death (RR 3.96,1.54–10.16) with an A1c of 5.9% to 6.4% in the first trimester.[50] Although consideration can be given to treatment of women with an HbA1c of 5.9% to 6.4% in the first trimester, whether intervention earlier in pregnancy makes a difference remains

unknown. Unfortunately, the lack of rigorous data has resulted in different professional groups and organizations having different criteria for diagnosis of early dysglycemia.[51,52] All women with overt diabetes diagnosed during pregnancy should be retested postpartum, as up to 41% will return to normal postpartum.[53]

Reduce hypertensive disorders of pregnancy

Maternal obesity is associated with increased risk of preeclampsia and gestational hypertension, and the risk increases as BMI increases.[9,54,55] Observational studies demonstrate an inverse association between maternal exercise and preeclampsia risk[56,57]; the risk of maternal hypertension, but not preeclampsia specifically, was reduced in RCTs of diet and/or exercise interventions during pregnancy.[47] However, the role of exercise in pregnancy for preeclampsia prevention is thought to be unclear.[58,59] Strategies for prevention of preeclampsia should be considered, including recommending both acetylsalicylic acid 81 mg daily (taken orally at bedtime from the time pregnancy is diagnosed until 37 weeks' gestation) and adequate calcium intake.[59,60]

Improve fetal surveillance

Aneuploidy detection is now performed using either traditional first-trimester screening (Integrated Prenatal Screening or its variations) or noninvasive prenatal testing (NIPT). Interestingly, the risk of trisomy 21 is increased among women with obesity.[61] A higher BMI does not affect the rate of positive first-trimester screening,[61] making such testing appropriate. Fetal cell-free DNA levels are inversely proportional to gestational weight; mothers with obesity should be advised that there is a higher rate of insufficient DNA levels, necessitating a second blood draw for NIPT testing.[62]

The ability of screening ultrasound to detect genetics syndromes, fetal anomalies, and nonreassuring fetal well-being status is substantially reduced in this population. In the FaSTER trial, maternal obesity was associated with a 10% higher false-negative rate for the detection of 2 more soft markers of aneuploidy, a lower rate of detection of congenital anomalies in general (adjusted OR 0.7, 95% CI 0.6–0.9), and a lower detection rate of congenital heart anomalies (8.3% vs 21.6%).[63] There is often an inability to both image completely *and* detect anomalies of cardiac and craniospinal structures in this population.[64,65] The limitations of prenatal ultrasound screening should be recognized and the women counseled accordingly.

Fetal surveillance is often indicated in later gestation to ensure fetal well-being. Common indications include concurrent diabetes and hypertension; but consideration may also be given to performing biophysical profile or nonstress tests on women with obesity in general, given their increased risk of fetal distress and stillbirth. Although it may be more difficult to physically perform such testing on women with obesity, they are not more likely to have nonreactive nonstress tests or to require additional time to a normal nonstress test.

Minimize risk of preterm birth

The risks of both overall preterm births and extremely preterm births are increased among women with obesity. These preterm deliveries are often iatrogenic and related to need for delivery due to medical comorbidities like hypertension and diabetes. In general, obesity is associated with prolonged pregnancy; but there seems to be an interesting increase in spontaneous extremely preterm labor (<28 weeks' gestation).[66] This increase was attributed to increased inflammatory markers and increased risk of intrauterine bacterial infection/chorioamnionitis.

Evidence for prevention of preterm birth among women with obesity is limited. Optimizing underlying medical conditions like diabetes and hypertension and incorporating strategies for prevention of preeclampsia should be considered. In women who are symptomatic or who have had a prior preterm birth, confirmed bacterial vaginosis should be treated with oral metronidazole or clindamycin for 7 days.

Labor and Delivery

Reduce still birth risk through timing of delivery

Determining the optimal timing of delivery of women with obesity is complex. Multiple studies have now shown a consistent increase in the risk of stillbirth among women with obesity, at all gestational ages. Overall, a 10-unit increase in prepregnancy BMI seems to be associated with a 1.5- to 2.0-fold increase in stillbirth risk.[67] Rates increase proportionately to BMI from an OR of 1.37 (95% CI 1.02–1.85) for overweight women to an OR of 5.04 (1.79–14.07) for women with a BMI higher than 50.[68] The lowest rates of neonatal death and cerebral palsy are associated with delivery at 39 weeks' gestation.[69] The lowest rates of intrauterine demise and brachial plexus injury can be obtained by delivering earlier. A recent decision analysis suggested that the optimal gestational age of delivery may be 38 weeks; in the theoretic population of 100,000 singleton pregnancies in women with obesity, elective delivery at 38 weeks would prevent 203 intrauterine demises compared with expectant management until 41 weeks.[69]

When the decision to proceed with delivery, whether for medical indications or to reduce the risk of stillbirth, has been made, the mode of delivery must be considered. Among women who have obesity, term elective induction of labor seems to actually decrease the risk of cesarean delivery, particularly in multiparous women, without increasing the risk of adverse outcomes, including operative vaginal delivery, lacerations, or neonatal respiratory distress syndrome (Lee II).[70] Thus, induction of labor at 38 to 39 weeks is currently preferred to elective cesarean delivery for appropriate candidates.

Reduce surgical complications

Cesarean delivery is intuitively more difficult and risk prone in women with obesity. Preparation is crucial; in addition to the usual requirements for cesarean delivery, the availability of specialized equipment (eg, retractors) is beneficial to both surgical team and patients. Surgeons should be familiar with and respect the weight capacity of wheelchairs, operating tables, and other equipment, such as commodes. The presence of a large pannus can alter the anatomy of the abdominal wall considerably, and strategies are needed to reduce the risk (**Table 2**). As the umbilicus is usually more

Table 2
Useful strategies for cesarean delivery of women with obesity

Strategy	Result
Pretreatment of the skin under the pannus with antibacterial/antifungal dressings for 1–2 wk	Improved skin health and decreased bacterial load
Skin cleansing with iodine or chlorhexidine	Decreased bacterial load
Antibiotics within 60 min of incision	Lower wound infection rates
Closure of the subcutaneous tissue with sutures when the fat thickness exceeds 2 cm	Decreased wound disruption by 34%[151]
Retraction of the pannus cephalad	Improved ease of transverse skin incision
Suturing of the skin incision	Decreased wound infection and wound separation rates[152]

caudad than normal, the ideal position of the incision should be determined from more stable landmarks, including the symphysis pubis, the iliac wings, and the fundus. The ideal choice of skin incision is still debated and should be individualized. A transverse skin incision can be made above or below the pannus and offers increased wound strength, reduced postoperative pain, and improved respiratory status postpartum.[71,72] However, a transverse incision makes retraction and delivery of the fetus more difficult because of the pannus. The climate underneath the pannus also results in frequent wound infection. A vertical skin incision allows for better visualization of the surgical field and easier wound care postpartum but causes more pain, resulting in decreased respiratory effort.[73] Vertical incisions do not necessarily decrease the risk of wound infection.[73]

Improve safety of anesthesia

Anesthetic risks are increased in women with obesity, for both regional techniques (epidural and spinal) and general anesthesia. Consultation with anesthesia during the third trimester is often very helpful to allow for risk assessment, additional testing (such as electrocardiogram or sleep studies), and patient counseling and expectation setting.

Placement of regional techniques is often challenging because the usual landmarks may be difficult to find because of adiposity. These challenges may lead to multiple attempts at needle insertion and, ultimately, a higher failure rate. Ultrasound-guided neuraxial analgesia is sometimes helpful.

General anesthesia is avoided whenever possible but is more common with increasing obesity. Intubation is made more difficult by increased breast mass, increased chest diameter, and exaggerated airway edema. These features result in a diagnosis of difficult intubation in up to 33% of women with obesity.[74]

Postpartum

Reduce postpartum hemorrhage

The risk of postpartum hemorrhage is approximately doubled in women who are overweight or have obesity, an effect that is seen after both vaginal delivery (OR 2.11, 95% CI 1.54–2.89) and cesarean delivery (OR 1.73, 95% CI 1.32–2.28).[75] When the effects of perineal laceration and retained placenta are controlled for, the elevated risk can be attributed to uterine atony. The risk of postpartum hemorrhage is increased with increased infant birthweight, antepartum hemorrhage, and Asian ethnicity.

Before delivery, iron stores should be optimized by providing oral or parenteral iron as needed. In addition to the usual practices of active management of the third stage, increased vigilance and preparation for postpartum hemorrhage are advised and additional uterotonics should be available, including carbetocin, ergotamine, misoprostol, and carboprost tromethamine. Internal uterine compression is a third-line treatment option.

Prevent Venous Thromboembolism

Women with a prepregnancy BMI greater than 30 kg/m^2 who have undergone an emergency cesarean delivery are considered to be at high risk for postpartum venous thromboembolism (VTE).[76,77] Guidelines recommend that either prophylactic low-molecular-weight heparin (LMWH) or mechanical prophylaxis, such as elastic stockings or intermittent pneumatic compression, be used in this population while in the hospital following delivery.[76,77] In women with obesity who undergo a nonemergent cesarean delivery, VTE prophylaxis is recommended only in the presence of at least one additional risk factor for VTE, such as preeclampsia or fetal intrauterine growth restriction.[76,77] LMWH is considered to be safe in women who are breastfeeding.[76]

Improve breastfeeding rates

Guidelines recommend that babies be breastfed exclusively for the first 6 months of life, followed by ongoing breastfeeding up to at least 1 to 2 years of age.[78,79] Breastfeeding is particularly beneficial for mothers with obesity, as it is associated with improved future cardiovascular risk in mothers,[80] reduced risk of future T2DM,[81,82] and decreased visceral adiposity in later life.[83,84] Some,[83,85] but not all,[86,87] studies have reported less postpartum weight retention and future risk of obesity with breastfeeding.

Women with obesity are less likely than normal-weight women to both initiate and maintain breastfeeding.[88,89] This circumstance has been attributed to delayed onset of milk production, higher prevalence of insufficient breast glandular tissue, and psychosocial factors, such as reduced confidence to breastfeed.[90] There is some evidence that increased postpartum breastfeeding support can increase breastfeeding exclusivity and duration.[90] The potential for breastfeeding challenges should be discussed with women before delivery; resources, such as lactation consultant services, should be made available to assist with breastfeeding difficulties.

Reduce postpartum weight retention

Postpartum weight retention is of particular concern in women with obesity who are planning future pregnancies.[21] In a Swedish population-based cohort study that evaluated BMI changes between first and second pregnancies, the risk of stillbirth in the second pregnancy was found to increase linearly with an interpregnancy increase in BMI.[91] Similarly, interpregnancy weight gain is associated with an increased risk of gestational hypertension and preeclampsia.[92] Weight gain between pregnancies is associated with an increased risk of GDM in a subsequent pregnancy, whereas a weight loss of just 10 lb is associated with a reduced GDM risk.[93] Weight loss between pregnancies in women with obesity decreases the risk of having a large-for-gestational-age offspring in the next pregnancy[94] and improves chances of a vaginal delivery after a previous cesarean section.[95]

A recent systematic review found that dietary interventions and diet with exercise interventions improved postpartum weight loss, as opposed to exercise-only interventions.[96] There was no evidence that these interventions had any adverse effect on maternal breastfeeding success. It is recommended that postpartum contraception and planning for future pregnancies be encouraged in women with obesity so that weight can be optimized between pregnancies.[21]

NEW EVIDENCE LINKING MATERNAL OBESITY AND LONG-TERM IMPLICATIONS TO OFFSPRING

The number of *infants* and young children with overweight or obesity has tripled between 1990 and 2012[97] and is increasing in parallel with rates of maternal obesity. Given that half of childhood obesity occurs by 5 years of age, early life events may be contributing to pediatric obesity development.[98] Many studies have reported strong associations between intrauterine exposure to maternal obesity and excess GWG with adiposity at birth[99,100] and offspring development of obesity in childhood[101,102] and adulthood[103] (**Fig. 1**). For example, increased adiposity at birth (but not birth weight) was correlated to adiposity at 6 to 11 years of age by dual-energy x-ray absorptiometry in offspring from a cohort of 89 mothers with either normal glucose tolerance or GDM.[102] Childhood adiposity did not correlate with maternal

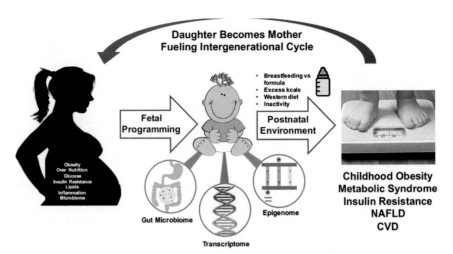

Fig. 1. The intrauterine environment is associated with adverse metabolic effects in offspring, promoting an intergenerational cycle of obesity. CVD, cardiovascular disease; NAFLD, nonalcoholic fatty liver disease.

GDM exposure but instead was strongly related to maternal obesity with an OR of approximately 5.5.

In utero exposure to maternal obesity also increases obesity comorbidities in offspring, such as insulin resistance and changes in mitochondrial function,[104–106] cardiovascular disease,[107,108] and nonalcoholic fatty liver disease (NAFLD).[109–111] NAFLD affects approximately 34% of children with obesity aged 3 to 18 years, and half have already progressed to the more severe NASH at the time of diagnosis.[112,113] Newborns at approximately 2 weeks of age who were born to mothers with obesity and mothers with GDM demonstrated 68% more intrahepatic fat compared with the newborns from normal-weight mothers and was correlated with maternal BMI ($r = 0.05$, $P = .02$).[110] Whether early deposition of lipid in the fetal liver could prime it to be more susceptible to the postnatal influences of an unhealthy lifestyle resulting in NAFLD is unknown. The powerful influence of an intrauterine environment characterized by nutrient excess and obesity is also underscored by the marked decrease in the risk of obesity in children born to women with obesity who underwent bariatric surgery before their pregnancy as compared with their siblings who were born before their mother received bariatric surgery.[114,115]

An intrauterine environment characterized by nutrient excess or obesity imparts long-term programming of offspring obesity risk,[116] especially in babies born large for gestational age. Umbilical cord–derived mesenchymal stem cells from infants born to mothers with obesity demonstrated greater capacity to develop into adipocytes. These findings suggest that progenitor cells that differentiate into various tissue types, such as adipose tissue, skeletal muscle, or chondrocytes, may already be detrimentally programmed in utero.[117]

Epigenetics as a Mechanism and Indicator of Fetal Programming

Metabolic programming can occur via gene-environment interactions that may produce epigenetic events. These intrauterine exposures may silence or augment gene expression to impact fetal brain function and organ development, which imparts a risk for developing chronic diseases.[118–121] Maternal nutrition can alter DNA methylation in infant tissues, such as buccal cells,[122] umbilical cord blood,[123,124] and umbilical cord.[125] Preconception maternal diet and nutritional status may be key determinants of the fetal epigenome.[126,127] Studies on mother-infant dyads in the Gambia found that seasonal variation (rainy vs dry) in maternal diet at the time of conception altered DNA methylation at metastable epi-alleles (MEs) in infants at 2 to 8 months of age.[126,127] These changes correlated with maternal plasma levels of key methyl-donor pathways (eg, methionine, choline, folate, homocysteine, B vitamins). DNA methylation at MEs is stochastically established during very early embryogenesis and is particularly sensitive to early maternal exposures, like nutrition and obesity. This early establishment of methyl groups at specific MEs allows methylation to be stably maintained systemically across cell lineages during differentiation. However, it still remains unclear whether maternal obesity, GWG, and maternal nutrition can permanently modify methylation patterns resulting in lasting changes in gene expression.

Potential Role of the Gut Microbiome in Maternal and Infant Obesity

Recently, the gut microbiome has garnered significant attention as another mode of transmitting obesity risk from mothers to offspring. A seminal study described the effect on a germ-free mouse when a first-trimester (insulin sensitive) versus third-trimester (insulin resistant) human microbiome was transplanted into a germ-free mouse.[128] The mouse receiving the third-trimester microbiome became fatter and demonstrated insulin resistance and gut dysbiosis compared with the mouse who received the first-trimester microbiome. The exposure of the fetal intestine to maternal microbes at childbirth and possibly through amniotic fluid is an important contributor to gut maturation and, by extension, to infant health. Animal and human data strongly suggest that the composition of the neonatal gut microbiota depends both on maternal obesity and maternal diet during pregnancy and lactation[129] as well as mode of delivery.[130]

The microbiome plays a major role in nutrition, extraction of energy, metabolism, protection against pathogens, resistance to infections, and immune system development. Studies in nonhuman primates have shown distinct effects of maternal high-fat diet on offspring microbiota as well as a decrease in overall bacterial diversity when compared with primates fed a control diet.[129,131,132] Although the exact implications of these changes in microbiota are not fully known, decreased bacterial diversity is associated with adiposity, insulin resistance, dyslipidemia, and low-grade inflammation in humans.[133,134] Another provocative study in primates has shown that after weaning, dysbiosis is only partially corrected by a controlled low-fat diet,[131,135] demonstrating the lasting effects of a high-fat maternal diet on the microbiome of the offspring. Human studies showed that the microbiome from newborns at 2 weeks of age born to mothers with obesity exhibited less Gammaproteobacteria, an early colonizing bacteria essential for the development of immune tolerance, and a higher trend in bacilli class in the Firmicutes phylum, a high consumer of choline, which may be highly relevant because low choline is associated with the development of NAFLD.[136] The breast milk of women with obesity contains higher levels of insulin and leptin, which may be able to pass through more permeable intestinal gap junctions in the newborn, potentially affecting appetite regulation, microbiome development, immune tolerance, and infant body composition and growth.[136]

Early microbes from infants born to women with obesity or GDM may contribute to long-term health risks by triggering proinflammatory remodeling of the innate and adaptive immune system as well as other organs and tissues in the neonate.[137] Dysbiosis of the gut microbiome has been correlated with NAFLD in children and adults.

However, if and how the early life microbial composition influences hepatic fat accumulation and inflammation before the disease occurs is unclear. Attempts to alter the infant microbiome by modifying the maternal microbiome by diet changes or prebiotics or probiotics in pregnancy have shown mixed results in prevention of GDM and GWG.[138,139] A large Australian RCT enrolling more than 500 women (SPRING Trial) was recently completed using the same probiotic, and the results should be available soon.[140]

It is clear the -omics, such as epigenetics, microbiome, and transcriptomics, can advance our understanding of how obesity risk is transmitted to offspring. Metabolomics is another increasing -omics platform that can provide information on macronutrient and micronutrient fluxes through metabolic pathways that can be altered by maternal diet or obesity, which could affect the offspring.[141,142] There is also emerging evidence driven by animal studies for paternal obesity influencing offspring risk.[143,144] Clinical studies suggest that sperm are altered by obesity[145] such that fathers may no longer be out of the loop in being metabolically accountable to their offspring.

SUMMARY

It is extremely important for clinicians to discuss pregnancy plans with women with obesity well in advance of conception in order to ensure that medical comorbidities and medications can be optimized before pregnancy. Weight management before pregnancy should be promoted with the aim of improving both maternal and fetal health. During pregnancy, careful screening for maternal and fetal complications should take place, with consideration given to preventative strategies where appropriate. Recognition of the increased risk of stillbirth in this population should lead to careful consideration of the risks and benefits of induction of labor around 38 to 39 weeks of gestation. In the postpartum period, promotion of breastfeeding and reducing postpartum weight retention should be recommended to women with obesity to improve future health and reduce adverse events in future pregnancies.

There is increasing recognition of the adverse metabolic effects on the offspring of women with obesity, which has large implications for future generations. Further research is needed to determine how best to attenuate these negative effects in order to halt and, it is hoped, reverse the increasing prevalence of obesity and metabolic disease.

REFERENCES

1. Flegal KM, Kruszon-Moran D, Carroll MD, et al. Trends in obesity among adults in the United States, 2005 to 2014. JAMA 2016;315(21):2284–91.
2. Kominiarek MA, Chauhan SP. Obesity before, during, and after pregnancy: a review and comparison of five national guidelines. Am J Perinatol 2016;33(5): 433–41.
3. Grohmann B, Brazeau-Gravelle P, Momoli F, et al. Obstetric healthcare providers' perceptions of communicating gestational weight gain recommendations to overweight/obese pregnant women. Obstet Med 2012;5(4):161–5.
4. Dinsdale S, Branch K, Cook L, et al. "As soon as you've had the baby that's it..." a qualitative study of 24 postnatal women on their experience of maternal obesity care pathways. BMC Public Health 2016;16:625.
5. Heslehurst N, Lang R, Rankin J, et al. Obesity in pregnancy: a study of the impact of maternal obesity on NHS maternity services. BJOG 2007;114(3): 334–42.

6. Mills A, Schmied VA, Dahlen HG. 'Get alongside us', women's experiences of being overweight and pregnant in Sydney, Australia. Matern Child Nutr 2013; 9(3):309–21.

7. Canadian Obesity Network. 5 A's of healthy pregnancy weight gain. Available at: http://www.obesitynetwork.ca/pregnancy. Accessed May 27, 2017.

8. Gesink Law DC, Maclehose RF, Longnecker MP. Obesity and time to pregnancy. Hum Reprod 2007;22(2):414–20.

9. Nohr EA, Timpson NJ, Andersen CS, et al. Severe obesity in young women and reproductive health: the Danish National Birth Cohort. PLoS One 2009;4(12): e8444.

10. van der Steeg JW, Steures P, Eijkemans MJ, et al. Obesity affects spontaneous pregnancy chances in subfertile, ovulatory women. Hum Reprod 2008;23(2): 324–8.

11. Alvarez-Blasco F, Botella-Carretero JI, San Millan JL, et al. Prevalence and characteristics of the polycystic ovary syndrome in overweight and obese women. Arch Intern Med 2006;166(19):2081–6.

12. Rotterdam ESHRE/ASRM-sponsored PCOS consensus working group. Revised 2003 consensus on diagnostic criteria and long-term health risks related to polycystic ovary syndrome. Fertil Steril 2004;81(1):19–25.

13. Metwally M, Ong KJ, Ledger WL, et al. Does high body mass index increase the risk of miscarriage after spontaneous and assisted conception? A meta-analysis of the evidence. Fertil Steril 2008;90(3):714–26.

14. Rittenberg V, Seshadri S, Sunkara SK, et al. Effect of body mass index on IVF treatment outcome: an updated systematic review and meta-analysis. Reprod Biomed Online 2011;23(4):421–39.

15. Sim KA, Partridge SR, Sainsbury A. Does weight loss in overweight or obese women improve fertility treatment outcomes? A systematic review. Obes Rev 2014;15(10):839–50.

16. Mutsaerts MA, van Oers AM, Groen H, et al. Randomized trial of a lifestyle program in obese infertile women. N Engl J Med 2016;374(20):1942–53.

17. Legro RS, Dodson WC, Kunselman AR, et al. Benefit of delayed fertility therapy with preconception weight loss over immediate therapy in obese women with PCOS. J Clin Endocrinol Metab 2016;101(7):2658–66.

18. Milone M, De Placido G, Musella M, et al. Incidence of successful pregnancy after weight loss interventions in infertile women: a systematic review and meta-analysis of the literature. Obes Surg 2016;26(2):443–51.

19. Mechanick JI, Youdim A, Jones DB, et al. Clinical practice guidelines for the perioperative nutritional, metabolic, and nonsurgical support of the bariatric surgery patient–2013 update: cosponsored by American Association of Clinical Endocrinologists, The Obesity Society, and American Society for Metabolic & Bariatric Surgery. Obesity (Silver Spring) 2013;21(Suppl 1):S1–27.

20. American College of Obstetricians and Gynecologists. ACOG practice bulletin no. 105: bariatric surgery and pregnancy. Obstet Gynecol 2009;113(6): 1405–13.

21. American College of Obstetricians and Gynecologists. ACOG practice bulletin no. 156: obesity in pregnancy. Obstet Gynecol 2015;126(6):e112–126.

22. Practice Committee of the American Society for Reproductive Medicine. Obesity and reproduction: a committee opinion. Fertil Steril 2015;104(5):1116–26.

23. Yi XY, Li QF, Zhang J, et al. A meta-analysis of maternal and fetal outcomes of pregnancy after bariatric surgery. Int J Gynaecol Obstet 2015;130(1):3–9.

24. Kjaer MM, Lauenborg J, Breum BM, et al. The risk of adverse pregnancy outcome after bariatric surgery: a nationwide register-based matched cohort study. Am J Obstet Gynecol 2013;208(6):464.e1-5.

25. Roos N, Neovius M, Cnattingius S, et al. Perinatal outcomes after bariatric surgery: nationwide population based matched cohort study. BMJ 2013;347:f6460.

26. Simmons D. Prevention of gestational diabetes mellitus: where are we now? Diabetes Obes Metab 2015;17(9):824–34.

27. Lifestyle intervention in preparation for pregnancy. Available at: https://clinicaltrials.gov/ct2/show/NCT03146156?term=catalano&rank=4. Accessed May 29, 2017.

28. Royal College of Obstetricians and Gynaecologists. Scientific impact paper #17: the role of reproductive surgery in improving reproductive health. 2015. Available at: https://www.rcog.org.uk/globalassets/documents/guidelines/scientific-impact-papers/sip_17.pdf. Accessed April 27, 2017.

29. Madsen NL, Schwartz SM, Lewin MB, et al. Prepregnancy body mass index and congenital heart defects among offspring: a population-based study. Congenit Heart Dis 2013;8(2):131–41.

30. Stothard KJ, Tennant PW, Bell R, et al. Maternal overweight and obesity and the risk of congenital anomalies: a systematic review and meta-analysis. JAMA 2009;301(6):636–50.

31. Mills JL, Troendle J, Conley MR, et al. Maternal obesity and congenital heart defects: a population-based study. Am J Clin Nutr 2010;91(6):1543–9.

32. Brite J, Laughon SK, Troendle J, et al. Maternal overweight and obesity and risk of congenital heart defects in offspring. Int J Obes (Lond) 2014;38(6):878–82.

33. Masho SW, Bassyouni A, Cha S. Pre-pregnancy obesity and non-adherence to multivitamin use: findings from the National Pregnancy Risk Assessment Monitoring System (2009-2011). BMC Pregnancy Childbirth 2016;16(1):210.

34. Tinker SC, Hamner HC, Berry RJ, et al. Does obesity modify the association of supplemental folic acid with folate status among nonpregnant women of childbearing age in the United States? Birth Defects Res A Clin Mol Teratol 2012;94(10):749–55.

35. Royal College of Obstetricians and Gynaecologists. Management of women with obesity in pregnancy. Joint Guideline. 2010. Available at: https://www.rcog.org.uk/globalassets/documents/guidelines/cmacercogjointguidelinemanagementwomenobesitypregnancya.pdf. Accessed 27 May 2017.

36. Mojtabai R. Body mass index and serum folate in childbearing age women. Eur J Epidemiol 2004;19(11):1029–36.

37. Ferraro ZM, Contador F, Tawfiq A, et al. Gestational weight gain and medical outcomes of pregnancy. Obstet Med 2015;8(3):133–7.

38. Adamo KB, Ferraro ZM, Brett KE. Pregnancy is a critical period for prevention of obesity and cardiometabolic risk. Can J Diabetes 2012;36:133–41.

39. Weisman CS, Hillemeier MM, Downs DS, et al. Preconception predictors of weight gain during pregnancy: prospective findings from the Central Pennsylvania Women's Health Study. Womens Health Issues 2010;20(2):126–32.

40. Ferraro ZM, Barrowman N, Prud'homme D, et al. Excessive gestational weight gain predicts large for gestational age neonates independent of maternal body mass index. J Matern Fetal Neonatal Med 2012;25(5):538–42.

41. Institute of Medicine and National Research Council Committee to Reexamine IOM Pregnancy Weight Guidelines, Rasmussen KM, Yaktine AL, editors. Weight gain during pregnancy: reexamining the guidelines. Washington, DC: 2009.

42. Kapadia MZ, Park CK, Beyene J, et al. Can we safely recommend gestational weight gain below the 2009 guidelines in obese women? A systematic review and meta-analysis. Obes Rev 2015;16(3):189–206.
43. Bogaerts A, Ameye L, Martens E, et al. Weight loss in obese pregnant women and risk for adverse perinatal outcomes. Obstet Gynecol 2015;125(3):566–75.
44. Blomberg M. Maternal and neonatal outcomes among obese women with weight gain below the new Institute of Medicine recommendations. Obstet Gynecol 2011;117(5):1065–70.
45. American College of Obstetricians and Gynecologists. ACOG Committee opinion no. 548: weight gain during pregnancy. Obstet Gynecol 2013;121(1):210–2.
46. Davies GA, Maxwell C, McLeod L, et al. SOGC clinical practice guidelines: obesity in pregnancy. No. 239, February 2010. Int J Gynaecol Obstet 2010;110(2):167–73.
47. Muktabhant B, Lawrie TA, Lumbiganon P, et al. Diet or exercise, or both, for preventing excessive weight gain in pregnancy. Cochrane Database Syst Rev 2015;(6):CD007145.
48. American College of Obstetricians and Gynecologists. ACOG committee opinion no. 650: physical activity and exercise during pregnancy and the post-partum period. Obstet Gynecol 2015;126(6):e135–142.
49. McIntyre HD, Sacks DA, Barbour LA, et al. Issues with the diagnosis and classification of hyperglycemia in early pregnancy. Diabetes Care 2016;39(1):53–4.
50. Hughes RC, Moore MP, Gullam JE, et al. An early pregnancy HbA1c >/=5.9% (41 mmol/mol) is optimal for detecting diabetes and identifies women at increased risk of adverse pregnancy outcomes. Diabetes Care 2014;37(11):2953–9.
51. Barbour LA. Unresolved controversies in gestational diabetes: implications on maternal and infant health. Curr Opin Endocrinol Diabetes Obes 2014;21(4):264–70.
52. American College of Obstetricians and Gynecologists. Practice bulletin No. 137: gestational diabetes mellitus. Obstet Gynecol 2013;122(2 Pt 1):406–16.
53. Wong T, Ross GP, Jalaludin BB, et al. The clinical significance of overt diabetes in pregnancy. Diabet Med 2013;30(4):468–74.
54. Robinson HE, O'Connell CM, Joseph KS, et al. Maternal outcomes in pregnancies complicated by obesity. Obstet Gynecol 2005;106(6):1357–64.
55. O'Brien TE, Ray JG, Chan WS. Maternal body mass index and the risk of pre-eclampsia: a systematic overview. Epidemiology 2003;14(3):368–74.
56. Sorensen TK, Williams MA, Lee IM, et al. Recreational physical activity during pregnancy and risk of preeclampsia. Hypertension 2003;41(6):1273–80.
57. Saftlas AF, Logsden-Sackett N, Wang W, et al. Work, leisure-time physical activity, and risk of preeclampsia and gestational hypertension. Am J Epidemiol 2004;160(8):758–65.
58. American College of Obstetricians and Gynecologists. Task force on hypertension in pregnancy. Hypertension in pregnancy. Obstet Gynecol 2013;122(5):1122–31.
59. Magee LA, Pels A, Helewa M, et al. Diagnosis, evaluation, and management of the hypertensive disorders of pregnancy: executive summary. J Obstet Gynaecol Can 2014;36(7):575–6.
60. Cantu JA, Jauk VR, Owen J, et al. Is low-dose aspirin therapy to prevent pre-eclampsia more efficacious in non-obese women or when initiated early in pregnancy? J Matern Fetal Neonatal Med 2015;28(10):1128–32.

61. Hildebrand E, Kallen B, Josefsson A, et al. Maternal obesity and risk of Down syndrome in the offspring. Prenat Diagn 2014;34(4):310–5.
62. Wang E, Batey A, Struble C, et al. Gestational age and maternal weight effects on fetal cell-free DNA in maternal plasma. Prenat Diagn 2013;33(7):662–6.
63. Aagaard-Tillery KM, Flint Porter T, Malone FD, et al. Influence of maternal BMI on genetic sonography in the FaSTER trial. Prenat Diagn 2010;30(1):14–22.
64. Dashe JS, McIntire DD, Twickler DM. Effect of maternal obesity on the ultrasound detection of anomalous fetuses. Obstet Gynecol 2009;113(5):1001–7.
65. Dashe JS, McIntire DD, Twickler DM. Maternal obesity limits the ultrasound evaluation of fetal anatomy. J Ultrasound Med 2009;28(8):1025–30.
66. Cnattingius S, Villamor E, Johansson S, et al. Maternal obesity and risk of preterm delivery. JAMA 2013;309(22):2362–70.
67. Carmichael SL, Blumenfeld YJ, Mayo J, et al. Prepregnancy obesity and risks of stillbirth. PLoS One 2015;10(10):e0138549.
68. Jacob L, Kostev K, Kalder M. Risk of stillbirth in pregnant women with obesity in the United Kingdom. Obes Res Clin Pract 2016;10(5):574–9.
69. Lee VR, Liu B, Anjali K, et al. Optimal timing of delivery in obese women: a decision analysis. Obstet Gynecol 2014;123(S1):152S–3S.
70. Lee VR, Darney BG, Snowden JM, et al. Term elective induction of labour and perinatal outcomes in obese women: retrospective cohort study. BJOG 2016; 123(2):271–8.
71. Alanis MC, Villers MS, Law TL, et al. Complications of cesarean delivery in the massively obese parturient. Am J Obstet Gynecol 2010;203(3):271.e1-7.
72. Alexander CI, Liston WA. Operating on the obese woman–a review. BJOG 2006; 113(10):1167–72.
73. Wall PD, Deucy EE, Glantz JC, et al. Vertical skin incisions and wound complications in the obese parturient. Obstet Gynecol 2003;102(5 Pt 1):952–6.
74. Tan T, Sia AT. Anesthesia considerations in the obese gravida. Semin Perinatol 2011;35(6):350–5.
75. Fyfe EM, Thompson JM, Anderson NH, et al. Maternal obesity and postpartum haemorrhage after vaginal and caesarean delivery among nulliparous women at term: a retrospective cohort study. BMC Pregnancy Childbirth 2012;12:112.
76. Bates SM, Greer IA, Middeldorp S, et al. VTE, thrombophilia, antithrombotic therapy, and pregnancy: antithrombotic therapy and prevention of thrombosis, 9th ed: American College of Chest Physicians evidence-based clinical practice guidelines. Chest 2012;141(2 Suppl):e691S–736S.
77. Chan WS, Rey E, Kent NE, et al. Venous thromboembolism and antithrombotic therapy in pregnancy. J Obstet Gynaecol Can 2014;36(6):527–53.
78. World Health Organization. Breastfeeding. health topics. Available at: http://www.who.int/topics/breastfeeding/en/. Accessed December 6, 2016.
79. American Academy of Pediatrics. Breastfeeding and the use of human milk. Pediatrics 2012;129:e827–41.
80. Schwarz EB, Ray RM, Stuebe AM, et al. Duration of lactation and risk factors for maternal cardiovascular disease. Obstet Gynecol 2009;113(5):974–82.
81. Stuebe AM, Rich-Edwards JW, Willett WC, et al. Duration of lactation and incidence of type 2 diabetes. JAMA 2005;294(20):2601–10.
82. Liu B, Jorm L, Banks E. Parity, breastfeeding, and the subsequent risk of maternal type 2 diabetes. Diabetes Care 2010;33(6):1239–41.
83. Natland ST, Nilsen TI, Midthjell K, et al. Lactation and cardiovascular risk factors in mothers in a population-based study: the HUNT-study. Int Breastfeed J 2012; 7(1):8.

84. McClure CK, Schwarz EB, Conroy MB, et al. Breastfeeding and subsequent maternal visceral adiposity. Obesity (Silver Spring) 2011;19(11):2205–13.
85. Baker JL, Gamborg M, Heitmann BL, et al. Breastfeeding reduces postpartum weight retention. Am J Clin Nutr 2008;88(6):1543–51.
86. Coitinho DC, Sichieri R, D'Aquino Benicio MH. Obesity and weight change related to parity and breast-feeding among parous women in Brazil. Public Health Nutr 2001;4(4):865–70.
87. Palmer JR, Kipping-Ruane K, Wise LA, et al. Lactation in relation to long-term maternal weight gain in African-American women. Am J Epidemiol 2015; 181(12):932–9.
88. Thompson LA, Zhang S, Black E, et al. The association of maternal pre-pregnancy body mass index with breastfeeding initiation. Matern Child Health J 2013;17(10):1842–51.
89. Amir LH, Donath S. A systematic review of maternal obesity and breastfeeding intention, initiation and duration. BMC Pregnancy Childbirth 2007;7:9.
90. Bever Babendure J, Reifsnider E, Mendias E, et al. Reduced breastfeeding rates among obese mothers: a review of contributing factors, clinical consider-ations and future directions. Int Breastfeed J 2015;10:21.
91. Cnattingius S, Villamor E. Weight change between successive pregnancies and risks of stillbirth and infant mortality: a nationwide cohort study. Lancet 2016; 387(10018):558–65.
92. Villamor E, Cnattingius S. Interpregnancy weight change and risk of adverse pregnancy outcomes: a population-based study. Lancet 2006;368(9542): 1164–70.
93. Glazer NL, Hendrickson AF, Schellenbaum GD, et al. Weight change and the risk of gestational diabetes in obese women. Epidemiology 2004;15(6):733–7.
94. Jain AP, Gavard JA, Rice JJ, et al. The impact of interpregnancy weight change on birthweight in obese women. Am J Obstet Gynecol 2013;208(3):205.e1-7.
95. Callegari LS, Sterling LA, Zelek ST, et al. Interpregnancy body mass index change and success of term vaginal birth after cesarean delivery. Am J Obstet Gynecol 2014;210(4):330.e1-7.
96. Amorim AR, Linne YM, Lourenco PM. Diet or exercise, or both, for weight reduc-tion in women after childbirth. Cochrane Database Syst Rev 2007;(3):CD005627.
97. Cunningham SA, Kramer MR, Narayan KM. Incidence of childhood obesity in the United States. N Engl J Med 2014;370(17):1660–1.
98. Ogden CL, Carroll MD, Kit BK, et al. Prevalence of childhood and adult obesity in the United States, 2011-2012. JAMA 2014;311(8):806–14.
99. Starling AP, Brinton JT, Glueck DH, et al. Associations of maternal BMI and gestational weight gain with neonatal adiposity in the Healthy Start study. Am J Clin Nutr 2015;101(2):302–9.
100. Nicklas JM, Barbour LA. Optimizing weight for maternal and infant health - tenable, or too late? Expert Rev Endocrinol Metab 2015;10(2):227–42.
101. Olson CM, Strawderman MS, Dennison BA. Maternal weight gain during preg-nancy and child weight at age 3 years. Matern Child Health J 2009;13(6): 839–46.
102. Catalano PM, Farrell K, Thomas A, et al. Perinatal risk factors for childhood obesity and metabolic dysregulation. Am J Clin Nutr 2009;90(5):1303–13.
103. Reynolds RM, Osmond C, Phillips DI, et al. Maternal BMI, parity, and pregnancy weight gain: influences on offspring adiposity in young adulthood. J Clin Endo-crinol Metab 2010;95(12):5365–9.

104. Catalano PM, Presley L, Minium J, et al. Fetuses of obese mothers develop insulin resistance in utero. Diabetes Care 2009;32(6):1076–80.

105. Nicholas LM, Morrison JL, Rattanatray L, et al. The early origins of obesity and insulin resistance: timing, programming and mechanisms. Int J Obes (Lond) 2016;40(2):229–38.

106. Barbour LA. Changing perspectives in pre-existing diabetes and obesity in pregnancy: maternal and infant short- and long-term outcomes. Curr Opin Endocrinol Diabetes Obes 2014;21(4):257–63.

107. Singhal A, Lucas A. Early origins of cardiovascular disease: is there a unifying hypothesis? Lancet 2004;363(9421):1642–5.

108. Reynolds RM, Allan KM, Raja EA, et al. Maternal obesity during pregnancy and premature mortality from cardiovascular event in adult offspring: follow-up of 1 323 275 person years. BMJ 2013;347:f4539.

109. McCurdy CE, Bishop JM, Williams SM, et al. Maternal high-fat diet triggers lipotoxicity in the fetal livers of nonhuman primates. J Clin Invest 2009;119(2): 323–35.

110. Brumbaugh DE, Tearse P, Cree-Green M, et al. Intrahepatic fat is increased in the neonatal offspring of obese women with gestational diabetes. J Pediatr 2013;162(5):930–6.e1.

111. Wesolowski SR, Kasmi KC, Jonscher KR, et al. Developmental origins of NAFLD: a womb with a clue. Nat Rev Gastroenterol Hepatol 2017;14(2):81–96.

112. Newton KP, Feldman HS, Chambers CD, et al. Low and high birth weights are risk factors for nonalcoholic fatty liver disease in children. J Pediatr 2017;187: 141–6.e1.

113. Goyal NP, Schwimmer JB. The progression and natural history of pediatric nonalcoholic fatty liver disease. Clin Liver Dis 2016;20(2):325–38.

114. Kral JG, Biron S, Simard S, et al. Large maternal weight loss from obesity surgery prevents transmission of obesity to children who were followed for 2 to 18 years. Pediatrics 2006;118(6):e1644–1649.

115. Smith J, Cianflone K, Biron S, et al. Effects of maternal surgical weight loss in mothers on intergenerational transmission of obesity. J Clin Endocrinol Metab 2009;94(11):4275–83.

116. Barker DJ, Winter PD, Osmond C, et al. Weight in infancy and death from ischaemic heart disease. Lancet 1989;2(8663):577–80.

117. Boyle KE, Patinkin ZW, Shapiro AL, et al. Mesenchymal stem cells from infants born to obese mothers exhibit greater potential for adipogenesis: the Healthy Start BabyBUMP Project. Diabetes 2016;65(3):647–59.

118. Heerwagen MJ, Miller MR, Barbour LA, et al. Maternal obesity and fetal metabolic programming: a fertile epigenetic soil. Am J Physiol Regul Integr Comp Physiol 2010;299(3):R711–22.

119. El Hajj N, Schneider E, Lehnen H, et al. Epigenetics and life-long consequences of an adverse nutritional and diabetic intrauterine environment. Reproduction 2014;148(6):R111–20.

120. Ganu RS, Harris RA, Collins K, et al. Maternal diet: a modulator for epigenomic regulation during development in nonhuman primates and humans. Int J Obes Suppl 2012;2(Suppl 2):S14–8.

121. Teh AL, Pan H, Chen L, et al. The effect of genotype and in utero environment on interindividual variation in neonate DNA methylomes. Genome Res 2014;24(7): 1064–74.

122. Ollikainen M, Smith KR, Joo EJ, et al. DNA methylation analysis of multiple tissues from newborn twins reveals both genetic and intrauterine components to

variation in the human neonatal epigenome. Hum Mol Genet 2010;19(21): 4176–88.

123. Cooper WN, Khulan B, Owens S, et al. DNA methylation profiling at imprinted loci after periconceptional micronutrient supplementation in humans: results of a pilot randomized controlled trial. FASEB J 2012;26(5):1782–90.

124. Khulan B, Cooper WN, Skinner BM, et al. Periconceptional maternal micronutrient supplementation is associated with widespread gender related changes in the epigenome: a study of a unique resource in the Gambia. Hum Mol Genet 2012;21(9):2086–101.

125. Lin X, Lim IY, Wu Y, et al. Developmental pathways to adiposity begin before birth and are influenced by genotype, prenatal environment and epigenome. BMC Med 2017;15(1):50.

126. Waterland RA, Kellermayer R, Laritsky E, et al. Season of conception in rural Gambia affects DNA methylation at putative human metastable epialleles. PLoS Genet 2010;6(12):e1001252.

127. Dominguez-Salas P, Moore SE, Baker MS, et al. Maternal nutrition at conception modulates DNA methylation of human metastable epialleles. Nat Commun 2014; 5:3746.

128. Koren O, Goodrich JK, Cullender TC, et al. Host remodeling of the gut microbiome and metabolic changes during pregnancy. Cell 2012;150(3):470–80.

129. Chu DM, Meyer KM, Prince AL, et al. Impact of maternal nutrition in pregnancy and lactation on offspring gut microbial composition and function. Gut Microbes 2016;7(6):459–70.

130. Brumbaugh DE, Arruda J, Robbins K, et al. Mode of delivery determines neonatal pharyngeal bacterial composition and early intestinal colonization. J Pediatr Gastroenterol Nutr 2016;63(3):320–8.

131. Prince AL, Antony KM, Ma J, et al. The microbiome and development: a mother's perspective. Semin Reprod Med 2014;32(1):14–22.

132. Chu DM, Antony KM, Ma J, et al. The early infant gut microbiome varies in association with a maternal high-fat diet. Genome Med 2016;8(1):77.

133. Cotillard A, Kennedy SP, Kong LC, et al. Dietary intervention impact on gut microbial gene richness. Nature 2013;500(7464):585–8.

134. Le Chatelier E, Nielsen T, Qin J, et al. Richness of human gut microbiome correlates with metabolic markers. Nature 2013;500(7464):541–6.

135. Ma J, Prince AL, Bader D, et al. High-fat maternal diet during pregnancy persistently alters the offspring microbiome in a primate model. Nat Commun 2014;5: 3889.

136. Lemas DJ, Young BE, Baker PR 2nd, et al. Alterations in human milk leptin and insulin are associated with early changes in the infant intestinal microbiome. Am J Clin Nutr 2016;103(5):1291–300.

137. Soderborg TK, Borengasser SJ, Barbour LA, et al. Microbial transmission from mothers with obesity or diabetes to infants: an innovative opportunity to interrupt a vicious cycle. Diabetologia 2016;59(5):895–906.

138. Luoto R, Laitinen K, Nermes M, et al. Impact of maternal probiotic-supplemented dietary counselling on pregnancy outcome and prenatal and postnatal growth: a double-blind, placebo-controlled study. Br J Nutr 2010; 103(12):1792–9.

139. Wickens KL, Barthow CA, Murphy R, et al. Early pregnancy probiotic supplementation with Lactobacillus rhamnosus HN001 may reduce the prevalence of gestational diabetes mellitus: a randomised controlled trial. Br J Nutr 2017; 117(6):804–13.

140. Nitert MD, Barrett HL, Foxcroft K, et al. SPRING: an RCT study of probiotics in the prevention of gestational diabetes mellitus in overweight and obese women. BMC Pregnancy Childbirth 2013;13:50.
141. Sandler V, Reisetter AC, Bain JR, et al. Associations of maternal BMI and insulin resistance with the maternal metabolome and newborn outcomes. Diabetologia 2017;60(3):518–30.
142. Hellmuth C, Lindsay KL, Uhl O, et al. Association of maternal prepregnancy BMI with metabolomic profile across gestation. Int J Obes (Lond) 2017;41(1): 159–69.
143. Ng SF, Lin RC, Laybutt DR, et al. Chronic high-fat diet in fathers programs beta-cell dysfunction in female rat offspring. Nature 2010;467(7318):963–6.
144. de Castro Barbosa T, Ingerslev LR, Alm PS, et al. High-fat diet reprograms the epigenome of rat spermatozoa and transgenerationally affects metabolism of the offspring. Mol Metab 2016;5(3):184–97.
145. Donkin I, Versteyhe S, Ingerslev LR, et al. Obesity and bariatric surgery drive epigenetic variation of spermatozoa in humans. Cell Metab 2016;23(2):369–78.
146. Balserak B. Sleep disordered breathing in pregnancy. Breathe (Sheff) 2015; 11(4):268–77.
147. Rice JR, Larrabure-Torrealva GT, Luque Fernandez MA, et al. High risk for obstructive sleep apnea and other sleep disorders among overweight and obese pregnant women. BMC Pregnancy Childbirth 2015;15:198.
148. Louis J, Auckley D, Miladinovic B, et al. Perinatal outcomes associated with obstructive sleep apnea in obese pregnant women. Obstet Gynecol 2012; 120(5):1085–92.
149. Dietrich P, Hellerbrand C. Non-alcoholic fatty liver disease, obesity and the metabolic syndrome. Best Pract Res Clin Gastroenterol 2014;28(4):637–53.
150. Hagstrom H, Hoijer J, Ludvigsson JF, et al. Adverse outcomes of pregnancy in women with non-alcoholic fatty liver disease. Liver Int 2016;36(2):268–74.
151. Chelmow D, Rodriguez EJ, Sabatini MM. Suture closure of subcutaneous fat and wound disruption after cesarean delivery: a meta-analysis. Obstet Gynecol 2004;103(5 part 1):974–80.
152. Tuuli MG, Rampersad RM, Carbone JF, et al. Staples compared with subcuticular suture for skin closure after cesarean delivery: a systematic review and meta-analysis. Obstet Gynecol 2011;117(3):682–90.

Dietary Management of Obesity

Cornerstones of Healthy Eating Patterns

Alissa D. Smethers, MS, RD, Barbara J. Rolls, PhD*

KEYWORDS

- Weight management • Dietary strategies • Energy density • Satiety
- Dietary patterns

KEY POINTS

- Multiple dietary patterns are effective for weight management, with energy density as a unifying factor across patterns.
- There are several evidence-based strategies to lower energy intake, reduce dietary energy density, and improve diet quality that can be applied to individualized eating patterns for weight management.
- A variety of tools to help manage energy intake can be incorporated into personalized eating patterns to facilitate weight management.

INTRODUCTION

The recent surge in rates of obesity is driven by eating behaviors and food choices that promote excessive energy intake.[1–8] The current recommendations for weight management emphasize the importance of healthy eating patterns that include a variety of nutrient-dense foods, limit portions of energy-dense foods, and reduce overall energy density.[8] Several dietary patterns that reduce energy intake in relation to energy expenditure lead to similar weight loss. A unifying factor for weight loss across dietary patterns is energy density. Reducing a diet's energy density allows individuals to consume satisfying amounts of food for fewer calories. Strategies that lower energy density are flexible and can be applied to multiple dietary patterns to match differences in energy needs, taste preferences, eating behaviors, food accessibility, and cultural backgrounds.[8,9] This article discusses the current evidence related to dietary

Disclosure Statement: This work was supported by the National Institute of Diabetes and Digestive and Kidney Diseases (grant Nos DK059853 and DK082580) and by the US Department of Agriculture, National Institute of Food and Agriculture (grant No. 2011-67001-30117).
Conflict of Interest: B.J. Rolls receives royalties from the Volumetrics Books.
Department of Nutritional Sciences, The Pennsylvania State University, 226 Henderson Building, University Park, PA 16802-6501
* Corresponding author.
E-mail address: bjr4@psu.edu

approaches for weight management and provides strategies and tools to create lower-energy-dense eating patterns that can be tailored to the individual to achieve a sustainable and healthy weight management program.

CURRENT EVIDENCE ON DIETARY PATTERNS FOR WEIGHT LOSS
Macronutrient Patterns for Weight Loss

Advice to alter the proportion of the macronutrients consumed has been the foundation for many weight loss diets.[10] Fat, carbohydrate, and protein have all been highlighted at different times as the key to weight loss.[11–13] There continues to be controversy over whether a low-fat or low-carbohydrate diet is better for weight loss or whether the increased satiating effects of a higher-protein diet help to sustain weight loss.[10,14] An evidence-based report from the American College of Cardiology/American Heart Association Task Force on Practice Guidelines and The Obesity Society supports several energy-restricted dietary approaches for weight loss that focus on the macronutrients, including low-fat, lower-carbohydrate, moderate- and higher-protein, and macronutrient-targeted diets.[15] Although such diets can be effective, several systematic studies indicate that focusing on a particular macronutrient for weight loss is not necessary. Different macronutrient recommendations have all led to similar clinically significant weight loss at 6 months, 1 year, and even 2 years.[12,16,17]

One large clinical trial that compared 4 diets with different proportions of macronutrients, the Preventing Overweight Using Novel Dietary Strategies (POUNDS LOST) study, found that weight loss was similar across the diets (**Fig. 1**).[12] Although the macronutrient composition did not affect weight loss or maintenance of lost weight, regression analysis showed that reductions in dietary energy density and increases in fiber intake were strong predictors for 6-month weight loss in all diet groups.[18–20] The fundamental dietary advice given to participants on all diets included strategies to lower the energy density of the diet, such as increasing vegetable and fruit consumption and decreasing consumption of high-calorie foods.[12,21] These results suggest that regardless of macronutrient composition, a goal for weight loss should be to adopt a pattern of eating that is lower in energy density.

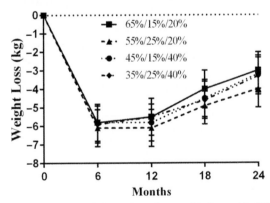

Fig. 1. Weight loss over 2 years in adults assigned to 1 of 4 diets with different proportions of carbohydrate/protein/fat as listed. There was no significant difference in weight loss related to the macronutrient composition. (*Data from* Sacks FM, Bray GA, Carey VJ, et al. Comparison of weight-loss diets with different compositions of fat, protein, and carbohydrates. N Engl J Med 2009;360(9):859–73.)

Food-Based Patterns for Weight Loss

In recent years, dietary guidance has emphasized the importance of considering whole diets and patterns of consumption rather than a reductionist approach that focuses on single foods or nutrients.[22] For example, the 2015 Dietary Advisory Committee recommends that individuals who have overweight and obesity achieve weight loss by adopting a healthy eating pattern. Examples of such patterns are the Healthy US-Style Eating Pattern, which represents the Dietary Approaches to Stop Hypertension (DASH) diet, and the Healthy Mediterranean-Style Eating Pattern.[8] The DASH eating pattern recommends reducing intake of the less healthy fats and keeping total fat intake to less than 25% of the diet's energy as well as increasing the proportion of low-energy-dense foods, such as vegetables and fruits (9–12 servings per day) and low-fat dairy products (2–3 servings per day).[23] The DASH diet is a lower-energy-dense pattern of eating that allows individuals to consume less energy without reducing the weight of food they typically eat.[24] The Mediterranean eating pattern also emphasizes intake of low-energy-dense fruits, vegetables, legumes, seafood, and dairy foods.[25] However, higher amounts of fat (30%–40% of total energy), especially from olive oil, are recommended with the Mediterranean pattern.[25] Even with this level of healthy fats, the high proportion of vegetables and fruits included in this pattern can help to keep the overall diet relatively low in energy density.[26] **Table 1** provides guidance on food groups and amounts in several healthy eating patterns.

Table 1
Recommended daily amounts of food from each food group for the US Healthy Eating Pattern (Dietary Approaches to Stop Hypertension) and the Mediterranean Eating Pattern at 2 calorie levels

	Healthy US-Style Eating Pattern		Healthy Mediterranean-Style Eating Pattern	
	1400 calories	1800 calories	1400 calories	1800 calories
Food Group	Daily amount from each food group			
Vegetables[a]	1.5 c	2.5 c	1.5 c	2.5 c
Fruits[b]	1.5 c	1.5 c	1.5 c	2.0 c
Grains[c]	5 oz	6 oz	5 oz	6 oz
Dairy[d]	2.5 c	3.0 c	2.5 c	2.0 c
Protein Foods[e]	4 oz	5 oz	4 oz	6 oz
Oils	17 g	24 g	17 g	24 g

[a] All fresh, frozen, and canned vegetables. Choose a variety, including dark green vegetables, red and orange vegetables, legumes, and starchy vegetables. A serving or 1.0-c equivalent for vegetables is 1.0 c raw or cooked vegetables, 1.0 c vegetable juice, and 2.0 c salad greens.
[b] All fresh, frozen, canned, and dried fruits and fruit juices. A serving or 1.0-c equivalent for fruits is 1.0 c raw or cooked fruit, 1.0 c fruit juice, or 0.5 c dried fruit.
[c] Choose whole grains for at least half of the grain servings. A serving or 1.0-oz equivalent for grains is 0.5 c cooked grain, 1 medium slice of bread, or 1.0 c of ready-to-eat-cereal.
[d] Includes all milk and fortified soy beverages, yogurt, frozen yogurt, dairy desserts, and cheeses. Most choices should be fat free or low fat. A serving or 1.0-c equivalent for dairy is 1.0 c of milk or yogurt or 1.5 oz of cheese.
[e] All seafood, meats, poultry, eggs, soy products, nuts, and seeds. Meats and poultry should be lean or low fat. A serving or 1.0-oz equivalent of protein is 1.0 oz lean meat, poultry, or seafood; 1 egg; 0.25 c cooked beans or tofu; 1.0 tbsp peanut butter; or 0.5 oz nuts or seeds.
Adapted from US Department of Health and Human Services and US Department of Agriculture. 2015–2020 Dietary guidelines for Americans. 8th edition. 2015. Available at http://health.gov/dietaryguidelines/2015/guidelines/. Accessed February 11, 2017.

The Influence of Energy Density on Weight Management

A key question is whether shifting to a healthy eating pattern that encourages individuals to lower the energy density of their diet will facilitate weight management.[24,27] This question was examined in the large multicenter PREMIER trial in which 3 intervention groups received information on diet and weight loss, with one group counseled to consume the DASH dietary pattern. Despite differences in treatment, after 6 months, all 3 groups experienced similar weight loss. Although the average change in energy density of the 3 groups was similar, there was considerable variability within groups, making it possible to determine whether changes in energy density were related to weight loss. In a secondary analysis that combined the participants from all 3 groups, results showed that participants with larger reductions in dietary energy density lost more weight than those who had smaller reductions in energy density.[24] Furthermore, those who had large or moderate reductions in energy density consumed a greater weight of food and improved diet quality by increasing vegetable and fruit consumption.[24] Thus, the adoption of strategies that lowered energy density had a greater impact on weight loss than the specific dietary advice given to the 3 intervention groups.

Other clinical trials confirm that a lower-energy-dense eating pattern is an effective strategy for weight management.[28,29] In one trial that compared the incorporation of either a low- or high-energy-dense food into a reduced-calorie diet, the reduction in dietary energy density was the main predictor of weight loss during the first 2 months of the study.[28] Over the year of the trial, the daily consumption of the low-energy-dense food (soup) instead of higher-energy-dense dry snacks with the same calorie content increased the magnitude of weight loss.[28] Encouraging regular consumption of low-energy-dense foods can reduce overall dietary energy density and can be an effective strategy for weight management.

Another clinical trial further explored the effectiveness of reducing energy density for weight management by comparing 2 energy density reduction strategies: reduced fat or reduced fat plus increased low-energy-dense vegetables and fruits.[29] There were no specific goals for energy intake. After 1 year, participants in the group focused on eating more vegetables and fruits lost more weight, had a lower dietary energy density, consumed a greater weight of food (especially vegetables and fruits), and reported less hunger compared with participants focused just on fat reduction.[29] An increase in the amount of food consumed when managing energy intake will likely improve the long-term acceptability of a low-energy-dense eating pattern because it could help to control hunger.

Lowering dietary energy density can also help patients maintain their weight loss.[30,31] In a clinic-based weight loss program that encouraged consumption of low-energy-dense foods, individuals who maintained their weight loss after 2 years reported eating a lower-energy-dense diet than those who regained 5% or more of their body weight.[32] In another trial, instruction on reducing dietary energy density led to sustained weight loss 36 months after the start of the intervention.[33]

Patients need education on implementing changes in their diet to lower energy density and replicating this in their personal food environment.[33] The strategies individuals use to reduce energy density can fit with a variety of healthy dietary approaches that are popular for weight loss. The next section focuses on dietary energy density, with more in-depth discussion of evidence-based principles that individuals can use to lower energy density and create sustainable eating patterns for weight management.

UNIFYING PRINCIPLE OF DIETARY PATTERNS: ENERGY DENSITY

The energy density of a food or beverage can range from 0 calories per gram to 9 calories per gram and varies based on the proportions of water (0 calories per gram), fiber (2 calories per gram), carbohydrate (4 calories per gram), protein (4 calories per gram), alcohol (7 calories per gram), and fat (9 calories per gram). Fat is the most energy-dense macronutrient, so when the fat content of a food is reduced, energy density also decreases. Water, however, has the biggest influence on energy density because it adds weight to food without adding calories. The more water a food contains, regardless of the fat content, the lower the energy density of the food. Low-energy-dense foods can help to reduce energy intake by enhancing satiation and satiety through psychological and physiologic mechanisms. This satiety leads to terminating a meal sooner, prolonging the time until the next eating occasion, and reducing intake at the next meal.[34,35]

The energy density of a food or beverage determines the portion size that can be eaten for a given number of calories: the lower the energy density, the larger the portion for the same number of calories. **Fig. 2** provides a visual example of how the portion size of a 100-calorie snack can vary based on the energy density of the food. For instance, a 100-calorie portion of raisins is about 0.25 c, whereas the same 100-calorie portion of cherry tomatoes is around 4.0 c. As seen in **Fig. 2**, energy density can be explained visually to patients to help them understand the relationship between energy density and the portions that can be consumed. To help further understand this concept, energy density can be divided into 4 categories: very low energy density, low energy density, medium energy density, and high energy density (**Table 2**).[34] No matter what dietary pattern an individual uses for weight loss, the energy density of the foods they choose influences the amount of food they can eat to stay within their calorie goals. For weight loss, patients need to be encouraged to regularly make simple healthy shifts within their habitual eating pattern so that a reduction in dietary energy density leads to lower energy intake.[35,36]

PRACTICAL DIETARY STRATEGIES FOR WEIGHT MANAGEMENT

Research shows that a variety of eating patterns that include a reduction in energy intake can work for weight management, but patients may not know which foods to choose or nutrients to emphasize to build their own healthy pattern.[8] In order to create a sustainable dietary pattern for weight loss, patients need to make changes that manage energy intake while receiving optimal nutrition, controlling hunger, and promoting satiety. This section discusses evidence-based strategies that individuals can use to lower dietary energy density, promote satiety, and meet nutrient recommendations.

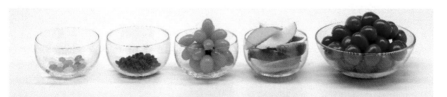

Fig. 2. The portion size of a 100-calorie snack varies depending on the energy density (ED) of the food. Jelly beans (ED 4.0 calories per gram) and raisins (ED 3.1 calories per gram) are high in ED and provide small portions. Grapes (ED 0.69 kcal/g), apples (ED 0.53 kcal/g), and cherry tomatoes (ED 0.18 kcal/g) are lower in ED and provide much bigger portions. (*Courtesy of* The Penn State Laboratory for the Study of Human Ingestive Behavior, University Park, PA.)

Table 2
Energy density categories and examples of foods in each category

Energy Density Category	Energy Density Range (Calories per Gram)	How to Eat	Examples of Foods
Very low energy density	0.0–0.6	Free foods to eat anytime	Most fruits and vegetables, broth-based soups, nonfat milk
Low energy density	0.6–1.5	Eat reasonable portions	Cooked grains, low-fat meats, beans and legumes, low-fat mixed dishes, such as chili and pasta
Medium energy density	1.5–4.0	Manage portions	Meats, cheese, bread, snack foods such as popcorn and pretzels, mixed dishes such as pizza and macaroni and cheese
High energy density	4.0–9.0	Carefully manage portions and frequency of eating	Crackers, chips, cookies, nuts, butter, oils

Adapted from The Ultimate Volumetrics Diet: Smart, Simple, Science-Based Strategies for Losing Weight and Keeping it Off by Barbara Rolls, PhD with Mindy Hermann, RD. Copyright © 2012 by Barbara Rolls, PhD. *Courtesy of* HarperCollins Publishers.

Strategies to Increase the Proportion of Low-Energy-Dense Foods

Substitute lower-energy-dense foods for higher-energy-dense food

In order to emphasize the importance of eating low-energy-dense foods, the dietary guidelines include MyPlate to communicate to the public (https://www.choosemyplate.gov).[37] MyPlate reminds people that half of their meal should be vegetables and fruits. An advantage to emphasizing the proportions of dietary components that comprise a healthy diet is that the message can be applied regardless of absolute energy needs.

But does such advice affect behavior? Numerous studies show that the portion of a food that is served affects intake, such that the bigger the portion, the greater the intake.[4,38–41] Increasing the proportion and, thus, the portion size of vegetables and fruits can increase their intake; but it is important that they are relatively palatable compared with the other foods available.[42] Thus, when advising patients to adopt MyPlate, they should be encouraged to find strategies to increase the palatability while not greatly increasing the energy density of the vegetables and fruits. The addition of herbs and spices or the use of moderate amounts of healthy fats and sauces can encourage vegetable consumption.[43,44] Providing a variety of vegetables has been shown to increase vegetable intake compared with just offering one.[45] Although increasing the portion of vegetables at a meal can increase vegetable intake, it will not necessarily reduce energy intake. In order to decrease energy intake at the meal, larger portions of vegetables or fruits must be substituted for foods higher in energy density so that the overall energy density of the meal is lowered.[46] See **Fig. 3** for an example of how substituting lower-energy-dense foods for higher-energy-dense foods can create a more satisfying meal.

Decrease the energy density of the main course

Because the main course or entrée often contributes the most calories to a meal, a reduction in its energy density can significantly decrease energy intake at a meal. Importantly, studies show that lower-energy-dense entrées still satisfy hunger and

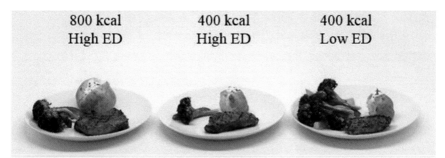

Fig. 3. These 3 plates all contain steak, a baked potato with toppings, and vegetables. The plate on the far left contains 800 calories, which is almost half of a day's worth. However, if as shown in the middle picture, the portions of all foods are decreased to provide a 400-calorie meal, they do not seem very satisfying. The picture on the right also provides 400 calories but provides a more satisfying meal by increasing the portions of low-energy-dense foods, reducing the fat content, and moderating the protein portion. ED, energy density. (*Courtesy of* The Penn State Laboratory for the Study of Human Ingestive Behavior, University Park, PA.)

do not lead to compensation by consuming more food later in the day.[47] Practical methods for modifying the energy density of an entrée include simple shifts, such as reducing unhealthy fat and substituting water-rich ingredients, such as fruits or vegetables for those higher in energy density.[48–50] For individuals who do not particularly like vegetables, the covert incorporation of vegetables into meals has been shown to improve diet quality and manage energy intake.[51,52]

Add a low-energy-dense first course
Another way to increase the proportion of low-energy-dense foods and reduce dietary energy density is through the addition of a low-energy-dense first course. "Filling up first" with a 100- to 150-calorie broth-based soup, leafy green salad, or whole fresh fruit before a meal is a simple strategy to lower the intake of higher-energy-dense main dishes and decrease meal energy intake.[34,38,53–57]

These strategies to increase the consumption of low-energy-dense foods and reduce those higher in energy density are flexible; patients can choose which foods to substitute and how the substitution will fit into their diet. They should be encouraged to try several strategies until they find an approach that they can sustain.

Strategies to Enhance Satiety and Meet Nutrient Needs with a Low-Energy-Dense Eating Pattern

Manage fat to lower energy density and moderate energy intake
For years, scientists thought reducing dietary fat was the key to weight management; but now evidence from multiple clinical trials shows that both low- and moderate-fat diets combined with an energy restriction can be used to achieve weight loss.[14,15,58] The government guidelines recommend a range of fat intake (**Table 3**) to meet daily energy requirements. The range allows individuals to make adjustments to fat intake in their dietary pattern based on food or cultural preferences in order to promote adherence.[8] Recent studies show success at weight loss at both the high and low ends of government-recommended fat intakes.[11,58]

Although there is a range in the amount of fat that is recommended in an eating pattern for weight loss, consuming too much fat can lead to a higher-energy-dense diet and weight gain.[7] Because of the high energy density of high-fat foods, their portion size needs to be moderated to stay within recommended energy intakes.

Table 3
Summary of nutritional goals and practical dietary strategies for weight loss

Element	Nutritional Goal	Recommendation
Fat	20%–35% of total calorie intake	Fat is high in energy density: Choose appropriate portions of healthy fats to improve diet quality and meet nutritional needs. • Substitute lower-fat foods for those higher in fat. • Include monounsaturated and polyunsaturated fats.
Protein	10%–35% of total calorie intake	Include protein to create satisfying meals and meet nutrient needs. • Include lean meats, poultry without skin, fish, eggs, legumes, tofu, and low-fat dairy products.
Carbohydrate	45%–65% of total calorie intake	Switch to whole grains instead of refined grains. • Examples include wheat, brown rice, oats, barley, and corn.
Fiber	20–35 g/d	Include fiber to help increase satiety. • Add legumes, fruits, vegetables, and whole grains.
Added sugar	Limit to <10% of total calorie intake	Limit foods and beverages containing added sugars. • Main sources of added sugars are snacks, sweets, and beverages. • Nonnutritive sweeteners can be a substitute.
Beverages	—	Select low-calorie beverages. • Water is the best choice. • Limit intake of alcoholic beverages.

Dietary Strategy	Recommendation
Monitor portions	Choose appropriately sized portions to help meet daily energy requirements. • Serve large portions of very-low- and low-energy-dense foods. • Serve smaller, less frequent portions of medium-energy-dense foods. • Limit portions of high-energy-dense foods.
Increase the proportion of lower-energy-dense foods	Lower-energy-dense foods provide satisfying portions to help increase satiety. • Fill half the plate with fruits and vegetables. • Start the meal with a first course broth-based soup or salad. • Substitute fruits and vegetables for higher-energy-dense ingredients.

Some methods for moderating fat intake at meals include switching to lower-fat alternatives, such as grilled chicken instead of fried chicken or low-fat Greek yogurt instead of sour cream. Shifts should also be made to decrease the amount of solid fats, which contain saturated and trans fat, and to substitute with oils containing polyunsaturated and monounsaturated fats to improve diet quality and overall health.[8] Patients should focus on using healthy fats in moderate amounts that improve their diet's palatability.

Include protein and fiber to create satisfying meals
Both protein and fiber have been suggested to promote satiety or feelings of fullness. Individuals are often reluctant to make changes to their dietary pattern because they

do not want to feel hungry, and higher protein intakes are frequently recommended to help manage hunger and increase satiety.[59–61] Protein is described as the most satiating macronutrient, and multiple studies suggest that incorporating more protein can increase satiety and decrease daily energy intake.[62,63] However, other laboratory-based studies have shown that when energy density is controlled, the amount of protein served during a meal had no influence on daily energy intake or satiety.[64] Research needs to continue to investigate the satiating properties of protein and to further evaluate the amounts and types of protein that show promise for body weight management.[14,62,63,65,66] Patients should be encouraged to incorporate recommended amounts of lean protein sources, such as grilled chicken breast, legumes, or low-fat dairy, to create satisfying low-energy-dense meals.[34] **Table 3** provides nutritional guidance on recommended amounts of protein and lean protein sources to include in a healthy eating pattern.

Dietary fiber is thought to promote feelings of fullness by increasing chewing time, promoting stomach expansion, and decreasing absorption efficiency.[67] Studies show that increasing fiber at meals can lead to decreased energy intake and increased ratings of fullness.[68,69] Population-based studies suggest that diets containing higher amounts of fiber are associated with lower body weights and reduced disease risks.[70] Some randomized controlled trials evaluating the addition of fiber-rich foods, such as legumes, have also found increased fiber to be beneficial for weight management.[68] Fiber is often found in foods low in energy density, such as fruits and vegetables; choosing fiber-rich foods can help enhance satiety, improve overall health, and support weight management (see **Table 3**).[34,70]

Manage added sugar intake and consider nonnutritive sweeteners

A goal to reduce consumption of foods and beverages containing added sugars should be a part of every weight loss program.[34] The main sources of added sugars are beverages (which are discussed next), snacks, and sweets.[8] Foods such as fruits, vegetables, and dairy products also contain sugar; but these items contain natural sugars, and the recommendations limit added sugars typically found in nutrient-poor, higher-energy-dense foods and beverages.[8,71]

One option to help manage added sugar and energy intake is the use of nonnutritive sweeteners.[71,72] Although observational studies suggest a link between nonnutritive sweeteners and weight gain, randomized controlled trials have consistently found nonnutritive sweeteners to support weight loss.[72,73] Multiple organizations support the use of nonnutritive sweeteners to help moderate energy intake when they are substituted for a higher-energy-dense food, like sugar.[71]

Choose water and other low-calorie beverages to satisfy thirst

Even though most beverages are low in energy density because of their high water content, added sugar or fat can quickly increase the number of calories a beverage contains. This means that patients should be encouraged to choose water and other low-calorie beverages in place of higher-calorie beverages. Beverages have been suggested to have low satiating properties, in that people do not reduce their food intake to compensate for calories in beverages.[34,74,75] This point reinforces the importance of messages to patients emphasizing that drinking caloric beverages can lead to increased energy intake.[34,74] Eliminating or reducing caloric beverage consumption is a promising strategy for weight management; research suggests substituting water or diet beverages for caloric beverages can improve weight loss.[72,73]

Beverages that individuals may be unwilling to eliminate from their dietary pattern are those containing alcohol. Alcoholic beverages can be included in moderation within recommended calorie limits.[8] Individuals need to be aware that energy from alcohol is poorly compensated for, meaning that they are unlikely to eat less because alcohol has been consumed at a meal or snack. So if having an alcoholic drink, they should consume lower-energy-dense foods to help control energy intake.[34,75,76] When consuming alcoholic beverages, patients should make sure the energy content fits within their own personal eating pattern for weight management.[8,75,77]

Daily Intake Patterns That can Help to Lower Dietary Energy Density

Breakfast

The pattern of food consumption over a day as either meals or snacks could affect weight management. Most members of the National Weight Control Registry, people who have lost 30 lb or more and kept it off for at least a year, report eating breakfast every day as a strategy to help with maintenance of weight loss.[78] Epidemiologic studies have also found breakfast consumption to be associated with lower body weights and lower daily energy density.[78–81] However, controlled intervention trials have not found that consistently eating breakfast leads to greater weight loss than skipping the meal.[81,82] If individuals are habitual breakfast eaters, including higher amounts of protein and fiber during breakfast may help increase satiety, decrease energy intake, and lower dietary energy density.[80,81]

Snacking

The definition of snacking varies, but it commonly refers to the consumption of foods and beverages between regular meals.[83] Research suggests that eating more than the standard 3 times per day has minimal influence on energy intake but that eating less than 3 times per day may negatively influence energy regulation.[84] However, as the frequency of eating or snacking increases, the energy consumed from snacks high in energy density can also increase.[85] Patients should moderate their intake from medium- and high-energy-dense snacks (like chips, pretzels, and confectionary) to keep snack intake less than 200 calories per day and stay within energy needs.[8,34] They should instead choose lower-energy-dense snacks so that they can have a larger, more satisfying portion for the same 200 calories, while also enhancing satiety and improving diet quality.[83] Evidence on the influence of snacking on body weight is mixed; but it does indicate that choosing low-energy-dense snacks, such as vegetables and fruits, helps moderate energy intake.[83,86]

TOOLS TO ACHIEVE HEALTHY DIETARY PATTERNS

Providing individuals with tools and resources for managing portion sizes can help them make sustainable changes to their dietary patterns. Tools can promote additional structure or provide visual cues to help individuals manage energy intake in the current obesogenic environment. This section discusses current tools that patients can use to help support weight loss and weight loss maintenance.

Incorporate Preportioned Foods or Meal Replacements

The use of preportioned foods and meal replacements can help moderate intake by providing a structured meal plan with appropriate portion sizes.[87–89] Preportioned foods include liquid meal replacements, single-serving snacks, and frozen entrées packaged and portioned for consumption at a single meal. Several randomized controlled trials show that replacing one or 2 meals a day with liquid and solid preportioned foods can lead to substantial weight loss.[82,87,88,90]

Although preportioned foods and meal replacements have proven to be effective for weight loss, they have only recently been compared with other portion-control strategies. The Portion Control Strategies Trial compared the effectiveness of 3 diet strategies (standard advice, portion selection, and preportioned foods) in a behavioral weight loss trial.[91] The trial found that the preportioned foods group lost weight at a faster rate but also regained weight at a greater rate compared with the other groups.[91] Adherence to the preportioned foods strategy declined over time, possibly because of an increase in feelings of deprivation or to a decrease in the provision of vouchers for the preportioned foods.[91] Further development is needed to determine the most effective strategies for incorporating preportioned foods in diets for weight management.

Include Portion-Control Tools

Portion-control tools, such as plates, bowls, scales, serving spoons, measuring cups, and photographs, may help individuals to moderate energy intake by providing visual cues and teaching appropriate serving sizes.[87] The use of smaller dishware and utensils has been promoted; however, simply using smaller plates has not consistently been found to decrease energy intake and has not been tested for weight loss.[92–94] Interventions have found that using plates designed to teach appropriate proportions to control energy intake (such as those based on MyPlate) promotes weight loss.[95–97] The studies found that the portion-control plate groups achieved greater short-term weight loss at 6 months than the control groups.[95–97] However, the studies reported poor compliance and high attrition rates, indicating that strategies are needed to maintain continued use of these portion-control tools.

Smartphone applications provide another tool that may help control energy intake by providing a platform for individuals to monitor their dietary intake.[98,99] Self-monitoring helps individuals become aware of the foods and portion sizes they are consuming and has been associated with increased and sustained weight loss.[100–102] Digital photography can be used to help monitor intake by providing estimates of food portion sizes.[103–105] However, using photographs with smartphone applications has limitations. It is difficult to measure and assess the energy density of the food in a photograph without knowing the recipes, and this limitation makes it challenging to estimate patients' energy intake. Portion-control tools using smartphone applications and photographs seem promising; but most are not evidenced based, so they require further development in order to be improved for use in weight loss interventions.[106]

Incorporate Government-Recommended Tools

A reduction in dietary energy intake is the foundation for all weight loss dietary patterns. Individuals are typically told to reduce energy intake by 30% or 500 to 750 calories per day.[15] On average, this equates to women consuming between 1200 to 1500 calories per day and men consuming 1500 to 1800 calories per day.[15] However, energy needs can vary widely based on body composition and physical activity level and must be reevaluated as weight is lost. To adjust for changing energy requirements, the National Institutes of Health has launched the Body Weight Planner based on mathematical models to create personalized energy prescriptions according to an individual's eating and exercise habits (refer to Ch14 in this book).[107,108] The Body Weight Planner can be used in combination with the US Department of Agriculture's Super Tracker and MyPlate to help individuals create personalized eating patterns and monitor food intake.[109]

FUTURE DIRECTIONS

Over the past several decades, obesity research has debated what the optimal diet is for weight loss and weight maintenance. Emerging research indicates that diet recommendations should consider the variability that stems from individual character-istics.[110,111] For example, individuals with high insulin secretion or high fasting plasma glucose may achieve greater weight loss on a diet with a low glycemic load compared with normoglycemic individuals.[111–113] Future research should take a more personal-ized approach to determine how individuals' behaviors, genes, or metabolic profiles influence their weight.[110,111] The rapid advances in technology and biology will pro-vide exciting new opportunities to collect information that will allow dietary patterns to be individually tailored for effective and sustainable weight loss.

SUMMARY

Obesity is a multifactorial disease, with both individual and environmental factors influ-encing dietary adherence.[114,115] Dietary approaches with a reduction in energy intake that have led to success at weight loss have focused on macronutrient composition and food patterns. A unifying principle for weight loss across eating patterns is dietary energy density.[12,16,116–118] There is a variety of strategies and tools that individuals can use to achieve a personalized healthy eating pattern, and physicians or nutrition professionals can provide support and specific dietary advice on changes to improve an individual's eating behaviors.[8] **Table 3** provides a summary of nutritional goals and recommendations that can be used to help patients create sustainable and satisfying low-energy-dense eating patterns for weight loss.

REFERENCES

1. Ogden CL, Carroll MD, Fryar CD, et al. Prevalence of obesity among adults and youth: United States, 2011–2014. NCHS data brief, no 219. Hyattsville (MD): Na-tional Center for Health Statistics; 2015.
2. World Health Organization. Global Health Observatory data: overweight and obesity. Revised 2017. Available at: www.who.int/gho/ncd/risk_factors/overweight/en/. Accessed April 2, 2017.
3. World Health Organization. Diet, nutrition and the prevention of chronic diseases (WHO Technical Report Series, No. 916). Report of the joint WHO/FAO expert consultation. Published 2014. Geneva (Switzerland): World Health Organization; 2003. Available at: http://www.who.int/dietphysicalactivity/publications/trs916/summary/en/. [Accessed 2 April 2017].
4. Rolls BJ, Morris EL, Roe LS. Portion size of food affects energy intake in normal-weight and overweight men and women. Am J Clin Nutr 2003;76(6):1207–13.
5. Karl JP, Roberts SB. Energy density, energy intake, and body weight regulation in adults. Adv Nutr 2014;5(6):835–50.
6. Livingstone MBE, Pourshahidi LK. Portion size and obesity. Adv Nutr 2014;5(6): 829–34.
7. Vernarelli JA, Mitchell DC, Rolls BJ, et al. Dietary energy density is associated with obesity and other biomarkers of chronic disease in US adults. Eur J Nutr 2015;54(1):59–65.
8. U.S. Department of Health and Human Services and U.S. Department of Agriculture. 2015–2020 Dietary guidelines for Americans. 8th edition. Pub-lished December 2015. Available at: http://health.gov/dietaryguidelines/2015/guidelines/. Accessed February 11, 2017.
9. Drewnowski A. Taste preferences and food intake. Annu Rev Nutr 1997;17(1): 237–53.
10. Bray GA, Siri-Tarino PW. The role of macronutrient content in the diet for weight management. Endocrinol Metab Clin North Am 2016;45(3):581–604.

11. Hooper L, Abdelhamid A, Moore HJ, et al. Effect of reducing total fat intake on body weight: systematic review and meta-analysis of randomised controlled trials and cohort studies. BMJ 2012;35:e7666.

12. Sacks FM, Bray GA, Carey VJ, et al. Comparison of weight-loss diets with different compositions of fat, protein, and carbohydrates. N Engl J Med 2009; 360(9):859–73.

13. Fogelholm M, Anderssen S, Gunnarsdottir I, et al. Dietary macronutrients and food consumption as determinants of long-term weight change in adult population: a systematic literature review. Food Nutr Res 2012;56. https://doi.org/10.3402/fnr.v56i0.19103.

14. Makis A, Foster GD. Dietary approaches to the treatment of obesity. Psychiatr Clin North Am 2011;34(4):813–27.

15. Jensen MD, Ryan DH, Apovian CM, et al. 2013 AHA/ACC/TOS guideline for the management of overweight and obesity in adults: a report of the American College of Cardiology/American Heart Association Task Force on Practice Guidelines and the Obesity Society. Circulation 2014;129(25 Suppl 2):S102–38.

16. Schwingshackl L, Hoffmann G. Long-term effects of low-fat diets either low or high in protein on cardiovascular and metabolic risk factors: a systematic review and meta-analysis. Nutr J 2013;12:48.

17. Foster GD, Wyatt HR, Hill JO, et al. Weight and metabolic outcomes after 2 years on a low-carbohydrate versus low-fat diet: a randomized trial. Ann Intern Med 2010;153(3):147–57.

18. Champagne C, Burton J, DeCesare L, et al. Energy density and adherence as predictors of weight loss in the POUNDS LOST study. FASEB J 2015;29(1). 117.5.

19. Champagne CM, Bray G, Sacks F, et al. Fiber intake, dietary energy density, and diet-type predict 6-month weight-loss in free-living adults who adhered to prescribed macronutrient and energy composition of varying diets. FASEB J 2017;31(1). 796.3.

20. Miketinas D, Bray G, Sacks F, et al. Fiber intake, dietary energy density, and adherence to diet assignment are positively associated with weight-loss in free-living adults consuming calorie-restricted diets at 6-month follow-up: the POUNDS LOST study. FASEB J 2017;31(1). 796.2.

21. American Heart Association. The American Heart Association's diet and lifestyle recommendations. Revised August 2015. Available at: http://www.heart.org/HEARTORG/HealthyLiving/HealthyEating/Nutrition/The-American-Heart-Associations-Diet-and-Lifestyle-Recommendations_UCM_305855_Article.jsp#.WROI51LMzus. Accessed May 10, 2017.

22. Thorning TK, Bertram HC, Bonjour JP, et al. Whole dairy matrix or single nutrients in assessment of health effects: current evidence and knowledge gaps. Am J Clin Nutr 2017;105(5). https://doi.org/10.3945/ajcn.116.151548.

23. Karanja NM, Obarzanek E, Lin PH, et al. Descriptive characteristics of the dietary patterns used in the dietary approaches to stop hypertension trial. DASH Collaborative Research Group. J Am Diet Assoc 2005;99:S19–27.

24. Ledikwe JH, Rolls BJ, Smiciklas-Wright H, et al. Reductions in dietary energy density are associated with weight loss in overweight and obese participants in the PREMIER trial. Am J Clin Nutr 2007;85(5):1212–21.

25. Davis C, Bryan J, Hodgson J, et al. Definition of the Mediterranean diet: a literature review. Nutrients 2015;7(11):9139–53.

26. Ledikwe JH, Blanck HM, Khan LK, et al. Dietary energy density is associated with energy intake and weight status in U.S. adults. Am J Clin Nutr 2006;83: 1362–8.

27. Fung TT, Pan A, Hou T, et al. Long-term change in diet quality is associated with body weight change in men and women. J Nutr 2015;145(8):1850–6.

28. Rolls BJ, Roe LS, Beach AM, et al. Provision of foods differing in energy density affects long-term weight loss. Obes Res 2005;13(6):1052–60.

29. Ello-Martin JA, Roe LS, Ledikwe JH, et al. Dietary energy density in the treatment of obesity: a year-long trial comparing 2 weight loss diets. Am J Clin Nutr 2007;85:1465–77.

30. Raynor HA, Anderson AM, Miller GD, et al. Partial meal replacement plan and quality of the diet at 1 year: action for health in diabetes (Look AHEAD) trial. J Acad Nutr Diet 2015;115(5):731–42.

31. Stelmach-Mardas M, Rodacki T, Dobrowolska-Iwanek J, et al. Link between food energy density and body weight changes in obese adults. Nutrients 2016;8(4):229.

32. Greene LF, Malpede CZ, Henson CS, et al. Weight maintenance 2 years after participation in a weight loss program promoting low energy dense foods. Obesity 2006;14(10):1795–801.

33. Lowe MR, Butryn ML, Thomas JG, et al. Meal replacements, reduced energy density eating, and weight loss maintenance in primary care patients: a randomized controlled trial. Obesity 2014;22(1):94–100.

34. Rolls BJ. The ultimate volumetrics diet. New York: Morrow; 2012.

35. Rolls BJ. The relationship between dietary energy density and energy intake. Physiol Behav 2009;97(5):609–15.

36. Centers for Disease Control Prevention and Health Promotion, Division of nutrition, physical activity, and obesity, low energy dense foods and weight management: cutting calories while controlling hunger. Available at: https://www.cdc.gov/nccdphp/dnpa/nutrition/pdf/r2p_energy_density.pdf. Accessed February 23, 2017.

37. United States Department of Agriculture. Choose MyPlate. Available at: https://www.choosemyplate.gov. Accessed June 1, 2017.

38. Rolls BJ, Roe LS, Meengs JS. Salad and satiety: energy density and portion size of a first course salad affect energy intake at lunch. J Am Diet Assoc 2004;104: 1570–6.

39. Rolls BJ, Roe LS, Kral TVE, et al. Increasing the portion size of a packaged snack increases energy intake in mean and women. Appetite 2004;42(1):63–9.

40. Flood JE, Roe LS, Rolls BJ. The effects of beverage type and portion size on beverage consumption and lunch intake. Appetite 2005;44:350.

41. Rolls BJ, Roe LS, Meengs JS. The effect of large portion size on energy intake is sustained for 11 days. Obesity 2007;15(6):1535–43.

42. Roe LS, Kling SM, Rolls BJ. What is eaten when all of the foods at a meal are served in large portions? Appetite 2016;99:1–9.

43. Peters JC, Polsky S, Stark R, et al. The influence of herbs and spices on overall liking of reduced fat food. Appetite 2014;79:183–8.

44. Zhaoping L, Krak M, Zerlin A, et al. The impact of spices on vegetable consumption: a pilot study. Food Nutr Sci 2015;6:437–44.

45. Meengs JS, Roe LS, Rolls BJ. Vegetable variety: an effective strategy to increase vegetable intake in adults. J Acad Nutr Diet 2012;112(8):1211–5.

46. Rolls BJ, Roe LS, Meengs JS. Portion size can be used strategically to increase vegetable consumption in adults. Am J Clin Nutr 2010;91:913–22.

47. Bell EA, Castellanos VH, Pelkman CL, et al. Energy density of foods affects energy intake in normal-weight women. Am J Clin Nutr 1998;67(3):412–20.
48. Blatt AD, Roe LS, Rolls BJ. Hidden vegetables: an effective strategy to reduce energy intake and increase vegetable intake in adults. Am J Clin Nutr 2011; 93(4):756–63.
49. Williams RA, Roe LS, Rolls BJ. Comparison of three methods to reduce energy density. Effects on daily energy intake. Appetite 2013;66:75–83.
50. Chang UJ, Hong YH, Suh HJ, et al. Lowering the energy density of parboiled rice by adding water-rich vegetables can decrease total energy intake in a parboiled rice-based diet without reducing satiety on healthy women. Appetite 2010;55:338–42.
51. Appleton KM, Hemingway A, Saulais L, et al. Increasing vegetable intakes: rationale and systematic review of published interventions. Eur J Nutr 2016; 55(3):869–96.
52. Appleton KM, McGill R, Neville C, et al. Barriers to increasing fruit and vegetable intakes in the older population of Northern Ireland: low levels of liking and low awareness of current recommendations. Public Health Nutr 2010;13(4):514.
53. Buckland NJ, Finlayson G, Hetherington MM. Slimming starters. Intake of a diet-congruent food reduces meal intake in active dieters. Appetite 2013;71:430–7.
54. Flood-Obbagy JE, Rolls BJ. The effect of fruit in different form on energy intake and satiety at a meal. Appetite 2009;52:416–22.
55. Rolls BJ, Bell EA, Thorwart ML. Water incorporated into food but not served with a food decreases energy intake in lean women. Am J Clin Nutr 1999;70:448–55.
56. Flood JE, Rolls BJ. Soup preloads in a variety of forms reduce meal energy intake. Appetite 2007;49:626–34.
57. Roe LS, Meengs JS, Rolls BJ. Salad and satiety: the effect of timing of salad consumption on meal energy intake. Appetite 2012;58(1):242–8.
58. Tobias D, Chen M, Manson JE, et al. Effect of low-fat vs other diet interventions on long-term weight change in adults: a systematic review and meta-analysis. Lancet Diabetes Endocrinol 2015;3(12):968–79.
59. Westerterp-Plantenga MS, Lemmens SG, Wetserterp KR. Dietary protein- its role in satiety, energetics, weight loss, and health. Br J Nutr 2012;108:S105–12.
60. Bellisimo N, Akhavan T. Effect of macronutrient composition on short-term food intake and weight loss. Adv Nutr 2015;6:302S–8S.
61. Hetherington MM, Cunningham K, Dye L, et al. Potential benefits of satiety to the consumer: scientific considerations. Nutr Res Rev 2013;26:22–38.
62. Dhillion J, Craig BA, Leidy HJ, et al. The effects of increased protein intake on fullness: a meta-analysis and its limitations,. J Acad Nutr Diet 2016;116:968–83.
63. Leidy HJ, Clifton PM, Astrup A, et al. The role of protein in weight loss and maintenance. Am J Clin Nutr 2015;101(6):1320S–9S.
64. Blatt AD, Roe LS, Rolls BJ. Increasing the protein content of meals and its effect on daily energy intake. J Am Diet Assoc 2011;111:290–4.
65. Chambers L, McCrickerd K, Yeomans MR. Optimising foods for satiety. Food Sci Tech 2015;41:149–60.
66. Clifton PM, Condo D, Keogh JB. Long term weight maintenance after advice to consume low carbohydrate, higher protein diets- a systematic review and meta-analysis. Nutr Metab Cardiovasc Dis 2014;24:224–5.
67. Slavin JL. Dietary fiber and body weight. Nutrition 2005;21:411–8.
68. Kim SJ, de Souza RJ, Choo VL, et al. Effects of dietary pulse consumption on body weight: a systematic review and meta-analysis of randomized controlled trials. Am J Clin Nutr 2016;103:1213–23.

69. Wanders AJ, van den Borne JJ, de Graff C, et al. Effects of dietary fibre on subjective appetite, energy intake and body weight: a systematic review of randomized control trials. Obes Rev 2011;12(9):724–36.

70. Dahl WJ, Stewart ML. Position of the academy of nutrition and dietetics: health implications of dietary fiber. J Acad Nutr Diet 2015;115(11):1861–70.

71. Fitch C, Keim KS, Academy of Nutrition and Dietetics. Position of the Academy of Nutrition and Dietetics: use of nutritive and nonnutritive sweetners. J Acad Nutr Diet 2012;112:739–58.

72. Peters JC, Beck J. Low calorie sweetener (LCS) use and energy balance. Physiol Behav 2016;164:524–8.

73. Bellisle F. Intense sweeteners, appetite for the sweet taste, and relationship to weight management. Curr Obes Rep 2015;4:106–10.

74. De Graaf C. Why liquid energy results in overconsumption. Proc Nutr Soc 2011; 70:162–70.

75. Poppitt SD. Beverage consumption: are alcoholic and sugary drinks tipping the balance towards overweight and obesity? Nutrients 2015;7:6700–18.

76. Caton SJ, Nolan LJ, Hetherington MM. Alcohol, appetite and loss of restraint. Curr Obes Rep 2015;4:99–105.

77. Traversy G, Chaput JP. Alcohol consumption and obesity: an update. Curr Obes Rep 2015;4:122–30.

78. Hill JO, Thompson H, Wyatt H. Weight maintenance: what's missing? J Am Diet Assoc 2005;105:S63–6.

79. Wing RR, Phelan S. Long-term weight loss maintenance. Am J Clin Nutr 2005; 82:222S–5S.

80. Kant AK, Andon MB, Angelopoulous TJ, et al. Association of breakfast energy density with diet quality and body mass index in American adults: National Health and Nutrition Examination Surveys, 1999-2004. Am J Clin Nutr 2008; 88(5):1396–404.

81. Leidy HJ, Gwin JA, Roenfeldt CA, et al. Evaluating the intervention-based evidence surrounding the causal role of breakfast on markers of weight management, with specific focus on breakfast composition and size. Adv Nutr 2016;7: 563S–75S.

82. Raynor HA, Champagne CM. Position of the Academy of Nutrition and Dietetics: interventions for the treatment of overweight and obesity in adults. J Acad Nutr Diet 2016;116(1):129–47.

83. Njike VY, Smith TM, Shuval O, et al. Snack food, satiety, and weight. Adv Nutr 2016;7:866–78.

84. Leidy HJ, Campbell WW. The effect of eating frequency on appetite control and food intake: brief synopsis of controlled feeding studies. J Nutr 2011;141(1): 154–7.

85. Bes-Rastrollo M, Sanchez-Villegas A, Basterra-Gortari FJ, et al. Prospective study of self-reported usual snacking and weight gain in a Mediterranean cohort: the SUN project. Clin Nutr 2010;29(3):323–30.

86. Bellisle F. Meals and snacking, diet quality and energy balance. Physiol Behav 2014;132:38–43.

87. Rolls BJ. What is the role of portion control in weight management? Int J Obes 2014;38:S1–8.

88. Wing RR, Jeffery RW, Burton LR, et al. Food provision vs structured meal plans in the behavioral treatment of obesity. Int J Obes Relat Metab Disord 1996;20(1): 56–62.

89. Heymsfield S, Van Mierlo C, Van Der Knaap H, et al. Weight management using a meal replacement strategy: meta and pooling analysis from six studies. Int J Obes 2003;27:537–49.

90. Raynor HA, Anderson AM, Miller GD, et al. Partial Meal Replacement Plan and Quality of the Diet at 1 Year: Action for Health in Diabetes (Look AHEAD) Trial. J Acad Nutr Diet 2015;115(5):731–42. https://doi.org/10.1016/j.jand.2014.11.003.

91. Rolls BJ, Roe LS, James BL, et al. Does the incorporation of portion-control strategies in a behavioral program improve weight loss in a 1-year randomized controlled trial? Int J Obes 2017;41:434–42.

92. Rolls BJ, Roe LS, Halverson KH, et al. Using a smaller plate did not reduce energy intake at meals. Appetite 2007;49(3):652–60.

93. Robinson E, Nolan S, Tuber-Smith C, et al. Will smaller plates lead to smaller waists? A systematic review and meta-analysis of the effect that experimental manipulation of dishware size has on energy consumption. Obes Rev 2014; 15(10):812–21.

94. Ayaz A, Akyol A, Cetin C, et al. Effect of plate size on meal energy intake in normal weight women. Nutr Res Pract 2016;10(5):524–9.

95. Pedersen SD, Kang J, Kline GA. Portion control plate for weight loss in obese patients with type 2 diabetes mellitus: a controlled clinical trial. Arch Intern Med 2007;167(12):1277–83.

96. Kesman RL, Ebbert JO, Harris KI, et al. Portion control for the treatment of obesity in the primary care setting. BMC Res Notes 2011;4:346.

97. Huber JM, Shapiro JS, Wieland ML, et al. Telecoaching plus a portion control plate for weight care management: a randomized trial. Trials 2015;16:323.

98. Wharton CM, Johnston CS, Cunningham BK, et al. Dietary self-monitoring, but not dietary quality, improves with use of smartphone app technology in an 8-week weight loss trial. J Nutr Educ Behav 2014;46(5):440–4.

99. Sutton EF, Redman LM. Smartphone applications to aid weight loss and management: current perspectives. Diabetes Metab Syndr Obes 2016;9:213–6.

100. Fuller NR, Fong M, Gerofi J, et al. Comparison of an electronic versus traditional food diary for assessing dietary intake—a validation study. Obes Res Clin Pract 2017. https://doi.org/10.1016/j.orcp.2017.04.001.

101. Burke LE, Wang J, Sevick MA. Self-monitoring in weight loss: a systematic review of the literature. J Am Diet Assoc 2011;111(1):92–102.

102. Goldstein CM, Thomas JG, Wing RR, et al. Successful weight loss maintainers use health-tracking smartphone applications more than a nationally representative sample: comparison of the National Weight Control Registry to pew tracking for health. Obes Sci Pract 2017. https://doi.org/10.10002/osp4.102.

103. Jia W, Chen H-C, Yue Y, et al. Accuracy of food portion size estimation from digital pictures acquired by a chest-worn camera. Public Health Nutr 2014;17(8): 1671–81.

104. Martin CK, Nicklas T, Gunturk B, et al. Measuring food intake with digital photography. J Hum Nutr Diet 2014;27(Suppl 1):72–81.

105. Williamson DA, Allen HR, Martin PD, et al. Comparison of digital photography to weighed and visual estimation of portion sizes. J Am Diet Assoc 2003;103(9): 1139–45.

106. Rivera J, McPherson A, Hamilton J, et al. Mobile apps for weight management: a scoping review. JMIR Mhealth Uhealth 2016;4(3):e87.

107. Hall KD, Sacks G, Chandramohan D, et al. Quantification of the effect of energy imbalance on bodyweight. Lancet 2011;378. https://doi.org/10.1016/S0140-6736(11)60812-X.

108. National Institute of Diabetes and Digestive and Kidney Diseases. Body weight planner. Available at: https://www.niddk.nih.gov/health-information/health-topics/weight-control/body-weight-planner/Pages/bwp.aspx. Accessed May 8, 2017.

109. United States Department of Agriculture. Super tracker. Available at: https://www.supertracker.usda.gov/foodtracker.aspx. Accessed May 8, 2017.

110. Qi L. Personalized nutrition and obesity. Ann Med 2014;46(5):247–52.

111. Hjorth MF, Ritz C, Blaak EE, et al. Pretreatment fasting plasma glucose and insulin modify dietary weight loss success: results from 3 randomized clinical trials. Am J Clin Nutr 2017. https://doi.org/10.3945/ajcn.117.155200.

112. Pittas AG, Das SK, Hajduk CL, et al. A low-glycemic load diet facilitates greater weight loss in overweight adults with high insulin secretion but not in overweight adults with low insulin secretion in the CALERIE Trial. Diabetes Care 2005;28: 2939–41.

113. Ebbeling CB, Leidig MM, Feldman HA, et al. Effects of a low-glycemic load vs low-fat diet in obese young adults: a randomized trial. JAMA 2007;297: 2092–102.

114. Schwartz MB, Just DR, Chriqui JF, et al. Appetite self-regulation: environmental and policy influences on eating behaviors. Obesity 2017;25:S26–38.

115. Stevenson RJ, Mahmut M, Rooney K. Individual differences in the interoceptive states of hunger, fullness, and thirst. Appetite 2015;95:44–57.

116. Tapsell LC, Neale EP, Nolan-Clark DJ. Dietary patterns may sustain weight loss among adults. Curr Nutr Rep 2014;3(1):35–42.

117. Johnston BC, Kanters S, Bandayrel K, et al. Comparison of weight loss among named diet programs in overweight and obese adults. JAMA 2014;312(9): 923–33.

118. Raben A, Agerholm-Larson L, Flint A, et al. Meals with similar energy densities but rich in protein, fat, carbohydrate, or alcohol have different effects on energy expenditure and substrate metabolism but not on appetite or energy intake. Am J Clin Nutr 2003;77(1):99–100.

The Role of Behavioral Medicine in the Treatment of Obesity in Primary Care

Scott Kahan, MD, MPH[a,b,]*, Dawn K. Wilson, PhD[c],
Allison M. Sweeney, PhD[c]

KEYWORDS

- Behavioral medicine • Counseling • Motivational interviewing • Behavior change

KEY POINTS

- Behavioral medicine provides a framework for supporting patients to achieve changes in target health behaviors, such as smoking cessation or dietary and physical activity changes.
- Behavioral medicine fits alongside traditional medical treatments, such as pharmacotherapy and surgery, and in many cases can minimize the need for more intensive medical treatments, improve outcomes of these treatments, and improve adherence to medication prescriptions or postsurgical recommendations.
- Health care providers should be familiar with target behaviors for weight regulation and behavioral medicine techniques for behavior change counseling.

INTRODUCTION

Improving the quality of health care and population health are national public health priorities.[1] Although medical treatment is a central component of health care, it is estimated that access to health care explains just 10% of the variance in health outcomes and premature death, whereas behavioral patterns account for 40%, with the remaining variance being explained by environmental exposure (5%), social circumstances (15%), and genetic predispositions (30%).[2] Thus, modifying health-related behaviors through behavioral medicine should be a key component of optimal health care, especially with respect to the treatment of obesity and related chronic diseases. Behavioral medicine provides a framework for supporting patients to achieve changes in target health behaviors, such as smoking cessation or dietary and physical activity changes.

Disclosure Statement: None.
[a] Johns Hopkins Bloomberg School of Public Health, Baltimore, MD, USA; [b] George Washington University School of Medicine, 1020 19th Street NW, Suite 450, Washington, DC 20036, USA; [c] Department of Psychology, Barnwell College, University of South Carolina, 1512 Pendleton Street, Columbia, SC 29208, USA
* Corresponding author. 1020 19th Street NW, suite 450, Washington, DC 20036.
E-mail address: kahan@gwu.edu

Behavioral medicine fits alongside traditional medical treatments, such as pharmaco-therapy or surgery, and may minimize the need for more intensive medical treatments, and improve adherence to medication prescriptions or postsurgical recommendations.

Increasing evidence from randomized controlled trials suggests that improving self-regulation is an effective approach for promoting changes in health-related be-haviors, such as increasing physical activity and improving dietary intake. In essence, self-regulation is a system of conscious personal management that involves a process of guiding one's own thoughts, behaviors, and feelings to reach goals, using a range of behavioral strategies, such as self-monitoring, action planning, goal setting, and prob-lem solving. In this paper, we provide an overview of behavioral medicine counseling for obesity management in primary care, rooted in the "5 As" approach[3] to health behavior change, and then offer a basic outline of behavioral skills interventions (including positive communication skills) in which health care providers (HCPs) can use self-regulatory and behavioral strategies as a method for improving health-related behaviors among patients with obesity.

OVERVIEW OF TARGET BEHAVIOR AND RANDOMIZED CONTROLLED TRIALS FOR BEHAVIORAL INTERVENTIONS

A range of target behaviors have been identified as effective for weight regulation. Many of these come from the National Weight Control Registry, a two decades–old database of successful weight losers, and other investigations of long-term weight management. Some of the behaviors that are associated with successful weight loss and weight loss maintenance include[4–6]

- Self-monitoring and self-weighing
- Reduced calorie intake, initially focused on low-fat diets, but more recently shown that most dietary patterns intended to reduce caloric intake lead to near-equivalent weight loss magnitude
- Smaller and more frequent meals/snacks throughout the day
- Increased physical activity, which has some contribution to initial weight loss but has been shown to be one of the most consistent predictors of long-term weight loss maintenance
- Eating breakfast
- More frequent at-home meals compared with restaurant and fast-food meals
- Reducing screen time
- Use of portion-controlled meals or meal substitutes
- Reducing sweetened beverage intake

These and other behavioral goals have been studied in several large randomized controlled trials that incorporate a range of behavioral skills training approaches to help patients achieve and maintain target behaviors. A seminal example is the Dia-betes Prevention Program (DPP).[7,8] The DPP was a 27-center randomized controlled trial that compared the effectiveness of a weight loss–focused lifestyle intervention with a metformin group and a placebo group, for preventing the onset of type 2 dia-betes among high-risk individuals with prediabetes and obesity. Participants in the lifestyle intervention group set weight loss and physical activity goals. They worked individually with a case manager who delivered a core curriculum of behavior change counseling and behavioral skills training. The tailored counseling visits consisted of a weigh-in, review of self-monitoring records, presentation of educational information, identification of barriers to weight loss and physical activity, and the development of a weekly action plan for meeting the behavioral and weight loss goals.

Across a 3-year follow-up period, diabetes incidence was lowest among the lifestyle-intervention group, with the lifestyle-intervention group showing a reduced risk of onset of 58% and the medication group showing a reduced risk of 31%, relative to the control group. In a follow-up study that evaluated outcomes 10 years later, the cumulative incidence of diabetes remained lowest among individuals assigned originally to the lifestyle-intervention group, despite the counseling ending after 3 years.[9] Of note, in line with research suggesting that chronic illnesses cluster,[10] the lifestyle changes made by participants in the DPP seem to have also influenced their risk for developing cardiovascular disease.[11] Over the 10-year follow-up period, all three groups showed a significant reduction in systolic blood pressure, diastolic blood pressure, and low-density lipoprotein cholesterol, although the lifestyle intervention group achieved these benefits with less use of lipid and blood pressure medications.

Several other randomized controlled trials have reported significant effects of behavioral counseling for weight loss, diabetes prevention, and other health outcomes.[12,13] Weight loss–focused behavioral counseling also improves health outcomes among patients who already have chronic illnesses. The Look AHEAD (Action for Health in Diabetes) study[14] was the first randomized controlled trial to provide direct evidence about the longitudinal health benefits of behavioral counseling and lifestyle changes among patients with a chronic illness. The Look AHEAD trial evaluated the outcomes of behavioral counseling and intentional weight loss among individuals with obesity and type 2 diabetes. Participants were randomly assigned to complete a diabetes support and educational program or an intensive lifestyle intervention program that included targeting behavioral skills for weight loss designed to help patients lose at least 7% of their initial weight and to increase physical activity to at least 175 minutes per week.

The lifestyle intervention was consistent with the methods used in the DPP, but adapted for individuals already diagnosed with type 2 diabetes. Phase one of the program was designed to help patients achieve initial weight loss through weekly on-site sessions with a behavioral counselor during the first 6 months and three sessions per month during months 7 to 12. Via a mixture of group and individual sessions, participants received information and counseling about behavioral change and weight management. Participants were instructed to track their daily caloric intake and were provided with a portion-controlled meal plan or meal replacement options. Individualized support was offered to help patients identify problem behaviors and barriers, develop behavior change plans with specific goals and action plans, and assist with problem solving.

During Years 2 to 4, phase two of the program was designed to help patients maintain their weight loss and consisted of bimonthly individual sessions in which a behavioral counselor would reinforce strategies introduced in Year 1 (eg, reviewing self-monitoring records, problem solving, goal setting). Participants had the opportunity to participate in a refresher group program and a reunion group program to reconnect with acquaintances from phase one. During phase three of the program (Year 5 and beyond), participants were encouraged to attend monthly, individual on-site sessions with a behavioral counselor. The purpose of these sessions was to help review successes and challenges in maintaining weight and physical activity goals, and to provide support for dietary and physical activity lapses and weight regain. Participants were followed for 13.5 years.[15]

The behavioral intervention was highly effective at helping patients to change behaviors and lose weight. In the first year, there was an average weight loss of 8.6% in the intensive lifestyle intervention program, compared with just 0.7% weight loss in the diabetes support and education group.[16] By the end of the fifth year, patients in the intervention group maintained about half of their lost weight, and tended to remain at that weight for the rest of the trial.[15] The control group displayed small decreases in weight across all years; however, at each time point the intervention group displayed a significantly greater change in weight loss than the control group. Importantly, patients in the intervention group reported greater practice of target behaviors and weight control activities, including increasing physical activity, reducing caloric intake and fat intake, using meal replacements, and regular self-weighing.[15]

Although there was no difference in cardiovascular deaths between the intervention and control groups after 8 years, there were numerous improvements in health outcomes, including improved glycemic control, blood pressure, and lipid profile.[17] Participants in the intervention group reduced their use of glucose-lowering and antihypertensive medications, were less likely to be diagnosed with metabolic syndrome, and had a greater rate of remission of type 2 diabetes.[16,17] Furthermore, patients who completed the lifestyle intervention had fewer hospitalizations, lower health care costs, and required less medication relative to patients in the control group.[18] These and other high-quality trials provide evidence that behavioral counseling to achieve moderate weight loss is feasible and leads to substantial health benefits (and likely cost reductions), and should be a standard part of HCP practice for patients with excess weight and obesity-related comorbid conditions.

BEHAVIORAL SKILLS COUNSELING AND BEHAVIORAL CHANGE PRACTICE CONCEPTS

Several well-studied theories of behavior change can serve as a platform for HCP approaches to behavior change and obesity counseling.[19–21] These theories describe key correlates of successful behavior change. Although numerous theories have been proposed, we believe that those described next are particularly germane for long-term weight loss counseling.

Social cognitive theory (SCT) assumes that individual cognitive factors, environmental events, and behavior are interacting and reciprocal determinants of each other.[19] SCT provides the framework for building skills and self-efficacy (self-confidence, competence, and self-regulation) through developing action plans that target goal setting, monitoring, and positive feedback within the context of providing support. Behavioral strategies from SCT, including self-monitoring, goal-setting, and skill building, are also important elements for promoting long-term lifestyle changes by targeting increases in self-efficacy and mastery (self-confidence, self-regulation skills). SCT proposes that self-efficacy, or an individual's belief in his or her capacity to carry out behaviors needed to attain a desired outcome, plays a central role in how people approach goals.[20] Specifically, people high in self-efficacy tend to be more likely to believe that they can master challenging problems and recover quickly from setbacks, skills that may be especially important among people seeking to change health behaviors.[19] However, few studies have integrated choice and autonomy into the development of self-monitoring plans, which, as described next, may be critical for long-term adherence in behavior change.[22,23]

Self-determination theory (SDT) argues for a social-contextual approach to motivation by encouraging patients to have input and choice (autonomy support) in making healthy lifestyle choices.[21] SDT postulates that experiences that are enjoyable and self-initiated through autonomy-supportive interactions promote and sustain behavior change, and that in particular behavior changes that are motivated by intrinsic factors, such as novel, enjoyable, self-driven, and satisfying experiences, are more likely to be sustained over the long term.[24] In addition to autonomy, a key component of SDT is competence, which is similar to the concept of self-efficacy described in SCT. In a recent meta-analysis of 184 intervention studies, an SDT-focused framework was shown to be effective at improving a broad range of physical and mental health outcomes including exercise, weight loss, diet, depression, and quality of life.[25] Previous studies have also provided evidence for the importance of choice and self-initiated behavior change on increasing intrinsic motivation for engaging in physical activity among individuals including underserved ethnic minorities.[26–28] Of note, motivational interviewing is a counseling process closely aligned with SDT. Motivational interviewing is a patient-centered communication style that uses specific techniques, such as open-ended questioning, reflective listening, autonomy support, shared decision-making, and eliciting change talk. Motivational interviewing has been shown to be effective across a range of behavioral change areas, including weight management.[29,30] A basic Google search for motivational interviewing videos offers a range of examples for clinical guidance.

THE 5 AS MODEL FOR WEIGHT MANAGEMENT COUNSELING IN PRIMARY CARE

Behavioral medicine for obesity management uses the insights of behavior change theories to promote a positive social climate, autonomy support, and self-efficacy as part of a structured model for behavior change and obesity counseling. We describe here an adaptation of the "5 As" framework for behavior change counseling, which was initially developed for tobacco smoking cessation counseling and has since been adapted for several other areas of behavior change including alcohol use and weight management.[3] This approach can help HCPs structure their clinical interactions and maximize their impact on obesity treatment.

Assess

Assess and screen for weight status, obesity-associated comorbid conditions that require management (eg, obstructive sleep apnea, diabetes, hypertension, liver disease) and conditions that may interfere with weight loss (eg, binge eating disorder, insomnia, chronic pain, attention-deficit/hyperactivity disorder), and patients' willingness to engage in behavioral change and weight management. A variant of the first "A" is "Ask." To support patient autonomy and ease what is often a sensitive topic, we recommend asking permission before discussing weight. A simple way to do so can be: "I noticed that your weight has been increasing over the years, and this can lead to several health problems. If you're open to it, I would like to offer myself as a resource so that we can work together on this. Would it be okay if we talked about weight today?" In our experience, most patients feel empowered by this nonjudgmental, patient-centered approach and open to engaging with the HCP. Even if not interested, this signals to patients that their autonomy will be respected and that when they are ready the HCP is interested and able to support their behavioral change and weight management attempts. For patients who are open to discussing their weight, HCPs should assess prior weight loss attempts, current strategies and barriers, and personal goals and motivations for weight loss.

Advise

Advise patients on the risks associated with obesity. Although some patients are not aware of these risks, many patients have already been inundated with "gloom and doom" messages about developing diabetes and other obesity-associated health risks. It may be more valuable in many cases to advise patients of the benefits of small behavioral changes and moderate weight losses. For example, just 2% to 3% weight loss begins to improve glycemic control; 5% weight loss further improves glycemic control, and lipids and other risk factors; and 7% weight loss is associated with 58% reduction in development of diabetes.[31] Many patients may benefit from informing them that many preconceived notions about dieting and weight loss are untrue. For example, there is no "magic diet"; caloric intake being equal, many dietary patterns are effective for weight loss, and patients should consider plans that fit their tastes and personal preferences.[31] Also, neither slow nor fast weight loss is necessarily better than the other, so again appealing to patients' preferences is important and empowering. For patients who are ready to engage in behavioral changes, offer options for target behaviors to begin working toward, as described in the previous section.

Agree

Work with patients collaboratively to agree on a set of goals for behavior change. Behavior change goals should be specific, measurable, attainable, relevant, and time-based:

- Specific: Make goals clear and include specific details. "Exercise a lot" is too vague. Instead, a patient might aim to walk more by going for a 20-minute walk after lunch 3 days per week.
- Measurable: Define a metric (measure) that lets you know when you have been successful. "Exercise a lot" is also not measurable. Instead, aiming for an increase of 500 steps per day is a measurable goal.
- Attainable: Set a goal that is realistic for to achieve. Running a marathon by next week is unrealistic for most, but aiming to walk for 20 minutes after lunch may be more achievable.
- Relevant: Create a goal that is consistent with the outcome you want to achieve.
- Time-bound: Set goals that can be completed in a specific amount of time.

Thinking through goals using this framework helps to minimize the likelihood of unrealistic goals and helps to create a structure on how patients can achieve these goals.

Assist

Assist patients to make progress toward their goals and to identify barriers that are limiting their progress. Numerous free patient education materials are helpful, such as the Dietary Guidelines for Americans (https://health.gov/dietaryguidelines) and the associated Choose My Plate site (https://www.choosemyplate.gov). Free self-monitoring apps are widely available, such as My Fitness Pal and Lose It. A central part of behavioral counseling involves regular interaction and teamwork to engage in problem solving to overcome barriers and pitfalls. Problem solving includes normalizing the patient's situation ("It's common to run into some struggles with weight loss, let's see if we can figure this out together"), helping patients identify the specific barrier, general alternate solutions, and experimenting with trying out the solutions.

Arrange

Arrange regular interaction with patients, and consider referrals as necessary. One of the most consistent predictors of weight loss progress is having regular, ongoing interaction with an HCP or group. Be sure to arrange regular follow-up appointments with HCPs or physician extenders to help patients continue their progress. During these appointments, one can check in on a patient's progress, review self-monitoring records, engage in problem solving, and continue to offer guidance and support. As appropriate, consider referral to specialists, such as registered dieticians, behavioral psychologists, or obesity medicine physicians, or community-based weight loss groups, such as DPP, which are now covered by Medicare.

Several considerations are foundational to each of the 5 As steps. Autonomy-supportive counseling should be respectful and supportive. HCPs should recognize that weight management is especially challenging in our society, in which structural and economic settings, social norms, and national and local policies generally push eating more and moving less. Neither failure to lose or maintain lost weight in the past, nor hesitancy to engage in further weight management attempts because of low confidence or prior negative experiences should be interpreted as the patient lacking willpower or personal responsibility. Acknowledging the challenge of managing weight can begin to ease patients' fears and build rapport. Using patient-centered language can support motivation and engender a positive and respectful HCP-patient climate. This includes people-first ("a patient with obesity," "a patient with diabetes," "a patient with cancer") rather than condition-first ("obese patient," "diabetic patient," "cancerous patient") language. Moreover, patient-preferred terminology, such as "unhealthy weight" is often considered motivating by patients, as opposed to such terms as "obese," "morbidly obese," or "fat."[32] These are small changes on the part of HCPs that can significantly improve HCP-patient interactions when discussing weight.

SUMMARY

Behavioral medicine may minimize the need for more intensive medical treatments, but counseling does not obviate the consideration for medical treatments, and in many cases behavioral medicine has been shown to improve the weight loss outcomes of medical treatments. Behavioral medicine provides an opportunity and framework for supporting patients to achieve changes in target health behaviors, including dietary and physical activity changes. Behavioral medicine can minimize the need for more intensive medical treatments, and can improve outcomes of these treatments and adherence to medication prescriptions or postsurgical recommendations. We have provided some practical guidelines based on large-scale evidenced-based national trials that are used easily in practice along with the 5 As model for communicating successfully with a target population.

REFERENCES

1. Stoto M. Population health in the affordable care act era. 1st edition. Washington, DC: Academy Health; 2013.

2. Schroeder S. We can do better: improving the health of the American people. N Engl J Med 2007;357(12):1221–8.

3. Fitzpatrick SL, Wischenka D, Appelhans BM, et al. An evidence-based guide for obesity treatment in primary care. Am J Med 2016;129(1):115.e1-e7.

4. Wing RR, Phelan S. Long-term weight loss maintenance. Am J Clin Nutr 2005; 82(1 Suppl):222S–5S.

5. Thomas JG, Bond DS, Phelan S, et al. Weight-loss maintenance for 10 years in the national weight control registry. Am J Prev Med 2014;46(1):17–23.

6. Wing RR, Hill JO. Successful weight loss maintenance. Annu Rev Nutr 2001;21: 323–41.

7. The Diabetes Prevention Program Research Group. The diabetes prevention program. Design and methods for a clinical trial in the prevention of type 2 diabetes. Diabetes Care 1999;22(4):623–34.

8. The Diabetes Prevention Program Research Group. Reduction in the incidence of type 2 diabetes with lifestyle intervention or metformin. N Engl J Med 2002; 346(6):393–403.

9. The Diabetes Prevention Program Research Group. 10-year follow-up of diabetes incidence and weight loss in the diabetes prevention program outcomes study. Lancet 2009;374(9702):1677–86.

10. Suhrcke M, Nugent R, Stuckler D, et al. Chronic disease: an economic perspective. London: Oxford Health Alliance; 2006.

11. The Diabetes Prevention Program Research Group. Long-term effects of the Diabetes prevention program interventions on cardiovascular risk factors: a report from the DPP outcomes study. Diabet Med 2013;30(1):46–55.

12. Pan XR, Li GW, Hu YH, et al. Effects of diet and exercise in preventing NIDDM in people with impaired glucose tolerance: the Da Qing IGT and diabetes study. Diabetes Care 1997;20(4):537–44.

13. Tuomilehto J, Indstrom J, Eriksson J, et al. Prevention of type 2 diabetes mellitus by changes in lifestyle among subjects with impaired glucose tolerance. N Engl J Med 2001;344(18):1343–50.

14. The Look AHEAD Research Group. The look AHEAD study: a description of the lifestyle intervention and the evidence supporting it. Obesity (Silver Spring) 2006; 14(5):737–52.

15. The Look AHEAD Research Group. Eight-year weight losses with an intensive lifestyle Intervention: the look AHEAD study. Obesity 2014;22(1):5–13.

16. The Look AHEAD Research Group. Reduction in weight and cardiovascular disease risk factors in individuals with type 2 diabetes: one-year results of the look AHEAD trial. Diabetes Care 2007;30(6):1374–83.

17. The Look AHEAD Research Group. Cardiovascular effects of intensive lifestyle intervention in type 2 diabetes. N Engl J Med 2013;369(2):145–54.

18. Espeland MA, Glick HA, Bertoni A, et al. Impact of an intensive lifestyle intervention on use and cost of medical services among overweight and obese adults with type 2 diabetes: the action for health in diabetes. Diabetes Care 2014; 37(9):2548–56.

19. Bandura A. Health promotion by social cognitive means. Heal Educ Behav 2004; 31(2):143–64.

20. Bandura A. Social foundations of thought and action: a social cognitive theory. New York: Prentice-Hall, Inc; 1986.

21. Ryan RM, Deci EL. Self-determination theory and the facilitation of intrinsic motivation, social development, and well-being. Am Psychol 2000;55(1):68–78.

22. Kitzman-Ulrich H, Wilson DK, St George SM, et al. The integration of a family systems approach for understanding youth obesity, physical activity, and dietary programs. Clin Child Fam Psychol Rev 2010;13(3):231–53.

23. Wilson DK. New perspectives on health disparities and obesity interventions in youth. J Pediatr Psychol 2008;34(3):231–44.

24. Silva MN, Vieira PN, Coutinho SR, et al. Using self-determination theory to promote physical activity and weight control: a randomized controlled trial in women. J Behav Med 2010;33(2):110–22.

25. Ng JY, Ntoumanis N, Thøgersen-Ntoumani C, et al. Self-determination theory applied to health contexts. Perspect Psychol Sci 2012;7(4):325–40.

26. Ferrer-Caja E, Weiss MR. Predictors of intrinsic motivation among adolescent students in physical education. Res Q Exerc Sport 2000;71(3):267–79.

27. Thompson CE, Wankel LM. The effects of perceived activity choice upon frequency of exercise behavior. J Appl Soc Psychol 1980;10(5):436–43.

28. Wilson DK, Van Horn ML, Kitzman-Ulrich H, et al. Results of the "Active by Choice Today" (ACT) randomized trial for increasing physical activity in low-income and minority adolescents. Health Psychol 2011;30(4):463–71.

29. Resnicow K, Gobat N, Naar S. Intensifying and igniting change talk in motivational interviewing: a theoretical and practical framework. Eur Heal Psychol 2015;17(3):102–10.

30. Martins R, McNeil D. Review of motivational interviewing in promoting health behaviors. Clin Psychol Rev 2009;29(4):283–93.

31. Jensen MD, Ryan DH, Apovian CM, et al. 2013 AHA/ACC/TOS guideline for the management of overweight and obesity in adults: a report of the American College of Cardiology/American Heart Association Task Force on Practice Guidelines and The Obesity Society. Circulation 2014;129(25 Suppl 2):S102–38.

32. Puhl R, Peterson JL, Luedicke J. Public perceptions of weight-related language used by health providers. Int J Obes 2013;37:612–9.

Obesity Pharmacotherapy

Katherine H. Saunders, MD, DABOM*, Devika Umashanker, MD, MBA,
Leon I. Igel, MD, DABOM, Rekha B. Kumar, MD, MS, DABOM,
Louis J. Aronne, MD, DABOM, FTOS

KEYWORDS

- Obesity • Weight management • Pharmacotherapy • Orlistat
- Phentermine/topiramate • Lorcaserin • Naltrexone/bupropion • Liraglutide

KEY POINTS

- Although diet, physical activity, and behavioral modifications are the cornerstones of weight management, weight loss achieved by lifestyle modifications alone is often limited and difficult to maintain.
- Pharmacotherapy for obesity can be considered if patients have a body mass index (BMI) of 30 kg/m^2 or greater or a BMI of 27 kg/m^2 or greater with weight-related comorbidities.
- The 6 most commonly used antiobesity medications are phentermine, orlistat, phentermine/topiramate extended release, lorcaserin, naltrexone sustained release (SR)/bupropion SR, and liraglutide 3.0 mg.
- It is important for primary care providers to be familiar with the pharmacotherapy available to patients who cannot lose weight and sustain weight loss with lifestyle interventions alone.
- Successful pharmacotherapy for obesity depends on tailoring treatment to patients' behaviors and comorbidities as well as close monitoring of efficacy, safety, and tolerability.

INTRODUCTION

Diet, physical activity, and behavioral modifications are the cornerstones of weight management.[1] However, weight loss achieved by lifestyle modifications alone is often limited and difficult to maintain. Reduced caloric intake and increased energy

Disclosure Statement: K.H. Saunders, D. Umashanker, and L.I. Igel have no conflicts of interest. R.B. Kumar is a speaker for Janssen Pharmaceuticals and Novo Nordisk A/S. She is a shareholder in Zafgen, VIVUS, and MYOS Corporation. L.J. Aronne has received research funding from Aspire Bariatrics, Eisai, and Takeda Pharmaceuticals. He declares consultant/advisory board work with Jamieson Labs, Pfizer Inc, Novo Nordisk A/S, Eisai, VIVUS, GI Dynamics, JOVIA Health, and Gelesis. He is a shareholder of Zafgen, Gelesis, MYOS Corporation, and Jamieson Labs, and he is on the board of directors of MYOS Corporation and Jamieson Labs.
Comprehensive Weight Control Center, Division of Endocrinology, Diabetes, and Metabolism, Weill Cornell Medicine, 1165 York Avenue, New York, NY 10065, USA
* Corresponding author.
E-mail address: kph2001@med.cornell.edu

expenditure are counteracted by adaptive physiologic responses.[2] Not only does appetite increase but resting metabolic rate slows out of proportion to what would be expected based on changes in body composition.[3] This phenomenon, called adaptive thermogenesis or metabolic adaptation, impedes weight loss and contributes to weight regain.[4,5]

Antiobesity pharmacotherapy is one strategy to offset the adaptive changes in appetite and energy expenditure that occur with weight loss and to improve adherence to lifestyle interventions.[3] According to the 2013 American College of Cardiology/American Heart Association/The Obesity Society's guideline for the management of overweight and obesity in adults and the Endocrine Society's clinical practice guidelines on the pharmacologic management of obesity, pharmacotherapy for obesity can be considered if patients have a body mass index (BMI) of 30 kg/m^2 or greater or a BMI of 27 kg/m^2 or greater with weight-related comorbidities, such as hypertension, dyslipidemia, type 2 diabetes, and obstructive sleep apnea.[1,6]

As obesity is a chronic disease, most antiobesity medications are approved for long-term treatment. Until a few years ago, phentermine (and other sympathomimetic amines) and orlistat were the only antiobesity medications approved by the Food and Drug Administration (FDA). In 2012, phentermine/topiramate extended release (ER) and lorcaserin were approved; in 2014, naltrexone sustained release (SR)/bupropion SR and liraglutide 3.0 mg were approved.

In this article, the authors review the 6 most widely used antiobesity medications (**Table 1**). The authors present efficacy and safety findings, discuss how to best select agents for each patient, and provide advice on how to manage patients who do not respond to medications. Although referral to an obesity medicine specialist is an option for some primary care providers, there are not enough obesity medicine specialists to address the obesity epidemic. Therefore, it is important for primary care providers to be familiar with the pharmacotherapy available to patients who are unable to lose weight and sustain weight loss with lifestyle interventions alone.

PHENTERMINE

Phentermine was approved by the FDA in 1959 and has been the most commonly prescribed medication for obesity in the United States. It is an adrenergic agonist that increases resting energy expenditure and suppresses appetite. Phentermine is indicated for short-term use (3 months), as there are no long-term safety trials of phentermine monotherapy; but it was approved in combination with topiramate ER for long-term therapy. Many practitioners prescribe phentermine for greater than 3 months as off-label therapy for ongoing weight management.

Two other sympathomimetic amines, diethylpropion and phendimetrazine, are also available in the United States; but data on these agents are minimal, and they are prescribed much less frequently.

Until recently, the available doses of phentermine were 15.0, 30.0, and 37.5 mg.[7-9] As prescribing practices should be individualized to determine the lowest effective dose, many practitioners recommend using quarter or half tablets of these formulations. In 2016, the FDA approved an 8-mg formulation, which can be prescribed up to 3 times daily.[10] Administration of the last dose late in the day should be avoided to prevent insomnia. Phentermine is a schedule IV controlled substance.

In a 28-week randomized controlled trial comparing phentermine, topiramate ER, and the combination of the two agents, phentermine 15 mg daily produced an average 6.0-kg weight loss compared with a 1.5-kg weight loss with placebo.[11] Forty-six percent of participants assigned to phentermine lost at least 5% of initial body weight

Table 1
Antiobesity medications

Medication	Mechanism, Dosage, and Available Formulations	Trial and Duration	Trial Arms	Weight Loss (%)	Most Common Adverse Events	Consider This Medication in These Patients	Avoid This Medication in These Patients
Phentermine[7–10] Schedule IV controlled substance NOTE: approved for short-term use	Adrenergic agonist 8.0 mg–37.5 mg daily (8-mg dose can be prescribed up to TID) Capsule, tablet	Aronne LJ, et al[11] 28 wk	15 mg daily 7.5 mg daily Placebo (topiramate ER and phentermine/ topiramate ER arms excluded)	6.06[a] 5.45[a] 1.71	Dry mouth, insomnia, dizziness, irritability	Younger patients who need assistance with appetite suppression	Patients with uncontrolled hypertension, active or unstable coronary disease, hyperthyroidism, glaucoma, anxiety, insomnia, or patients who are generally sensitive to stimulants; patients with a history of drug abuse or recent MAOI use; patients who are pregnant
Orlistat[14,15]	Lipase inhibitor 60–120 mg TID with meals Capsule	XENDOS[16] 208 wk	120 mg TID Placebo	9.6 (wk 52)[a] 5.25 (wk 208)[a] 5.61 (wk 52) 2.71 (wk 208)	Fecal urgency, oily stool, flatus with discharge, fecal incontinence	Patients with hypercholesterolemia and/or constipation who can limit their intake of dietary fat	Patients with malabsorption syndromes or other GI conditions that predispose to GI upset/diarrhea; patients who cannot modify the fat content of their diets; patients who are pregnant

(continued on next page)

Table 1
(continued)

Medication	Mechanism, Dosage, and Available Formulations	Trial and Duration	Trial Arms	Weight Loss (%)	Most Common Adverse Events	Consider This Medication in These Patients	Avoid This Medication in These Patients
Phentermine/topiramate ER[19] Schedule IV controlled substance	Adrenergic agonist/neuro-stabilizer 3.75/23–15/92 mg daily (dose titration) Capsule	EQUIP[21] 56 wk CONQUER[22] 56 wk SEQUEL[23] 108 wk (52-wk extension of CONQUER trial)	15/92 mg daily 3.75/23 mg daily Placebo 15/92 mg daily 7.5/46 mg daily Placebo 15/92 mg daily 7.5/46 mg daily Placebo	10.9[a] 5.1[a] 1.6 9.8[a] 7.8[a] 1.2 10.5[a] 9.3[a] 1.8 (wk 0–108)	Paresthesias, dizziness, dysgeusia, insomnia, constipation, dry mouth	Younger patients who need assistance with appetite suppression	Patients with uncontrolled hypertension, active or unstable coronary disease, hyperthyroidism, glaucoma, anxiety, insomnia, or patients who are generally sensitive to stimulants; patients with a history of drug abuse or recent MAOI use; patients with a history of nephrolithiasis; patients who are pregnant or trying to conceive

Drug / Mechanism / Dose	Trial (duration)	Dosing	Weight loss (%)	Side effects	Ideal candidates	Contraindications
Lorcaserin[25] Schedule IV controlled substance — Serotonin (5HT-2C) receptor agonist 10 mg BID or 20 mg XR daily Tablet	BLOOM[27] 52 wk	10 mg BID Placebo	5.8[a] 2.2	Headache, dizziness, fatigue, nausea, dry mouth, constipation	Patients who would benefit from appetite suppression	Patients on other serotonin-modulating medications and patients with known cardiac valvular disease; patients who are pregnant
	BLOSSOM[29] 52 wk	10 mg BID 10 mg daily Placebo	5.8[a] 4.7[a] 2.8			
	BLOOM-DM[28] 52 wk	10 mg BID 10 mg daily Placebo	4.5[a] 5.0[a] 1.5			
Naltrexone/ bupropion SR[43] — Opioid receptor antagonist/ dopamine and norepinephrine reuptake inhibitor 8/90 mg daily to 16/180 mg BID Tablet	COR-I[32] 56 wk	16/180 mg BID 8/180 mg BID Placebo	6.1[a] 5.0[a] 1.3	Nausea, vomiting, constipation, headache, dizziness, insomnia, dry mouth	Patients who describe cravings for food and/or addictive behaviors related to food; patients who are trying to quit smoking, reduce alcohol intake, and/or have concomitant depression	Patients with uncontrolled hypertension, uncontrolled pain, recent MAOI use, history of seizures, or any condition that predisposes to seizure, such as anorexia/bulimia nervosa, abrupt discontinuation of alcohol, benzodiazepines, barbiturates, or antiepileptic drugs; patients who are pregnant
	COR-II[33] 56 wk	16/180 mg BID Placebo	6.4[a] 1.2			
	COR-BMOD[34] 56 wk	16/180 mg BID Placebo	9.3[a] 5.1			
	COR-Diabetes[35] 56 wk	16/180 mg BID Placebo	5.0[a] 1.8			

(continued on next page)

Table 1
(continued)

Medication	Mechanism, Dosage, and Available Formulations	Trial and Duration	Trial Arms	Weight Loss (%)	Most Common Adverse Events	Consider This Medication in These Patients	Avoid This Medication in These Patients
Liraglutide 3.0 mg[44]	GLP-1 receptor agonist 0.6–3.0 mg daily Prefilled pen for subcutaneous injection	SCALE Obesity and Prediabetes[38] 56 wk	3.0 mg daily Placebo	8.0[a] 2.6	Nausea, vomiting, diarrhea, constipation, dyspepsia, abdominal pain	Patients who report inadequate meal satiety and/or have type 2 diabetes, prediabetes, or impaired glucose tolerance; patients requiring use of concomitant psychiatric medications	Patients with a history of pancreatitis, personal/family history of MTC or MEN2; patients with an aversion to needles; patients who are pregnant
		SCALE Diabetes[37] 56 wk	3.0 mg daily 1.8 mg daily Placebo	6.0[a] 4.7[a] 2.0			
		SCALE Maintenance[39] 56 wk (after initial ≥5% weight loss with LCD)	3.0 mg daily Placebo	6.2[a] 0.2			

Abbreviations: BID, twice daily; 5HT, 5-hydroxytryptamine; GI, gastrointestinal; GLP-1, glucagonlike peptide-1; LCD, low-calorie diet; MAOI, monoamine oxidase inhibitor; MEN2, multiple endocrine neoplasia syndrome type 2; MTC, medullary thyroid carcinoma; TID, 3 times daily; XR, extended release.

[a] P <.001 versus placebo.

Adapted from Igel LI, Kumar RB, Saunders KH, et al. Practical use of pharmacotherapy for obesity. Gastroenterology 2017;152(7):1765–79; and Saunders KH, Kumar RB, Igel LI, et al. Pharmacologic approaches to weight management: recent gains and shortfalls in combating obesity. Curr Atheroscler Rep 2016;18(7):36; with permission.

and 20.8% lost at least 10% of initial body weight, whereas 15.5% and 6.8% of subjects assigned to placebo achieved at least 5% and 10% weight loss, respectively. Interestingly, there seems to be no advantage of continuous compared with intermittent phentermine treatment, at least on a short-term basis. A 36-week, double-blind, placebo-controlled trial compared continuous phentermine, continuous placebo, and alternating phentermine/placebo every 4 weeks.[12] The mean weight loss was 12.2 kg and 13.0 kg in patients who received phentermine continuously and intermittently, respectively, compared with 4.8-kg weight loss in the placebo group. The weight loss in this study was higher than expected, as data were presented for completers only.

The most common treatment-emergent adverse events (TEAEs) include headache, dry mouth, insomnia, dizziness, irritability, nausea/vomiting, diarrhea, and constipation. Phentermine should not be prescribed in combination with other sympathomimetic amines or with monoamine oxidase inhibitors (MAOIs). Contraindications include pregnancy/nursing, history of cardiovascular disease or drug abuse, hyperthyroidism, glaucoma, and agitated states.

ORLISTAT

Before 2012, the only antiobesity medicine approved for long-term use was orlistat, which was approved by the FDA in 1999. Orlistat is indicated for obesity management including weight loss and weight maintenance when used in conjunction with a reduced-calorie diet. It is also indicated to reduce the risk of weight regain after prior weight loss.

Orlistat promotes weight loss by inhibiting pancreatic and gastric lipases, thereby decreasing the absorption of fat from the gastrointestinal tract. On average, 120 mg of orlistat taken 3 times per day with meals decreases fat absorption by 30%.[13]

The recommended dosage of orlistat is one 120-mg capsule or one 60-mg capsule 3 times per day with each meal containing fat.[14,15] The medication can be taken during a meal or up to 1 hour after food consumption. Patients on orlistat should be advised to follow a nutritionally balanced, reduced-calorie diet with approximately 30% of calories from fat. The daily intake of fat, carbohydrate, and protein should be distributed over 3 meals. Patients should take a multivitamin (separately from the medication) while on orlistat, as it can decrease the absorption of fat-soluble vitamins (A, D, E, K).

In a double-blind prospective study that randomized 3305 patients with a BMI of 30 kg/m^2 or greater to lifestyle changes with either orlistat 120 mg or placebo 3 times daily, the mean weight loss was significantly greater with orlistat (5.8 kg) than with placebo (3.0 kg) after 4 years.[16] Fifty-three percent of the patients assigned to orlistat lost 5% or greater of their initial body weight, and 26.2% lost 10% or greater of their initial body weight.

In addition to promoting weight loss, orlistat lowers serum glucose levels and improves insulin sensitivity. The cumulative incidence of diabetes in the XENical in the Prevention of Diabetes in Obese Subjects (XENDOS) trial was 6.2% with orlistat and 9.0% with placebo, which corresponds to a risk reduction of 37.3%. Orlistat has also been found to improve blood pressure, total cholesterol, and low-density lipoprotein cholesterol.[17]

Orlistat is not commonly used for obesity management because of the side effects of fecal urgency, oily stool, and fecal incontinence; but it may have a role as an additional medicine for patients who are constipated on other antiobesity pharmacotherapy. A slow dose titration or the addition of a psyllium fiber supplement can reduce side effects.

Orlistat should not be used in patients who are pregnant or who have chronic malabsorption syndromes or cholestasis. Orlistat can decrease the absorption of medications, such as cyclosporine, levothyroxine, warfarin, amiodarone, antiepileptic agents, and antiretroviral drugs.

PHENTERMINE/TOPIRAMATE EXTENDED RELEASE

In 2012, the FDA approved phentermine/topiramate ER for chronic weight management as an adjunct to a reduced-calorie diet and increased physical activity. The rationale for a combination medication is that appetite regulation involves multiple pathways, so targeting different mechanisms simultaneously can have an additive effect on body weight. Another benefit is that the smaller dose of each medication reduces the risk of TEAEs.

Topiramate was approved for epilepsy in 1996 and migraine prophylaxis in 2004. The medication's effect on caloric intake is thought to be mediated through modulation of gamma-aminobutyric acid receptors, inhibition of carbonic anhydrase, and antagonism of glutamate.[18]

Phentermine/topiramate ER is available in 4 doses (3.75/23 mg, 7.5/46 mg, 11.25/69 mg, and 15.0/92 mg), which are lower than the maximum doses of the individual agents.[19] The medication should be taken once daily in the morning with or without food. After 14 days of 3.75/23 mg daily, patients can progress to 7.5/46 mg daily. Phentermine/topiramate ER should be discontinued or the dose should be escalated if 3% weight loss is not achieved after 12 weeks. For escalation, a titration dose of 11.25/69 mg is taken daily for 2 weeks and then increased to 15/92 mg daily for maintenance. The medication should also be discontinued if 5% weight loss is not achieved after 12 additional weeks on 15/92 mg daily.

Phentermine/topiramate ER is a schedule IV controlled substance. The FDA requires a Risk Evaluation and Mitigation Strategy to inform prescribers and women of reproductive potential about the possible increased risk of orofacial clefts in infants exposed to phentermine/topiramate ER during the first trimester of pregnancy.[20]

Two randomized, double-blind, placebo-controlled trials, EQUIP and CONQUER, evaluated the efficacy of phentermine/topiramate ER over 56 weeks.[21,22] The CONQUER trial randomized 2487 patients with a BMI of 27 to 45 kg/m² and 2 or more comorbidities (hypertension, dyslipidemia, diabetes or prediabetes, or abdominal obesity) to phentermine/topiramate ER 15/92 mg, phentermine/topiramate ER 7.5/46 mg, or placebo. Compared with placebo, both doses resulted in significantly greater weight loss (9.8 kg with 15/92 mg, 7.8 kg with 7.5/46 mg, and 1.2 kg with placebo). Seventy percent of patients achieved at least 5% weight loss with 15/92 mg compared with 62% with 7.5/46 mg and 21% with placebo.

The SEQUEL trial evaluated ongoing weight loss with phentermine/topiramate ER for 52 weeks after completion of the CONQUER study.[23] The mean percentage reduction in body weight was found to be significantly greater in the treatment groups compared with placebo (10.5%, 9.3%, and 1.8% with 15/92 mg, 7.5/46 mg, and placebo, respectively). The study also reported a 76% reduction in the progression to diabetes in subjects receiving 15/92 mg and a 54% reduction in subjects receiving 7.5/46 mg compared with placebo.

The most common TEAEs with phentermine/topiramate ER include paresthesias, dizziness, dysgeusia, insomnia, constipation, and dry mouth. Contraindications include pregnancy (a pregnancy test is recommended before starting followed by monthly tests in appropriate patients), glaucoma, hyperthyroidism, and MAOI use.

LORCASERIN

Lorcaserin, a selective serotonin (5-hydroxytryptamine [5HT])-2C receptor agonist, was approved by the FDA in 2012 as a long-term treatment of obesity. Lorcaserin reduces appetite and increases satiety by binding to the 5HT-2C receptors on anorexigenic pro-opiomelanocortin (POMC) neurons in the hypothalamus. Because of its selective agonism of the serotonin 2C receptor, lorcaserin was designed to avoid cardiac valvular effects mediated through the 5HT-2B receptor. The development program has not observed an increased incidence of valvulopathy over 2 years, and long-term data are being collected in a 5-year cardiovascular outcome study.[24]

The recommended dosage of lorcaserin is 10 mg twice daily with or without food.[25] There is also a new 20-mg extended release tablet, which can be taken once daily.[26] The medication should be discontinued if 5% or less weight loss is achieved after 12 weeks. Lorcaserin is a schedule IV controlled substance.

The phase III double-blind placebo-controlled Behavioral Modification and Lorcaserin for Overweight and Obesity Management (BLOOM) trial included 3182 adults who were overweight or obese and received lorcaserin 10 mg twice daily or placebo for 52 weeks, in conjunction with diet and exercise.[27] At week 52, all subjects treated with lorcaserin were rerandomized to either placebo or lorcaserin for an additional year. At 1 year, the average placebo-subtracted weight loss was 3.6%, and 47% of the subjects taking lorcaserin lost at least 5.0% as compared with 20.5% in the control group. Subjects who showed a weight loss of at least 5% in year 1 and were maintained on lorcaserin treatment in year 2 were able to maintain their weight loss better than those who had been switched to placebo.

The Behavioral Modification and Lorcaserin for Obesity and Overweight Management in Diabetes Mellitus (BLOOM-DM) study was conducted in subjects with obesity and type 2 diabetes.[28] At 52 weeks, 37.5% of patients treated with lorcaserin 10 mg twice daily showed a weight loss of at least 5%, which was more than twice the percentage in the placebo group. There was a reduction of hemoglobin A1c (HbA1c) of 0.9% in those on lorcaserin as compared with a 0.4% reduction in the placebo group.

The most common TEAEs include headache, dizziness, fatigue, nausea, dry mouth, and constipation.[27–29] There is a theoretic interaction with other serotonergic drugs, as coadministration may lead to the development of serotonin syndrome or neuroleptic malignant syndromelike reactions.

NALTREXONE SUSTAINED RELEASE/BUPROPION

Naltrexone/bupropion was approved for the treatment of obesity in 2014. Bupropion is a dopamine and norepinephrine reuptake inhibitor that was FDA approved as an antidepressant in 1989 and as a smoking cessation aide in 1997. Naltrexone is an opioid antagonist that was FDA approved for the treatment of opioid dependence in 1984 and alcohol use disorder in 1994.

Together, naltrexone/bupropion has effects in 2 separate areas of the brain involved in the regulation of food intake. One region is the arcuate nucleus of the hypothalamus, which is integral to appetite regulation. The second region is the mesolimbic dopamine reward circuit. By increasing the firing rate of hypothalamic POMC neurons while simultaneously modulating the dopamine reward circuit, both appetite and food cravings are reduced.[30,31]

Each tablet of naltrexone/bupropion contains 8 mg of ER naltrexone and 90 mg of ER bupropion. The initial prescription should be for one tablet daily in the morning with instructions to increase by one tablet weekly to a therapeutic dosage of 2 tablets twice daily (32/360 mg). The medication should be discontinued if patients have achieved 5% or less weight loss at 16 weeks (after 12 weeks at the maintenance dose).

Four 56-week randomized double-blind placebo-controlled trials (COR-I, COR-II, Contrave Obesity Research Behavior Modification [COR-BMOD], and COR-Diabetes) were conducted to evaluate the effect of naltrexone/bupropion plus lifestyle modification in 4536 patients with overweight or obesity.[32–35] The COR-I, COR-II, and COR-BMOD trials enrolled patients with a BMI of 30 kg/m^2 or greater or a BMI of 27 kg/m^2 or greater and at least one weight-related comorbidity. The COR-Diabetes trial enrolled patients with a BMI of 27 kg/m^2 or greater with type 2 diabetes with or without hypertension and/or dyslipidemia.

In the COR-I trial, the mean weight loss of 6.1% was observed in patients receiving naltrexone/bupropion 360/32 mg compared with 1.3% in patients receiving placebo; 48% of naltrexone/bupropion patients lost greater than 5% body weight from baseline as compared with 16% of placebo patients. In the COR-Diabetes trial, 44.5% of patients receiving naltrexone/bupropion lost 5% or greater of their body weight after 56 weeks compared with 18.9% of patients receiving placebo. Patients receiving naltrexone/bupropion demonstrated a 0.6% reduction in HbA1c from baseline compared with a 0.1% reduction in patients receiving placebo.

The most common side effects of naltrexone/bupropion include nausea/vomiting, constipation, headache, dizziness, insomnia, and dry mouth. Administration of naltrexone/bupropion with high-fat meals should be avoided, as this significantly increases the systemic levels of both bupropion and naltrexone. Naltrexone/bupropion is contraindicated in patients taking MAOIs or chronic opioids and in patients with uncontrolled hypertension, history of seizures, or conditions that predispose to seizure, such as anorexia or bulimia nervosa, or abrupt discontinuation of alcohol, benzodiazepines, barbiturates, or antiepileptic drugs. Bupropion carries a black box warning (as do all antidepressants) related to a potential increase in suicidality in patients younger than 24 years during the early phase of treatment, so patients should be monitored closely for mood changes when initiating naltrexone/bupropion.

LIRAGLUTIDE 3.0 MG

Liraglutide 3.0 mg was the second agent approved by the FDA in 2014 for chronic weight management. Liraglutide mimics the gastrointestinal incretin hormone, glucagonlike peptide-1, which is released in response to food intake. It is also FDA approved for the treatment of type 2 diabetes in doses up to 1.8 mg. Among patients with obesity and without diabetes, liraglutide 3.0 mg daily was found to reduce hunger, decrease food intake, and delay gastric emptying.[36]

Liraglutide is administered as a subcutaneous injection once daily. The starting dosage is 0.6 mg daily for 1 week with instructions to increase by 0.6 mg weekly to a therapeutic dosage of 3.0 mg daily. Slower dose titration can reduce gastrointestinal side effects. The medication should be discontinued if patients have not achieved at least 4% weight loss at 16 weeks.

Two phase III trials, SCALE Diabetes and SCALE Obesity and Prediabetes, evaluated the effect of liraglutide 3.0 mg on subjects who were overweight or obese with and without diabetes, respectively.[37,38] Both 56-week, randomized, placebo-controlled, double-blind trials illustrated significantly greater mean weight loss than placebo. In SCALE Diabetes, the mean weight loss was 6.0% with 3.0 mg daily, 4.7% with 1.8 mg daily, and 2.0% with placebo. In SCALE Obesity and Prediabetes, participants assigned to 3.0 mg daily lost a mean of 8.0% body weight compared with 2.6% in the placebo group.

The efficacy of liraglutide for weight maintenance was investigated in the SCALE Maintenance study.[39] Four hundred twenty-two subjects who were overweight or obese and had lost at least 5% of their initial body weight on a low-calorie diet were randomly assigned to liraglutide 3.0 mg daily or placebo for 56 weeks. The mean weight loss on the initial diet was 6.0%. By the end of the study, participants in the liraglutide group lost an additional 6.2% compared with 0.2% with placebo.

The most common TEAEs include nausea, vomiting, diarrhea, constipation, dyspepsia, and abdominal pain. Liraglutide is contraindicated in patients who are pregnant or those with personal or family history of medullary thyroid carcinoma or multiple endocrine neoplasia syndrome type 2. Thyroid C-cell tumors were found in rodents given supratherapeutic doses of liraglutide; however, there is no evidence of liraglutide causing C-cell tumors in humans. Concomitant use of liraglutide with insulin or insulin secretagogues can increase the risk of hypoglycemia.

PRACTICAL TIPS FOR TREATMENT

Since 2012, 4 new antiobesity medications have been approved. When patients are unable to lose and maintain weight loss with lifestyle interventions alone, providers should consider the use of pharmacotherapy to counteract metabolic adaptation and improve adherence to diet and exercise.[1,6]

There are 2 important questions to ask when prescribing an antiobesity medication to patients. The first question is whether there are undesirable side effects, contraindications, or drug-drug interactions. For example, avoid orlistat if patients have a condition predisposing to malabsorption and avoid phentermine and phentermine/topiramate ER if patients have unstable coronary disease.

The second question is whether any of the medications could improve another symptom or condition. For example, consider phentermine/topiramate ER if patients have migraines or naltrexone SR/bupropion SR if patients also would like assistance with smoking cessation. **Table 1** provides examples of ideal and poor candidates for each medication.

Pharmacotherapy should not be prescribed in the absence of behavioral counseling focusing on diet, physical activity, and lifestyle modifications, which are the cornerstones of weight management. Patients should be monitored at least monthly for the first 3 months of treatment and then at least once every 3 months.[6] Efficacy and safety should be assessed and behavioral interventions should be reinforced at each visit.

If a medication is determined to be ineffective or if there are safety or tolerability concerns at any time, the medication should be discontinued and alternative medications or treatment approaches should be pursued.[6] Another agent with a different mechanism of action can be considered.

Obesity pharmacotherapy is intended for long-term use, as obesity is a chronic disease. Continued use of medication promotes sustained weight maintenance by offsetting increased appetite and reduced energy expenditure secondary to the metabolic adaptation that occurs with weight loss. Once a desired weight has been achieved, reducing the dose or frequency of medication is a possible strategy that requires further study.

FUTURE CONSIDERATIONS

Many patients require more than one medication to achieve clinically significant weight loss. By targeting multiple pathways simultaneously, combination therapy can have an additive or synergistic effect on body weight. In addition to phentermine/topiramate ER and naltrexone SR/bupropion SR, other combinations are under investigation, including phentermine/lorcaserin and phentermine/canagliflozin.[40,41] Instead of initiating 2 medications simultaneously, an alternative strategy is a stepwise approach in which an additional agent is added when patients reach a weight plateau.

Pharmacotherapy can be combined with bariatric surgery, both before and after the procedure. As weight regain after bariatric surgery is common, the addition of an antiobesity medication can be an effective tool to counteract recidivism and enhance weight maintenance.[42] Although data are limited, the optimal time to initiate antiobesity pharmacotherapy seems to be when patients reach a nadir weight instead of after weight regain has occurred. Finally, the combination of antiobesity pharmacotherapy with endoscopic procedures and devices is another area that requires further investigation.

REFERENCES

1. Jensen MD, Ryan DH, Apovian CM, et al. 2013 AHA/ACC/TOS guideline for the management of overweight and obesity in adults: a report of the American College of Cardiology/American Heart Association Task Force on Practice Guidelines and the Obesity Society. J Am Coll Cardiol 2014;63(25 Pt B):2985–3023.
2. Sumithran P, Prendergast LA, Delbridge E, et al. Long-term persistence of hormonal adaptations to weight loss. N Engl J Med 2011;365(17):1597–604.
3. Greenway FL. Physiological adaptations to weight loss and factors favouring weight regain. Int J Obes (Lond) 2015;39(8):1188–96.
4. Rosenbaum M, Leibel RL. Adaptive thermogenesis in humans. Int J Obes (Lond) 2010;34:S47–55.
5. Fothergill E, Guo J, Howard L, et al. Persistent metabolic adaptation 6 years after "The Biggest Loser" competition. Obesity (Silver Spring) 2016;24(8):1612–9.
6. Apovian CM, Aronne LJ, Bessesen DH, et al. Pharmacological management of obesity: an Endocrine Society clinical practice guideline. J Clin Endocrinol Metab 2015;100(2):342–62.
7. Adipex [package insert]. Tulsa, OK: Physicians Total Care, Inc; 2012.
8. Ionamin [package insert]. Rochester, NY: Celltech Pharmaceuticals, Inc; 2006.
9. Suprenza [package insert]. Cranford, NJ: Akrimax Pharmaceuticals, LLC; 2013.
10. Lomaira [package insert]. Newtown, PA: KVK-TECH, INC; 2016.
11. Aronne LJ, Wadden TA, Peterson C, et al. Evaluation of phentermine and topiramate versus phentermine/topiramate extended-release in obese adults. Obesity (Silver Spring) 2013;21(11):2163–71.
12. Munro JF, MacCuish AC, Wilson EM, et al. Comparison of continuous and intermittent anorectic therapy in obesity. Br Med J 1968;1(5588):352–4.
13. Zhi J, Melia AT, Guerciolini R, et al. Retrospective population-based analysis of the dose-response (fecal fat excretion) relationship of orlistat in normal and obese volunteers. Clin Pharmacol Ther 1994;56(1):82–5.
14. Xenical [package insert]. South San Francisco, CA: Genentech USA, Inc; 2015.
15. Alli [package insert]. Moon Township, PA: GlaxoSmithKline Consumer Healthcare, LP; 2015.
16. Torgerson JS, Hauptman J, Boldrin MN, et al. XENical in the prevention of diabetes in obese subjects (XENDOS) study: a randomized study of orlistat as an adjunct to lifestyle changes for the prevention of type 2 diabetes in obese patients. Diabetes Care 2004;27(1):155–61.
17. Rucker D, Padwal R, Li SK, et al. Long term pharmacotherapy for obesity and overweight: updated meta-analysis. BMJ 2007;335(7631):1194–9.

18. Kushner RF. Weight loss strategies for treatment of obesity. Prog Cardiovasc Dis 2014;56(4):465–72.
19. Qsymia [package insert]. Mountain View, CA: VIVUS, Inc; 2012.
20. Qsymia risk evaluation and mitigation strategy (REMS). VIVUS, Inc. Available at: http://www.qsymiarems.com/. Accessed February 20, 2017.
21. Allison DB, Gadde KM, Garvey WT, et al. Controlled-release phentermine/topiramate in severely obese adults: a randomized controlled trial (EQUIP). Obesity (Silver Spring) 2012;20(2):330–42.
22. Gadde KM, Allison DB, Ryan DH, et al. Effects of low-dose, controlled-release, phentermine plus topiramate combination on weight and associated comorbidities in overweight and obese adults (CONQUER): a randomised, placebo controlled, phase 3 trial. Lancet 2011;377(9774):1341–52.
23. Garvey WT, Ryan DH, Look M, et al. Two-year sustained weight loss and metabolic benefits with controlled-release phentermine/topiramate in obese and overweight adults (SEQUEL): a randomized, placebo-controlled, phase 3 extension study. Am J Clin Nutr 2012;95(2):297–308.
24. A study to evaluate the effect of long-term treatment with BELVIQ (Lorcaserin HCl) on the incidence of major adverse cardiovascular events and conversion to type 2 diabetes mellitus in obese and overweight subjects with cardiovascular disease or multiple cardiovascular risk factors (CAMELLIATIMI). Available at: https://clinicaltrials.gov/ct2/show/NCT02019264.
25. Belviq [package insert]. Zofingen, Switzerland: Arena Pharmaceuticals; 2012.
26. Belviq XR [package insert]. Zofingen, Switzerland: Arena Pharmaceuticals; 2016.
27. Smith SR, Weissman NJ, Anderson CM, et al. Multicenter, placebo-controlled trial of lorcaserin for weight management. N Engl J Med 2010;363(3):245–56.
28. O'Neil PM, Smith SR, Weissman NJ, et al. Randomized placebo-controlled clinical trial of lorcaserin for weight loss in type 2 diabetes mellitus: the BLOOM-DM study. Obesity (Silver Spring) 2012;20(7):1426–36.
29. Fidler MC, Sanchez M, Raether B, et al. A one-year randomized trial of lorcaserin for weight loss in obese and overweight adults: the BLOSSOM trial. J Clin Endocrinol Metab 2011;96(10):3067–77.
30. Greenway FL, Whitehouse MJ, Guttadauria M, et al. Rational design of a combination medication for the treatment of obesity. Obesity (Silver Spring) 2009;17(1): 30–9.
31. Contrave [package insert]. La Jolla, CA: Orexigen Therapeutics, Inc; 2016.
32. Greenway FL, Fujioka K, Plodkowski RA, et al. Effect of naltrexone plus bupropion on weight loss in overweight and obese adults (COR-I): a multicentre, randomised, double-blind, placebo-controlled, phase 3 trial. Lancet 2010;376(9741): 595–605.
33. Apovian CM, Aronne L, Rubino D, et al. A randomized, phase 3 trial of naltrexone SR/bupropion SR on weight and obesity-related risk factors (COR-II). Obesity (Silver Spring) 2013;21(5):935–43.
34. Wadden TA, Foreyt JP, Foster GD, et al. Weight loss with naltrexone SR/bupropion SR combination therapy as an adjunct to behavior modification: the COR-BMOD trial. Obesity (Silver Spring) 2011;19(1):110–20.
35. Hollander P, Gupta AK, Plodkowski R, et al. Effects of naltrexone sustained-release/bupropion sustained-release combination therapy on body weight and glycemic parameters in overweight and obese patients with type 2 diabetes. Diabetes Care 2013;36(12):4022–9.

36. Van Can J, Sloth B, Jensen CB, et al. Effects of the once-daily GLP-1 analog lir-aglutide on gastric emptying, glycemic parameters, appetite and energy metabolism in obese, non-diabetic adults. Int J Obes (Lond) 2014;38(6):784–93.

37. Davies MJ, Bergenstal R, Bode B, et al. Efficacy of liraglutide for weight loss among patients with type 2 diabetes: the SCALE Diabetes randomized clinical trial. JAMA 2015;314(7):687–99.

38. Pi-Sunyer X, Astrup A, Fujioka K, et al. A randomized, controlled trial of 3.0 mg of liraglutide in weight management. N Engl J Med 2015;373(1):11–22.

39. Wadden TA, Hollander P, Klein S, et al. Weight maintenance and additional weight loss with liraglutide after low-calorie-diet-induced weight loss: the SCALE Maintenance randomized study. Int J Obes (Lond) 2013;37(11):1443–51.

40. Smith SR, Garvey WT, Greenway FL, et al. Coadministration of lorcaserin and phentermine for weight management: a 12-week, randomized, pilot safety study. Obesity (Silver Spring) 2017;25(5):857–65.

41. Hollander P, Bays HE, Rosenstock J, et al. Coadministration of canagliflozin and phentermine for weight management in overweight and obese individuals without diabetes: a randomized clinical trial. Diabetes Care 2017;40(5):632–9.

42. Stanford FC, Alfaris N, Gomez G, et al. The utility of weight loss medications after bariatric surgery for weight regain or inadequate weight loss: a multi-center study. Surg Obes Relat Dis 2017;13(3):491–500.

43. Contrave [package insert]. Deerfield, IL: Takeda Pharmaceuticals America, Inc; 2014.

44. Saxenda [package insert]. Plainsboro, NJ: Novo Nordisk; 2014.

Medical Devices for Obesity Treatment
Endoscopic Bariatric Therapies

Eric J. Vargas, MD, Monika Rizk, BS, Fateh Bazerbachi, MD,
Barham K. Abu Dayyeh, MD, MPH*

KEYWORDS

- Endoscopy • Obesity • Treatment • Devices • Gastric balloon
- Endoscopic suturing

KEY POINTS

- Endoscopic bariatric therapies are effective and safe treatment options for obesity as part of a multifaceted approach in patients with normal gastrointestinal anatomy and motility.
- Gastric endoscopic interventions, such as intragastric balloons and remodeling techniques, alter gastric physiologic processes to enhance satiety and satiation, resulting in 10% to 20% total body weight loss.
- Small bowel interventions, such as bypass sleeves, duodenal mucosal resurfacing, and incisionless anastomoses systems, are effective for both weight loss and metabolic improvement and may offer a complementary role to gastric endoscopic interventions.

INTRODUCTION

The number of patients with obesity in the United States and worldwide that would benefit from bariatric/metabolic surgery is overwhelming. However, less than 2% of patients who are otherwise eligible receive these interventions.[1–3] This gap in care is likely multifactorial, owing to lack of appeal, costs, and morbidity and mortality associated with bariatric surgery. Thus, similar to other areas in medicine where a minimally invasive approach bridges the gap between medical and surgical management options,[4] endoscopic bariatric therapies (EBTs) have been developed to offer effective weight loss options by targeting gastric and small intestinal pathways similar to

Disclosure Statement: Drs E.J. Vargas, F. Bazerbachi, and Mrs M. Rizk have no financial disclosures. Dr B.K. Abu Dayyeh is a consultant for Apollo Endo Surgery, Boston Scientific, Olympus, and Metamodix. He has received research support from Aspire Bariatrics, Medtronic, Apollo Endosurgery, and GI Dynamics.
Division of Gastroenterology and Hepatology, Mayo Clinic, 200 First Street Southwest, Rochester, MN 55905, USA
* Corresponding author.
E-mail address: AbuDayyeh.Barham@mayo.edu

Med Clin N Am 102 (2018) 149–163
https://doi.org/10.1016/j.mcna.2017.08.013
0025-7125/18/© 2017 Elsevier Inc. All rights reserved.

bariatric/metabolic surgery with better safety profile afforded by their anatomy preserving and endoscopic nature.[5]

With recent US Food and Drug Administration (FDA) approvals, these devices/techniques are becoming popular across the nation, despite their current lack of insurance coverage. Therefore, primary care providers would benefit by becoming familiar with EBTs and when to use them. Thus, this clinical review focuses on the EBTs that are available in clinical practice or are in advanced stages of development, reviewing their efficacy and safety for primary care providers, with the goals of facilitating future patient discussions, ultimately assisting their decision to implement devices in their obesity management algorithm.

CONSIDERATIONS FOR PRIMARY CARE PROVIDERS
Why Endoscopic Bariatric Therapies for Managing Obesity

Current treatment options to lose weight for patients with obesity include lifestyle intervention, obesity pharmacotherapy, and bariatric surgery. The components of lifestyle intervention include diet, exercise, and behavior modification and should be considered the cornerstone of any obesity treatment. However, as a stand-alone therapy, even intensive lifestyle intervention is only modestly effective with an expected percent total body weight loss (%TBWL) <3%.[6]

The scientific literature is clear in showing that the magnitude of weight loss is strongly associated with prevention and improvement in obesity-related comorbidities, such as diabetes, blood pressure, hyperlipidemia, obstructive sleep apnea, and fatty liver disease. The odds of clinically significant improvements in obesity-related comorbidities are much higher when %TBWL exceeds 10%.[7,8]

Most patients with mild to moderate obesity (body mass index [BMI] 30–40 kg/m^2) do not qualify for bariatric surgery and are left without an effective management approach to their disease; therefore, both government agencies (Agency for Healthcare Research and Quality), and national societies (American Society of Bariatric and Metabolic Surgery and American Society of Gastrointestinal Endoscopy) now recognize that a significant management gap exists for patients with mild to moderate obesity (BMI between 30 and 40 kg/m^2) or those with severe obesity (BMI $\geq$ 40 mg/kg^2) who do not wish to pursue bariatric surgery.[9–11]

EBTs can achieve greater than 10% TBWL in most patients with excellent safety and lower cost than bariatric surgery. Furthermore, they are anatomy preserving and reversible, thus, well positioned to fill the gap in the management of obesity.

Despite their proven efficacy, weight loss produced by EBTs is temporary (as in the case of removable devices) or less durable (gastric remodeling techniques) than traditional bariatric surgery. Thus, EBTs should be viewed as effective weight loss tools, but a weight maintenance strategy is needed to maintain their effect long term to effectively impact obesity-related comorbidities. Therefore, primary care providers should embrace and get comfortable with a paradigm shift in managing obesity as a chronic disorder with an initial effective weight loss strategy followed by an aggressive weight maintenance phase that counteracts the physiologic and behavioral adaptations resulting from the weight loss phase using both obesity pharmacotherapies and behavioral interventions as detailed elsewhere in this issue.

Appropriate Candidates for Endoscopic Bariatric Therapies

Most of the devices and therapies mentioned in later discussion are approved or indicated for patients with a BMI between 30 and 40 kg/m^2 (1) who have not been able to lose weight or maintain weight loss though nonsurgical methods, such as moderate to intensive lifestyle interventions and/or pharmacologic interventions, or (2) who do not wish to undergo permanent surgical interventions. These therapies can also be used off-label as bridge therapy to nonbariatric surgical interventions, the outcomes of which are weight limited, such as orthopedic and transplant surgery. Generally, these therapies are contraindicated in those with prior gastroesophageal (GE) surgery, large hiatal hernias (>3 cm), or gastric motility disorders. Detailed contraindications can be found in **Box 1**. Following device placement or technique, symptoms are generally managed by the gastroenterologist or endoscopist. As described in later discussion, these EBTs have overall favorable safety profiles and result in meaningful weight loss for patients when combined with supervised weight loss programs.

GASTRIC ENDOSCOPIC BARIATRIC THERAPIES

Gastric volume reduction represents an important component of bariatric surgery. Anatomic manipulations of the stomach reduce the available area for caloric intake and induce satiety and satiation by altering gastric emptying and accommodation.[12-16] Thus, multiple EBTs have been developed that

1. Reduce the stomach's capacity via space-occupying devices, such as intragastric balloons (IGBs),
2. Remodel the stomach using endoscopic suturing/plication devices, such as endoscopic sleeve gastroplasty (ESG), and
3. Divert excess calories away from the stomach, such as aspiration therapy (AT).

Space-Occupying Devices

Space-occupying devices can be divided into balloon and nonballoon devices. At present, there are 3 FDA-approved IGBs (ReShape Duo, Orbera, Obalon) (**Table 1**) and 2 (Spatz3, Elipse) currently under investigation in the United States. Non–balloon-based devices include the TransPyloric Shuttle and the Full Sense that are under clinical investigation.

Box 1
Contraindications to intragastric balloon use

Prior bariatric, gastric, or esophageal surgery

Large hiatal hernia

Esophageal motility disorder

Esophageal strictures

Inflammatory bowel disease affecting the upper GI tract

Pregnancy

Higher risk of upper gastrointestinal bleeding (Gastric Antral Vascular Ectasias, Arteriovenous Malformations, varices, and so forth)

Concurrent use of anticoagulation or nonsteroidal anti-inflammatory drug therapy

Inability to use proton pump inhibitor

Coagulopathy

Uncontrolled psychiatric or drug/alcohol use disorder

Table 1
Intragastric balloons: outcomes in pivotal trials

IGB Name	Study Design	%TBWL	Outcome Assessment Time, mo	Placement/Removal	Reference
ReShape Duo	Pivotal randomized controlled trial (RCT)	8.4	6	Endoscopy	ASGE Bariatric Endoscopy Task Force et al,[11] 2015
Orbera	Pivotal RCT	10.2 + 6.6	6	Endoscopy	Peterli et al,[16] 2012
Obalon[a]	Pivotal RCT	6.8 ± 5	6	Capsule guided by fluoroscopy; endoscopy	FDA,[18] 2015
Spatz 3	Prospective single arm	14 (95% CI, −0.5–36.2)	6	Endoscopy	Wahlen et al,[19] 2001
Elipse	Prospective single arm	14.6 (95% CI −0.2% to 27.1%)	4	Capsule guided by fluoroscopy; pass through GI tract	Mion et al,[22] 2013

[a] Air-filled balloons; scuba diving and unpressured airplane cabins contraindicated.

Balloon space-occupying devices

ReShape Duo The ReShape Duo (ReShape Medical, San Clemente, CA, USA) device is a fluid-filled dual-balloon system that is interconnected by a flexible wire (**Fig. 1A**). The device requires endoscopic placement, and once placed, the 2 balloons are independently filled with up to 450 mL of normal saline each with methylene blue to detect early deflation. After 6 months, the balloon is removed endoscopically.

In a US pivotal multicenter randomized sham-controlled clinical trial, investigators compared 187 patients receiving balloon therapy plus lifestyle intervention to 139 patients receiving sham procedure in addition to lifestyle intervention. At 6 months, % TBWL in the ReShape Duo Group (n = 167) was 7.6% ± 5.5% compared with 3.6% ± 6.3% in the control group (n = 126).[17] Balloon intolerance rate necessitating early removal was 15%, with reports of device modification reducing this figure to 7.5%.

The dual-balloon system affords a lesser risk of balloon migration into the small bowel should 1 of the 2 balloons deflate (6% deflation rate). In the pivotal trial, gastric ulcers and erosions were initially frequent because of a design flaw that, once modified, reduced ulcer rates from 39.6% to 10.3% in study subjects.[18] There were no reported deaths, balloon migrations, obstructions, or gastric perforations. At device removal, 3 serious adverse events were reported involving an esophageal tear requiring endoscopic treatment, a contained cervical esophagus perforation that was managed with antibiotics, and one postretrieval aspiration pneumonitis that resolved without sequelae.[17,18]

Orbera Intragastric Balloon The Orbera Intragastric Balloon (Apollo EndoSurgery, Austin, TX, USA) is the most studied IGB for obesity, with favorable weight loss outcomes as demonstrated in multiple multinational research studies.[19,20] The device is a single fluid-filled spherical balloon system that requires endoscopy to confirm placement (see **Fig. 1B**). Once placed in the stomach, the balloon is filled with 450 to 700 mL of saline with optional methylene blue to detect spontaneous deflation.

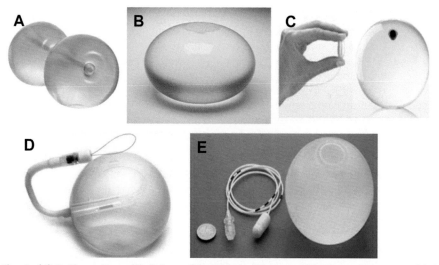

Fig. 1. (*A*) ReShape Duo. (*B*) Orbera. (*C*) Obalon. (*D*) Spatz. (*E*) Elipse. (*Courtesy of* [*A*] ReShape Medical, San Clemente, CA; [*B*] Apollo EndoSurgery, Austin, TX; [*C*] Obalon Therapeutics, Inc, Carlsbad, CA; [*D*] Spatz FGIA, Inc, Great Neck, NY; and [*E*] Allurion Technologies, Wellesley, MA.)

At 6 months, the balloon requires endoscopic removal. Balloon intolerance was reported to be 7.5%.[11,20]

A prior meta-analysis of 55 studies that included more than 6500 Orbera IGB placements worldwide demonstrated a pooled estimate of 13.2% TBWL at 6 months and 11.3% at 12 months.[20] In the following pivotal US multicenter randomized controlled clinical trial, investigators compared subjects (n = 125) who received 6 months of balloon therapy plus lifestyle intervention to those who received lifestyle intervention alone (n = 130). At time of removal (6 months), the %TBWL in the Orbera group (n = 116) was 10.2% ± 6.6% versus 3.3% ± 5% in the control group (n = 99). At 12 months, patients in the balloon arm maintained more than 70% of their weight lost at 6 months.[21]

In a meta-analysis of more than 65 studies, accommodative symptoms after placement, such as abdominal pain and nausea, were frequent side effects occurring in 29% to 34% of patients, but these symptoms mostly dissipated after a few days of therapy. Serious side effects, such as migration and gastric perforation, were 1.4% and 0.1% with the 50% of the perforations occurring in those with prior gastric surgery, which is a contraindication for placement in the United States.[20]

Obalon Balloon The Obalon Balloon (Obalon Therapeutics, Inc, Carlsbad, CA, USA) is an air-filled balloon system packaged within a gelatin capsule (see **Fig. 1C**).[22] Among the approved balloon devices, the Obalon Balloon is the only one that does not require endoscopic placement. The capsule contains a self-sealing valve that is connected to a thin catheter extending from the stomach to the mouth when the capsule is ingested. Capsule entry into the stomach is verified by fluoroscopy; upon entry into the stomach, the gelatin dissolves, freeing the balloon. The catheter is then used to inflate the balloon with nitrogen gas. The inflated balloon detaches from the catheter and remains in place until it is removed endoscopically after 12 to 26 weeks. Up to 3 capsules can be swallowed during the same session or preferably sequentially throughout therapy as weight loss plateaus.

In a US pivotal multicenter randomized sham-controlled clinical trial, investigators compared 185 patients receiving up the 3 consecutive balloon capsules plus lifestyle intervention to 181 patients receiving sham capsules in addition to lifestyle intervention. %TBWL after swallowing 3 consecutive balloon capsule (n = 185) was 6.8% ± 5.1% at 6 months from the first swallowed capsule compared with 3.65 ± 5.0% in the control group (n = 181). The safety profile of the Obalon Balloon system is favorable. In the pivotal trial, no unanticipated adverse device events occurred, and only one serious adverse event occurred, which was a gastric ulcer in the setting of nonsteroidal anti-inflammatory medication use. Nausea and abdominal cramping occurred in most (89%) subjects, but these were mostly (99.7%) rated as mild or moderate. The Obalon was approved September 2016.[23]

Spatz Adjustable Balloon The Spatz Adjustable Balloon (Spatz Medical, Great Neck, NY, USA) is an adjustable fluid-filled IGB placed endoscopically (see **Fig. 1D**). The balloon has an extractable thin, flexible tube that allows for endoscopic volume adjustment while the balloon is in place. The balloon volume may be decreased to improve tolerability or increased to aid in increased weight loss. Prior generations of the Spatz Adjustable Balloon resulted in up to 20% TBWL at 12 months but had device-related complications, such as ulcer formation and adjustment catheter impaction requiring surgical removal.[24] However, the new-generation device overcomes these design flaws and is approved for 12-month placement outside of the United States. The US multicenter pivotal trial is currently underway.

Elipse Balloon The Elipse Balloon (Allurion Technologies, Wellesley, MA, USA) is fluid-filled balloon that comes enclosed within a capsule attached to a long, thin catheter that extends from the stomach to the outside the mouth once the capsule is swallowed (see **Fig. 1**E).[25,26] Placement of the capsule in the stomach is then confirmed with fluoroscopy. Once the capsule enters the stomach, it degrades, freeing the balloon, and the catheter is used to fill the balloon with up to 550 mL of saline. After 4 months of therapy, the balloon valve opens, allowing the balloon to empty and the deflated balloon is excreted spontaneously from the gastrointestinal (GI) tract, thus eliminating the need for endoscopy for device placement or removal. Pilot data in 12 patients demonstrated 14.6% TBWL at 4 months and 5.9% TBWL at 12 months.[27] The Elipse balloon is approved for use outside of the United States, and the US pivotal trial is currently being planned.

Nonballoon space-occupying devices

The TransPyloric Shuttle The TransPyloric Shuttle (TPS; BAROnova, Goleta, CA, USA) is a nonballoon gastric-occupying device that is delivered through an overtube, a protective hollow tube, allowing safe passage of the device into the stomach, where it self-assembles. Composed of a greater spherical silicone orb that is attached to a lesser cylindrical silicone bulb by a flexible cord, the device's lesser bulb transverses the duodenum with natural peristalsis with the greater orb remaining behind the pylorus (**Fig. 2**A). This device creates an intermittent seal inducing satiety through gastric emptying delay. In the first feasibility study, 20 patients were randomized to TPS placement for either 3 or 6 months. Patients who had the device for 3 months experienced 25.1% excess weight loss (EWL), whereas those with the device for 6 months lost an average %EWL of 41%.[28] A pivotal multicenter randomized trial is currently underway in the United States to support the regulatory approval of this device.

The Full Sense The Full Sense Bariatric Device (Baker, Foote, Kemmeter, Walburn LLC, Grand Rapids, MI, USA) is both endoscopically placed and removed. This bariatric device is composed of an esophageal stent connected to a gastric disk via a strut (see **Fig. 2**B). By residing in the cardia, it induces satiety and feelings of fullness. Reportedly, unpublished human data with 3 subjects showed 28% EWL in 46 days. A median of 80% EWL has been reported during a 6-month trial in an unknown number of subjects. These results are reportedly backed by a randomized trial and follow-up crossover trial design.[29] The company is in the process of starting a large trial in hopes of regulatory approval.

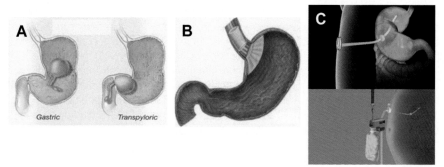

Fig. 2. (A) TransPyloric Shuttle. (B) Full Sense. (C) Aspiration therapy. (*Courtesy of* [A] BAR-Onova, Goleta, CA; [B] Baker, Foote, Kemmeter, Walburn LLC, Grand Rapids, MI; and [C] Aspire Bariatrics, King of Prussia, PA.)

Aspiration therapy

AT is another endoscopic treatment approach involving partial disposal of an ingested meal to reduce overall caloric intake through a modified percutaneous endoscopic gastrostomy (PEG) tube (see **Fig. 2**C). This device is FDA approved for use in the United States in patients with a BMI between 35 and 55 kg/m^2, a higher BMI range than for IGBs, for up to 5 years. It requires endoscopic replacement and removal, unlike standard PEG tubes.

The AT process uses a specifically designed percutaneous gastrostomy tube (A-Tube; Aspire Bariatrics, King of Prussia, PA, USA) made of silicone. The tube is inserted in a similar fashion as standard PEG tubes. After 2 weeks, the A-tube is shortened to the level of the skin and the skin port is attached. The skin port allows attachment to the aspiration device, which fits in a small zippered bag. Once the device is connected to the skin port, a water reservoir flushes tap water into the stomach to facilitate disposal of food. Patients are instructed to perform aspiration about 20 minutes after ingesting a meal, removing and discarding about one-third of the meal. The process takes about 10 to 15 minutes to complete. The device has a built in counter that locks the device to avoid overuse.

In a US pivotal, multicenter, randomized controlled trial, 111 subjects underwent AT with lifestyle intervention for 12 months compared with 60 subjects who underwent lifestyle intervention alone. At 12 months, %TBWL for those who completed AT (n = 82) was 14.2% ± 9.8% compared with 4.9% ± 7% in the control group (n = 31). Because aspiration removes around 30% of ingested calories, it is estimated that AT accounts for 80% of the reported weight loss. AT requires food to be chewed thoroughly and for patients to eat slower, potentially adapting new eating behaviors. As far as safety, the adverse events included stoma granulation tissue (40.5%), stoma infection (14.4%), peritonitis (0.9%), and gastric ulcer rates (0.9%). Careful review of disordered eating behavior questionnaires found no evidence of worsening eating behaviors with therapy.[30]

ENDOSCOPIC PLICATION PROCEDURES
Endoscopic Sleeve Gastroplasty

ESG is an incisionless gastric volume reduction technique that creates a restrictive endoscopic sleeve that delays gastric emptying and decreased the overall consumption of calories.[31] This endoscopic sleeve is achieved using a commercially available full-thickness suturing device (OverStitch; Apollo EndoSurgery) by placing a series of triangular full-thickness sutures through the gastric wall along the greater curvature of the stomach from the prepyloric antrum to the GE junction, leaving a small pouch in the fundus (**Fig. 3**A).[32,33] The procedure has been successfully performed across many centers inside and outside the United States, with reproducible results.[31,34–39] A recent multinational study with 245 patients revealed 24-month %TBWL of 18.6% (95% confidence interval [CI] 15.7–21.5) with greater than 84% and 53% of subjects achieving greater than 10% TBWL at 24 months on per protocol and intention-to-treat analyses, respectively.[40] Compared with space-occupying devices, these techniques seem to offer a larger magnitude of effect and durability, yet not as effective as vertical sleeve gastrectomy.

Procedure-related adverse events occurred in 5 subjects (2%), including 2 perigastric inflammatory fluid collections that resolved with percutaneous drainage and antibiotics, one self-limited extragastric hemorrhage that required blood transfusion, one pulmonary embolism 72 hours after the procedure, and one pneumoperitoneum and pneumothorax requiring chest tube placement. All patients recovered fully without surgical intervention, and most of these adverse events were mitigated with minor procedural adjustments, such as using CO_2 gas instead of air for the procedure.

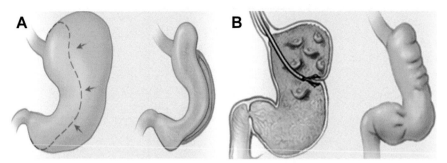

Fig. 3. (*A*) Endoscopic sleeve gastroplasty (ESG). (*B*) Primary obesity surgery endoluminal (POSE).

Primary Obesity Surgery Endoluminal

Primary obesity surgery endoluminal (POSE) uses a peroral incisionless operating platform (USGI Medical, San Clemente, CA, USA) to place transmural tissue anchor plications that reduce accommodation of the gastric fundus. Three additional plications are placed in the distal gastric body to delay gastric emptying (see **Fig. 3**B). POSE has been associated with both improved satiation and satiation gut neurohormonal response.[41]

A pivotal US multicenter, randomized blinded clinical trial compared 221 patients receiving POSE in addition to a low-intensity lifestyle intervention for 12 months to 111 patients receiving lifestyle intervention alone. The %TBWL at 12 months for the POSE group was 4.94% $\pm$ 7% compared with 1.38% $\pm$ 5.6% in the control group. The rate of serious adverse events was 4.7% (1.9% vomiting requiring longer hospital stay, 1.6% nausea requiring longer hospital stay, 0.4% pain requiring longer hospital stay, 0.4% extragastric bleeding requiring open surgical exploration, and 0.4% hepatic abscess requiring percutaneous drainage).[42] Prior open-label prospective and nonblinded randomized trials demonstrated better weight loss (>15% TBWL) at 6 to 12 months.[43,44] Further clinical trials are currently under development (**Table 2**).

SMALL BOWEL ENDOSCOPIC THERAPIES

The small intestine plays a major role in nutrient sensing and absorption. In response to luminal nutrients, the proximal small intestine's neuroendocrine cells release gut peptides and activate neuronal circuitry that have been implicated in satiety and glucose metabolism, thus partially contributing to the success of Roux-en-Y gastric bypass surgery in diabetes resolution.[4,45,46] EBTs targeting the small intestine and mimicking bypass physiology through (1) bypass linear, (2) resurfacing of the duodenal mucosa, and (3) incisionless anastomoses systems are under investigation.

EndoBarrier

The EndoBarrier (Endobarrier GI Dynamics, Lexington, MA, USA) is a 65-cm-long Teflon-coated duodenal jejunal bypass sleeve (DJBS) that allows undigested food to reach the jejunum, where it mixes with pancreaticobiliary juices (**Fig. 4**A). The device comes packaged in a delivery capsule that is endoscopically placed with the assistance of a stiff wire and fluoroscopy. Once the capsule reaches the duodenal bulb, the sleeve is advanced 65 cm into the small bowel, and the anchoring crown is deployed in the duodenal bulb. The device is designed to stay in place for 12 months, when it is

Table 2
Aspiration and gastric remodeling therapies: reported outcomes

IGB Name	Study Design	%TBWL	Outcome Assessment Time, mo	Placement/Removal	Reference
Aspiration therapy	Pivotal RCT	14.2 ± 9.8	12	Endoscopy	Machytka et al,[25] 2017
ESG	Multinational trial (retrospective)	18.6 (95% CI 15.7–21.5)	24	Endoscopy	Lopez-Nava Breviere et al,[35] 2016
POSE	Pivotal RCT	4.94 ± 7	12	Endoscopy	Sullivan et al,[37] 2017

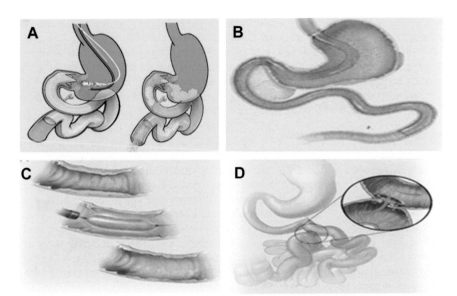

Fig. 4. (*A*) EndoBarrier. (*B*) Endoluminal bypass. (*C*) Duodenal mucosal resurfacing (DMR). (*D*) Incisionless magnetic anastomosis system (IMAS). (*Courtesy of* [*A*] Endobarrier GI Dynamics, Lexington, MA; [*B*] valenTx, Maple Grove, MN; [*C*] Fractyl, Lexington, MA; and [*D*] GI Windows, W. Bridgewater, MA.)

endoscopically removed using a custom device that allows the anchoring crown to collapse into a foreign body hood, minimizing any trauma to the GI tract during removal.

The device's efficacy has been demonstrated through a recent meta-analysis of the published literature. The EndoBarrier resulted in 35.3% (95% CI, 24.6%–46.1%) EWL at 12 months.[20] Four randomized controlled trials compared 12 to 24 weeks of treatment with the EndoBarrier (n = 90) with a sham or control arm (n = 84) with significant mean difference %EWL compared with the control group at 9.4% (95% CI, 8.26%–10.65%). The device also demonstrated an impact on diabetic control after implantation, with improvements in hemoglobin A1c (HgbA1c) from −0.7 (95% CI, −1.76–0.2; P = .16) at 12 weeks to −1.7 (95% CI, −2.5 to −0.86; P<.001) at 24 weeks, and −1.5 (95% CI, −2.2 to −0.78; P<.001) beyond 52 weeks from implantation. This improvement in HgbA1c was statistically significant compared with the sham or control diabetic group, where the EndoBarrier DJBS resulted in an additional −1% (95% CI, −1.67 to −0.4) (P = .001) reduction in HgbA1c. A pivotal multicenter double-blinded sham control trial in the United States was terminated early after enrollment of 325/500 patients owing to a 3.5% incidence of hepatic abscess formation. Despite only two-thirds enrollment, subjects who received the device lost significantly more weight at 12 months (TBWL 7.7% ± 9.6% vs 2.1% ± 5.4%, P<.0001) and had more significant improvement in HgbA1c (−1.1 ± 1.5 vs −0.3 ± 1.6) compared with control subjects. Early device retrieval owing to adverse events was performed in 10.9% of patients. Second-generation devices with atraumatic anchoring and retrieval systems are currently undergoing human clinical trials.

Endoluminal Bypass

The Endoluminal Bypass (valenTx, Maple Grove, MN, USA) is a 120-cm liner endoscopically placed from the GE junction to the small bowel mimicking the Roux-en-Y bypass surgery. It is designed to stay in place for 12 months when it is endoscopically removed (see **Fig. 4**B). In the pilot study, 12 patients had the device successfully placed, with 2 requiring early removal due to intolerance. The remaining 10 patients completed 12 months of therapy, with 60% of them having fully attached devices at 12 months. The remaining 40% experienced partial cuff detachment seen at follow-up endoscopy. Among the 6 patients who had fully intact and functional sleeves at 12 months, mean %EWL was 54% with improvement in obesity-related comorbidities. Clinical trials are currently undergoing consideration.[47]

Duodenal Mucosal Resurfacing

Duodenal mucosal resurfacing (DMR) (Fractyl, Lexington, MA, USA) is an endoscopic procedure that uses heated water to thermally ablate the superficial duodenal mucosa (see **Fig. 4**C). It is hypothesized that mucosal remodeling may reset duodenal stem and enteroendocrine cells that have become inactive, thus improving glucose metabolism.[48] A study of 39 patients with poorly controlled diabetes mellitus who underwent long-segment DMR (>9 cm; n = 28) or short-segment DMR (<6 cm; n = 11), showed improvement in HbA1c from 9.5% to 8.3% with greater improvements seen in the greater than 9 cm cohort compared with the less than 6-cm cohort.[49] Duodenal stenosis developed in 3 patients who were treated successfully with balloon dilation. A European multicenter trial is currently underway.

Incisionless Magnetic Anastomotic System

Designed to mimic duodenal switch and ileal transposition, the Incisionless Magnetic Anastomotic System (GI Windows, West Bridgewater, MA, USA) uses self-assembling magnets to create an anastomosis via incisionless magnetic compression. The technique requires simultaneous dual upper and lower endoscopy, whereby the self-assembling magnets are deployed from the working channel of each endoscope, forming magnetic octagons in the jejunum and ileum (see **Fig. 4**D). After a week, the anastomosis forms, and the coupled magnets pass spontaneously through the stool. Preliminary studies using 10 subjects showed 14.6 %TBWL at 1 year (range 0.3%-41.8%) with HbA1c levels improving from 6.6% ± 1.8% to 5.4% ± 0.5%.[50] More investigations and applications are underway.

FUTURE CONSIDERATIONS

EBTs are safe and effective treatments for obesity. The magnitude and duration of weight loss vary by device given their temporary nature. Therefore, weight recidivism should be expected and managed by a comprehensive team of primary care providers, gastroenterologists, nutritionists, dieticians, and behavioral therapy professionals. Moving forward, personalizing EBTs to each subject based on their physiology and clinical phenotype will be imperative.[51] The sequential and tandem use of EBTs in conjunction with pharmacotherapy and comprehensive lifestyle interventions remain to be investigated, which may yield the most robust and durable weight loss response, achieving a lasting effect on obesity and its comorbidities.

REFERENCES

1. Buchwald H, Oien DM. Metabolic/bariatric surgery worldwide 2011. Obes Surg 2013;23(4):427–36.

2. Sjoholm K, Anveden A, Peltonen M, et al. Evaluation of current eligibility criteria for bariatric surgery: diabetes prevention and risk factor changes in the Swedish Obese Subjects (SOS) study. Diabetes Care 2013;36(5):1335–40.

3. GBD 2015 Obesity Collaborators, Afshin A, Forouzanfar MH, Reitsma MB, et al. Health effects of overweight and obesity in 195 countries over 25 years. N Engl J Med 2017;377(1):13–27.

4. Schauer PR, Bhatt DL, Kirwan JP, et al. Bariatric surgery versus intensive medical therapy for diabetes - 5-year outcomes. N Engl J Med 2017;376(7):641–51.

5. Abu Dayyeh BK, Edmundowicz S, Thompson CC. Clinical practice update: expert review on endoscopic bariatric therapies. Gastroenterology 2017;152(4): 716–29.

6. Look AHEAD Research Group. Eight-year weight losses with an intensive lifestyle intervention: the look AHEAD study. Obesity (Silver Spring) 2014;22(1):5–13.

7. Daniel S, Soleymani T, Garvey WT. A complications-based clinical staging of obesity to guide treatment modality and intensity. Curr Opin Endocrinol Diabetes Obes 2013;20(5):377–88.

8. Vilar-Gomez E, Martinez-Perez Y, Calzadilla-Bertot L, et al. Weight loss through lifestyle modification significantly reduces features of nonalcoholic steatohepatitis. Gastroenterology 2015;149(2):367–78.e5.

9. ECRI Institute. AHRQ healthcare horizon scanning system potential high-impact interventions: priority area 10: obesity (Prepared by ECRI Institute under Contract No. HHSA290-2010-00006-C.). Rockville (MD): Agency for Healthcare Research and Quality; 2015. Available at: http://effectivehealthcare.ahrq.gov/index.cfm/.

10. Committee ASfMaBSCI. American Society for Metabolic and Bariatric Surgery position statement on intra-gastric balloon therapy. 2015. Available at: https:// asmbs.org/wp/uploads/2015/10/IntraGastricBalloon_Statement_DRAFT.pdf. Accessed December, 2016.

11. ASGE Bariatric Endoscopy Task Force, Sullivan S, Kumar N, et al. ASGE position statement on endoscopic bariatric therapies in clinical practice. Gastrointest Endosc 2015;82(5):767–72.

12. Aron-Wisnewsky J, Dore J, Clement K. The importance of the gut microbiota after bariatric surgery. Nat Rev Gastroenterol Hepatol 2012;9(10):590–8.

13. Cummings DE, Weigle DS, Frayo RS, et al. Plasma ghrelin levels after diet-induced weight loss or gastric bypass surgery. N Engl J Med 2002;346(21):1623–30.

14. Fruhbeck G, Diez Caballero A, Gil MJ. Fundus functionality and ghrelin concentrations after bariatric surgery. N Engl J Med 2004;350(3):308–9.

15. Li JV, Ashrafian H, Bueter M, et al. Metabolic surgery profoundly influences gut microbial-host metabolic cross-talk. Gut 2011;60(9):1214–23.

16. Peterli R, Steinert RE, Woelnerhanssen B, et al. Metabolic and hormonal changes after laparoscopic Roux-en-Y gastric bypass and sleeve gastrectomy: a randomized, prospective trial. Obes Surg 2012;22(5):740–8.

17. Ponce J, Woodman G, Swain J, et al. The REDUCE pivotal trial: a prospective, randomized controlled pivotal trial of a dual intragastric balloon for the treatment of obesity. Surg Obes Relat Dis 2015;11(4):874–81.

18. FDA. ReShape integrated dual balloon system: summary of safety and effectiveness data (SSED). 2015. Available at: http://www.accessdata.fda.gov/cdrh_docs/pdf14/P140012b.pdf. Accessed December 20, 2016.

19. Wahlen CH, Bastens B, Herve J, et al. The BioEnterics Intragastric Balloon (BIB): how to use it. Obes Surg 2001;11(4):524–7.

20. ASGE Bariatric Endoscopy Task Force and ASGE Technology Committee, Abu Dayyeh BK, Kumar N, Edmundowicz SA, et al. ASGE Bariatric Endoscopy Task Force systematic review and meta-analysis assessing the ASGE PIVI thresholds for adopting endoscopic bariatric therapies. Gastrointest Endosc 2015;82(3): 425–38.e5.

21. Courcoulas A, Abu Dayyeh BK, Eaton L, et al. Intragastric balloon as an adjunct to lifestyle intervention: a randomized controlled trial. Int J Obes (Lond) 2017; 41(3):427–33.

22. Mion F, Ibrahim M, Marjoux S, et al. Swallowable Obalon(R) gastric balloons as an aid for weight loss: a pilot feasibility study. Obes Surg 2013;23(5):730–3.

23. FDA. Obalon balloon system: summary of safety and effectiveness data 2016. Available at: http://www.accessdata.fda.gov/cdrh_docs/pdf16/P160001b.pdf. Accessed December 20, 2016

24. Brooks J, Srivastava ED, Mathus-Vliegen EM. One-year adjustable intragastric balloons: results in 73 consecutive patients in the U.K. Obes Surg 2014;24(5):813–9.

25. Machytka E, Gaur S, Chuttani R, et al. Elipse, the first procedureless gastric balloon for weight loss: a prospective, observational, open-label, multicenter study. Endoscopy 2017;49(2):154–60.

26. Machytka E, Chuttani R, Bojkova M, et al. Elipse, a procedureless gastric balloon for weight loss: a proof-of-concept pilot study. Obes Surg 2016;26(3):512–6.

27. Raftopoulos I, Giannakou A. The Elipse balloon, a swallowable gastric balloon for weight loss not requiring sedation, anesthesia or endoscopy: a pilot study with 12-month outcomes. Surg Obes Relat Dis 2017;13(7):1174–82.

28. Marinos G, Eliades C, Raman Muthusamy V, et al. Weight loss and improved quality of life with a nonsurgical endoscopic treatment for obesity: clinical results from a 3- and 6-month study. Surg Obes Relat Dis 2014;10(5):929–34.

29. Myall P. New endoscopic stent can lead to 100% EWL. 2012. Available at: http://www.bariatricnews.net/?q=node/102. Accessed October 11, 2016.

30. Thompson CC, Abu Dayyeh BK, Kushner R, et al. Percutaneous gastrostomy device for the treatment of class II and class III obesity: results of a randomized controlled trial. Am J Gastroenterol 2017;112(3):447–57.

31. Abu Dayyeh BK, Acosta A, Camilleri M, et al. Endoscopic sleeve gastroplasty alters gastric physiology and induces loss of body weight in obese individuals. Clin Gastroenterol Hepatol 2017;15(1):37–43.e1.

32. Lopez-Nava G, Galvao MP, da Bautista-Castano I, et al. Endoscopic sleeve gastroplasty for the treatment of obesity. Endoscopy 2015;47(5):449–52.

33. Abu Dayyeh BK, Rajan E, Gostout CJ. Endoscopic sleeve gastroplasty: a potential endoscopic alternative to surgical sleeve gastrectomy for treatment of obesity. Gastrointest Endosc 2013;78(3):530–5.

34. Sharaiha RZ, Kedia P, Kumta N, et al. Initial experience with endoscopic sleeve gastroplasty: technical success and reproducibility in the bariatric population. Endoscopy 2015;47(2):164–6.

35. Lopez-Nava Breviere G, Bautista-Castano I, Fernandez-Corbelle JP, et al. Endoscopic sleeve gastroplasty (the Apollo method): a new approach to obesity management. Rev Esp Enferm Dig 2016;108(4):201–6.

36. Galvao-Neto MD, Grecco E, Souza TF, et al. Endoscopic sleeve gastroplasty - minimally invasive therapy for primary obesity treatment. Arq Bras Cir Dig 2016;29(Suppl 1):95–7.

37. Sullivan S, Edmundowicz S. Early experience with endoscopic sleeve gastroplasty and hints at mechanisms of action. Clin Gastroenterol Hepatol 2017; 15(1):44–5.

38. Sharaiha RZ, Kumta NA, Saumoy M, et al. Endoscopic sleeve gastroplasty significantly reduces body mass index and metabolic complications in obese patients. Clin Gastroenterol Hepatol 2017;15(4):504–10.

39. Barola S, Chen YI, Ngamruengphong S, et al. Technical aspects of endoscopic sleeve gastroplasty. Gastrointest Endosc 2017;85(4):862.

40. Lopez-Nava G, Sharaiha RZ, Vargas EJ, et al. Endoscopic sleeve gastroplasty for obesity: a multicenter study of 248 patients with 24 months follow-up. Obes Surg 2017;27(10):2649–55.
41. Espinos JC, Turro R, Moragas G, et al. Gastrointestinal physiological changes and their relationship to weight loss following the pose procedure. Obes Surg 2016;26(5):1081–9.
42. Sullivan S, Swain JM, Woodman G, et al. Randomized sham-controlled trial evaluating efficacy and safety of endoscopic gastric plication for primary obesity: the ESSENTIAL trial. Obesity (Silver Spring) 2017;25(2):294–301.
43. Lopez-Nava G, Bautista-Castano I, Jimenez A, et al. The Primary Obesity Surgery Endolumenal (POSE) procedure: one-year patient weight loss and safety outcomes. Surg Obes Relat Dis 2015;11(4):861–5.
44. Miller K, Turro R, Greve JW, et al. MILEPOST multicenter randomized controlled trial: 12-month weight loss and satiety outcomes after pose SM vs. medical therapy. Obes Surg 2017;27(2):310–22.
45. Rubino F, Gagner M, Gentileschi P, et al. The early effect of the Roux-en-Y gastric bypass on hormones involved in body weight regulation and glucose metabolism. Ann Surg 2004;240(2):236–42.
46. Rubino F, Forgione A, Cummings DE, et al. The mechanism of diabetes control after gastrointestinal bypass surgery reveals a role of the proximal small intestine in the pathophysiology of type 2 diabetes. Ann Surg 2006;244(5):741–9.
47. Sandler BJ, Rumbaut R, Swain CP, et al. One-year human experience with a novel endoluminal, endoscopic gastric bypass sleeve for morbid obesity. Surg Endosc 2015;29(11):3298–303.
48. Garvey WT. Ablation of the duodenal mucosa as a strategy for glycemic control in type 2 diabetes: role of nutrient signaling or simple weight loss. Diabetes Care 2016;39(12):2108–10.
49. Rajagopalan H, Cherrington AD, Thompson CC, et al. Endoscopic duodenal mucosal resurfacing for the treatment of type 2 diabetes: 6-month interim analysis from the first-in-human proof-of-concept study. Diabetes Care 2016;39(12):2254–61.
50. Machytka E, Buzga M, Lautz DB, et al. 103 a dual-path enteral bypass procedure created by a novel incisionless anastomosis system (IAS): 6-month clinical results. Gastroenterology 150(4):S26.
51. Acosta A, Abu Dayyeh BK, Port JD, et al. Challenges and opportunities in management of obesity. Gut 2014;63(4):687–95.

Bariatric Surgery for Obesity

Carel W. le Roux, MD, PhD[a], Helen M. Heneghan, MD, PhD[b],*

KEYWORDS

- Obesity • Bariatric surgery • Metabolic surgery • Type 2 diabetes mellitus
- Gastric bypass • Sleeve gastrectomy

KEY POINTS

- Bariatric surgery is the most effective treatment for severe obesity. It is associated with significant and sustained weight loss and is more effective than lifestyle or medical management in achieving glycemic control and reductions in morbidity and mortality from cardiovascular disease and even cancer.
- The most commonly performed bariatric procedures are gastric banding, sleeve gastrectomy, Roux-en-Y gastric bypass, and biliopancreatic diversion (BPD), with or without duodenal switch. Most operations are successfully performed laparoscopically.
- Weight loss plays a major role in inducing improved glucose homeostasis following bariatric surgery, but there are several weight-independent mechanisms at play.
- Bariatric surgery has a very low mortality (0.04%–0.3%) and morbidity (4.3% incidence of major adverse events in the early postoperative period).
- Nutritional deficiencies are common following some bariatric procedures (gastric bypass and BPD). Lifelong supplementation of vitamins D and B12, folic acid, iron, and calcium, among others, is recommended.

INTRODUCTION

The rising prevalence of obesity, along with high numbers of nonresponders to medical weight-reduction programs, has led to the evolution and success of bariatric surgery.[1–3] Although this treatment was initially conceived purely for weight loss, bariatric surgery has since evolved into a treatment for health gain. Several randomized trials and prospective cohort studies have demonstrated that bariatric surgery is not only superior to usual medical care for weight loss but also, more importantly, translates into several health benefits, including improved glycemic control and reductions in

Disclosure Statement: The authors have no disclosures.
[a] Diabetes Complication Research Centre, UCD Conway Institute, School of Medicine and Medical Science, University College Dublin, Dublin, Ireland; [b] Department of Surgery, St Vincent's University Hospital, University College Dublin, Elm Park, Dublin, Ireland
* Corresponding author.
E-mail address: helenheneghan@hotmail.com

Med Clin N Am 102 (2018) 165–182
https://doi.org/10.1016/j.mcna.2017.08.011
0025-7125/18/© 2017 Elsevier Inc. All rights reserved.

morbidity and mortality from cardiovascular disease and even cancer.[4-9] Observing and investigating the significant metabolic impact of bariatric procedures have led to an understanding of several weight-independent mechanisms by which these procedures affect metabolic health. Indeed, many have embraced the term "metabolic surgery" to emphasize such effects.[10,11] Furthermore, surgical procedures have evolved and outcomes improved over the last decade, with the widespread adoption of minimally invasive techniques, enhanced recovery programs, and a commitment to data reporting.

Gastric banding, sleeve gastrectomy, Roux-en-Y gastric bypass (RYGB) and biliopancreatic diversion (BPD), with or without duodenal switch (DS), are the most commonly performed bariatric procedures at present. These operations have traditionally been categorized as restrictive (band and sleeve), malabsorptive (BPD, DS), or combined restrictive and malabsorptive (RYGB) procedures. However, this classification is unscientific, and an increasing body of literature demonstrates that mechanisms other than restriction and malabsorption are at play. It has emerged that procedure effects are largely determined by visceral signals, which occur as a result of anatomic alterations to the gut.[12,13] Gastric banding and sleeve gastrectomy only alter stomach anatomy, whereas RYGB and BPD involve anatomic alterations of both the stomach and the small bowel. The mechanism of action of each procedure results in unique outcomes and can give rise to a constellation of procedure-specific risks, merits, and limitations. In this review, the authors summarize the published outcomes of commonly performed bariatric procedures, including weight loss, perioperative morbidity and mortality, late complications, as well as the impact of bariatric surgery on comorbidities, cardiovascular risk, and mortality. The authors also briefly discuss the mechanisms by which bariatric/metabolic surgery causes such significant weight loss and health gain.

INDICATIONS FOR SURGERY

The eligibility criteria for bariatric surgery established by the National Institutes of Health in 1991 are widely used,[14] but are now being challenged. According to these criteria, patients are eligible if they have a body mass index (BMI) between 35 and 40 kg/m^2 as well as an obesity-related complication, such as diabetes mellitus, obstructive sleep apnea, or cardiovascular risk factors, or a BMI $\geq$40 kg/m^2, regardless of weight-related comorbidities. These criteria were based on risk-benefit evidence (risk of obesity vs surgical risk-benefit) at the time when most operations were not being done laparoscopically. The criteria reflect the consensus views of an expert group of surgeons, physicians, psychologists, and others that were expressed more than 25 years ago, whereas many of today's commonly used procedures were not in existence. Despite the time elapsed, many of the fundamental issues of bariatric surgery remain the same, although the widespread adoption of the laparoscopic approach to bariatric surgery and safer anesthetic techniques in these patients have reduced surgical risk significantly.

More recently, the International Diabetes Federation and more than 50 other organizations interested in the treatment of diabetes have recommended considering bariatric surgery for individuals with BMI less than 35 kg/m^2 and poorly controlled type 2 diabetes (T2D) despite best medical care.[15] If a candidate meets these eligibility criteria for surgery, then a multidisciplinary team assessment is made as to the suitability of the candidate. In some countries, this can be a complex process involving psychological, surgical, dietetic, and medical review to ensure that the individual is physically and psychologically fit to proceed to surgery[16]; however, many of these practices have evolved without an evidence base. There are also no evidence-based exclusion criteria, but the main contraindications in common use are psychological features that indicate that a patient would not be able to cope with the impact of the procedure, such as personality disorders, or that the procedures may put the patient at higher risk after surgery, such as alcohol addiction. Patient's fitness for surgery is assessed by the anesthetist on a case-by-case basis. The decision to operate will consider the candidate's potential benefit from surgery and the perioperative risks.

SURGICAL PROCEDURES

Over the last decade, bariatric surgical techniques have evolved and advanced. Recent data examining the utilization of laparoscopic bariatric procedures at academic medical centers in the United States reflect changing trends.[17] Vertical-banded gastroplasty was the prototype operation for many years, until acknowledgment of its high failure rates and long-term complications resulted in it being largely abandoned. Sleeve gastrectomy was initially used as the first component of a 2-stage DS procedure in high-risk patients, but has since been demonstrated to be effective as a stand-alone bariatric procedure and has now become the most commonly performed procedure in the United States, where it accounts for approximately 54% of all bariatric operations. Gastric bypass is the second most commonly performed procedure at present (approximately 23%), and gastric banding is much less commonly performed than previously (approximately 6% of all procedures). BPD and DS (**Fig. 1**) are infrequently performed in the United States (<1%), and revisional procedures are becoming increasingly common (13%) (ASMBS [American Society for Metabolic & Bariatric Surgery] data acquired from BOLD [Bariatric Outcomes Longitudinal Database], ACS/MBSAQIP [American College of Surgeons/Metabolic and Bariatric Surgery Accreditation and Quality Improvement Program], National Inpatient Sample data https://asmbs.org/resources/estimate-of-bariatric-surgery-numbers).

Novel endoscopic procedures are proposed alternatives to bariatric surgery and include intragastric balloons, duodenojejunal bypass liners such as the EndoBarrier, and endoscopic suturing platforms.[18,19] These largely experimental procedures are associated with a mean weight loss of 5% to 15% in the short term, and a complication rate of up to 20%. Given the lack of long-term data at present, the role for such devices remains to be determined. Most recently, The AspireAssist System has received approval from the US Food and Drug Administration and is in clinical trials. This device is a novel endoscopic weight-loss device composed of an endoscopically placed percutaneous gastrostomy tube and an external device to facilitate drainage of approximately one-third of the calories consumed in a meal. Pilot data from patients with this device demonstrate a total body weight loss of 12% at 1-year follow-up.

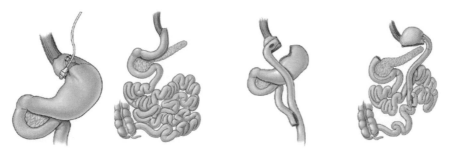

Gastric Banding   Sleeve gastrectomy   Roux-en-Y Gastric Bypass   BPD

Fig. 1. Common bariatric procedures. (Reprinted with permission, Cleveland Clinic Center for Medical Art & Photography © 2017. All Rights Reserved.)

OUTCOMES OF BARIATRIC SURGERY: BENEFITS
Weight Loss

Previously, the primary goal of bariatric procedures has been weight loss. Although the various procedures achieve this to different extents, the overall weight loss is reported to be 15% to 30% in the long term.[11,20,21] RYGB and BPD achieve greater and more durable weight loss compared with sleeve gastrectomy and gastric banding, although at the expense of higher nutritional complications. Patients undergoing gastric banding and sleeve gastrectomy may also have a greater risk of weight regain in long-term follow-up.[22,23]

Overall, up to 20% of all bariatric patients lose less than 20% of their weight and are considered by some as surgical failures. The cause of failed bariatric procedures is complex and multifactorial. Contributing factors include technical complications (rare), patients with complex and chronic obesity syndromes that do not respond to surgery (common), and specific postsurgical causes that attenuate the usual profound effect of bariatric surgery on appetite (common).[24] Attempts to identify factors predictive of weight loss failure have been rather futile thus far.[24,25] Careful patient selection, preoperative education, meticulous operative technique, and routine follow-up have been thought to contribute to a lower incidence of failure, but most studies have failed to prove causation between these factors and outcomes. Clinical research endeavors are focused on identifying clinical, biochemical, or molecular factors that may influence bariatric surgery outcomes and therefore have utility as prognostic tools to better select the right procedure for the right patient. Thus, far very few prognostic markers have been identified. Revisional bariatric surgery is a growing subspecialty, in response to the rapid increase worldwide of the numbers of primary bariatric procedures, a proportion of which will be unsuccessful. RYGB is the most commonly practiced revisional bariatric procedure and has been documented to achieve excellent rescue rates with up to 25% weight loss from original presurgical weight.[26,27] The morbidity and mortality rates for revisional bariatric surgery are higher than those of primary procedures, but are deemed acceptable when considered alongside the restored benefits of weight loss and comorbidity resolution.[28,29]

Impact on Complications of Obesity

In addition to substantial weight loss, bariatric surgery is known to have profound metabolic effects, the most striking of which is the marked resolution of obesity-associated complications, such as diabetes, hypertension, and dyslipidemia. The various procedures differ in the degree of improvement they impart on an individual's state of metabolic disarray, with RYGB and BPD demonstrating greatest benefit in this regard overall.[20]

A substantial body of evidence, including data from 16 randomized controlled trials (summarized in **Table 1**),[4,5,30–48] demonstrates that bariatric/metabolic surgery achieves superior glycemic control and reduction of cardiovascular risk factors in patients with T2D compared with various medical and lifestyle interventions. The first of these to clearly report on weight loss and diabetic outcomes, by Dixon and colleagues,[49] compared the 2-year outcomes of conventional medical treatment with gastric banding for the management of type 2 diabetes mellitus (T2DM), in 60 obese patients. More recently, Schauer and colleagues[5] and Mingrone and colleagues[4] evaluated the 12-, 24-, 36-, and 60-month effects of bariatric surgery (gastric bypass, sleeve gastrectomy, or BPD) compared with intensive medical therapy on diabetes management.[35–37] All 3 groups demonstrated that weight loss surgery was far more effective than medical therapy at inducing remission or improvement of

Table 1
Summary of all randomized controlled trials in the field of bariatric and metabolic surgery to date

Authors	Study Group	N	Mean (SD) Age (y)	Female (%)	Mean (SD) Preop BMI (kg/m²)	Follow-up Duration (mo)	Type 2 Diabetes Prevalence (%)	Type 2 Diabetes Duration (y)	Mean Weight Loss (kg)	Diabetes Remission[a]	Mean Decrease in HbA1C (% Points)
Petry, 2015	Bariatric surgery (DJBm)	10	47 (8)	nr	29.7 (1.9)	12	100	6 (3)	8 (nr)	0.0%	1.2 (nr)
	Control	7	44 (5)	nr	31.7 (3.5)	12	100	5 (3)	1 (nr)	0.0%	0.6 (nr)
Ding, 2015	Bariatric surgery (LAGB)	18	50.6 (12.6)	50.0%	36.4 (3.0)	12	100	10.4 (5.6)	13.5 (1.7)	5.6%	1.23 (0.3)
	Control	22	51.4 (7.5)	41.0%	36.7 (4.2)	12	100	8.4 (4.2)	8.5 (1.6)	0.0%	1.0 (0.3)
Courcoulas, 2014; Courcoulas, 2015	Bariatric surgery (RYGB + LAGB)	41	46.6 (7)	80.0%	35.7 (3)	36	100	6.9 (4.5)	19.8 (2.1)	10.0%	1.1 (0.3)
	Control	20	48.9 (4.7)	85.0%	35.7 (3.3)	36	100	5.7 (5.6)	5.0 (2.5)	0.0%	0.21 (0.4) increase
Cummings, 2016	Bariatric surgery (RYGB)	15	52.0 (8.3)	80.0%	38.3 (3.7)	12	100	11.4 (4.8)	28.1 (15.8)	60.0%	1.3 (nr)
	Control	17	54.6 (6.3)	64.7%	37.1 (3.5)	12	100	6.8 (5.2)	7.2 (6.5)	5.9%	0.4 (nr)
Halperin, 2014	Bariatric surgery (RYGB)	19	50.7 (7.6)	68.0%	36.0 (3.5)	12	100	10.6 (6.6)	27.8 (nr)	58.0%	nr
	Control	19	52.6 (4.3)	53.0%	36.5 (3.4)	12	100	10.2 (6.1)	7.6 (nr)	16.0%	nr
Mingrone et al,[48] 2012; Mingrone et al,[4] 2015	Bariatric surgery (BPD&RYGB)	40	43.4 (7.8)	55.0%	45.0 (6.5)	60	100	6	40.9 (18.1)	50.0%	2.3 (1.7)
	Control	20	43.5 (7.3)	50.0%	45.1 (7.8)	60	100	6	10.0 (12.2)	0.0%	1.6 (1.0)
Schauer et al,[37] 2012; Schauer et al,[36] 2014; Schauer et al,[5] 2017	Bariatric surgery (RYGB & SG)	100	48.1 (8.1)	68.0%	36.6 (3.6)	60	100	8	20.9 (8.6)	26.0%	2.1 (1.8)
	Control	50	49.7 (7.4)	62.0%	36.8 (3.0)	60	100	9	5.3 (10.8)	5%	0.3 (2.0)
Reis, 2010	Bariatric surgery (RYGB)	10	36.7 (11.5)	0.0%	55.7 (7.8)	24	nr	nr	36.1 (3.8)	nr	nr
	Control	10	42.2 (11.0)	0.0%	54.0 (6.1)	24	nr	nr	0.8 (1.7)	nr	nr

(continued on next page)

Table 1
(continued)

Authors	Study Group	N	Mean (SD) Age (y)	Female (%)	Mean (SD) Preop BMI (kg/m²)	Follow-up Duration (mo)	Type 2 Diabetes Prevalence (%)	Type 2 Diabetes Duration (y)	Mean Weight Loss (kg)	Diabetes Remission[a]	Mean Decrease in HbA1C (% Points)
Ikramuddin et al, 2013; Ikramuddin et al, 2015	Bariatric surgery (RYGB)	60	49 (9)	63.0%	34.9 (3.0)	24	100	8.9 (6.1)	nr	25.0%	3.2 (nr)
	Control	60	49 (8)	34.0%	34.3 (3.1)	24	100	9.1 (5.6)	nr	0.0%	1.2 (nr)
Liang, 2013	Bariatric surgery (RYGB)	31	50.8 (5.4)	29.0%	30.5 (0.9)	12	100	7.4 (1.7)	nr	90.3%	4.5 (1.5)
	Control[b]	70	51.4 (6.2)	31.0%	30.3 (1.7)	12	100	7.2 (1.7)	nr	0.0%	3.6 (1.4)
O'Brien, 2006	Bariatric surgery (LAGB)	40	41.8 (6.4)	75.0%	33.7 (1.8)	24	nr	nr	21.6 (8.2)	nr	nr
	Control	40	40.7 (7.0)	77.0%	33.5 (1.4)	24	nr	nr	4.1 (8.0)	nr	nr
O'Brien, 2010	Bariatric surgery (LAGB)	25	16.5 (1.4)	64.0%	42.3 (6.1)	24	nr	nr	34.6 (7.5)	nr	nr
	Control	25	16.6 (1.2)	72.0%	40.4 (3.1)	24	nr	nr	3.0 (9.5)	nr	nr
Dixon et al,[49] 2008	Bariatric surgery (LAGB)	30	46.6 (7.4)	50.0%	37 (2.7)	24	100	<2	20.3 (6.5)	75.9%	1.8 (1.2)
	Control	30	47.1 (8.7)	57.0%	37.2 (2.5)	24	100	<2	5.9 (8.0)	15.4%	0.4 (1.3)
Dixon, 2012	Bariatric surgery (LAGB)	30	47.4 (8.8)	43.0%	46.3 (6.0)	24	33	nr	27.8 (10.7)	nr	nr
	Control	30	50.0 (8.2)	40.0%	43.8 (4.9)	24	33	nr	5.1 (6.6)	nr	nr
Mingrone, 2002	Bariatric surgery (BPD)	46	37.4 (4.6)	85.0%	48.2 (5.0)	24	nr	nr	40.6 (8.2)	nr	nr
	Control	33	37.4 (4.6)	88.0%	48.2 (7.7)	24	nr	nr	7.8 (8.0)	nr	nr
Heindorff, 1997	Bariatric surgery (LAGB)	8	Range 22–41	75.0%	Range 43–54	10	nr	nr	26.0 (2.0)	nr	nr
	Control	8	Range 21–43	15.0%	Range 40–56	10	nr	nr	1.0 (2.0)	nr	nr

Abbreviations: BPD, Biliopancreatic diversion; DJBm, duodenal-jejunal bypass surgery with minimal gastric resection; nr, not reported; RYGB, Roux-en-Y gastric bypass; SG, Sleeve Gastrectomy; LAGB, Laparoscopic adjustable gastric banding.

[a] The definition of diabetes remission varied in the different studies. Complete remission rates are listed here.
[b] Control group consisted of a medical group with and without exenetide.

diabetes. A published meta-analysis of the data from 11 of these RCTs comparing multimodal medical therapy with bariatric surgery for management of T2DM indicates that weight loss was significantly greater in the surgical groups, and bariatric surgery patients had a higher remission rate of T2D (relative risk 22.1 [3.2–154.3]) and metabolic syndrome (relative risk 2.4 [1.6–3.6]), greater improvements in quality of life, and reductions in medicine use.[50] Other notable benefits in the surgical arms of these trials included significant decrease in plasma triglyceride concentrations and increase in high-density lipoprotein cholesterol concentrations.[50] Although not included in this meta-analysis because it was not a randomized trial, the noteworthy Swedish Obese Subjects (SOS) case-control study demonstrated a hazard ratio (HR) of 0.17 for diabetes incidence following assorted bariatric surgical interventions, illustrating how effectively bariatric surgery reduces progression from the prediabetic state.[51] The SOS studies have also shown that bariatric surgery is associated with a decreased incidence of diabetic microvascular complications (HR 0.44; 95% confidence interval [CI], 0.34–0.56; $P<.001$) and macrovascular complications (HR 0.68; 95% CI, 0.54–0.85; $P = .001$).[52]

The mechanisms by which gastrointestinal surgery leads to T2D remission are not completely understood. The contribution of weight loss to the metabolic benefits of bariatric surgery is critical. Observations supporting this statement include the fact that procedures, such as gastric banding and sleeve gastrectomy, achieve significant improvements in glycemic control, which correlate directly with the amount of weight lost. Buchwald's meta-analysis examining weight loss and diabetes resolution outcomes after bariatric surgery showed that diabetes mellitus resolution rates were proportional to the degree of weight loss.[11] It has also been observed that weight gain after bariatric surgery is associated with recurrence of metabolic comorbidities, including T2D. The reduction in volume of adipose tissue (particularly central adiposity), which occurs with weight loss, positively affects the inflammatory milieu and decreases intra-abdominal pressure, both of which are associated with metabolic benefits. Although weight loss certainly plays a major role in inducing improved glucose homeostasis following bariatric surgery, it appears that there are other mechanisms at play. Evidence to support this assertion includes the fact that leaner patients with T2D experience similar antidiabetic effects without significant weight loss, and most patients' glucose control improves or normalizes almost immediately after surgery, well before any significant weight loss takes place, but during the phase when calorie intake is significantly suppressed. Many patients with T2D can decrease, or even discontinue, insulin and oral hypoglycemic drugs just hours after undergoing RYGB.[53] Furthermore, the BPD and DS result in significantly greater remission of metabolic comorbidities such as T2DM, compared with other interventions with equivalent weight loss.

The various weight-independent mechanisms proposed to induce diabetes remission after bariatric/metabolic surgery include the following[54–56]:

- Increased postprandial secretion of gut hormones from intestinal L cells such as the incretin glucagon-like peptide 1 (GLP-1)
- Changes in intestinal nutrient-sensing mechanisms that affect insulin sensitivity
- Plasma bile acid alterations
- Changes in the gut microbiome
- Exclusion of the proximal duodenum and small intestine from nutrient flow, and possibly downregulation of an unidentified anti-incretin factor or factors

Diabetes remission is more likely in those with better preserved pancreatic function as indicated by lower glycosylated hemoglobin (HbA1c) levels preoperatively and shorter duration of diabetes (<5 years) and insulin independence at the time of surgery.[57,58] In those who do not achieve remission, bariatric procedures, including laparoscopic adjustable gastric banding (LAGB), facilitate better glycemic control and a reduced medication burden compared with intensive medical therapy.[4,37] Up to 25% of patients with initial resolution of their diabetes will have reoccurrence of glucose intolerance, insulin resistance, and T2D, although this phenomenon is often associated with failure to lose a significant amount of weight primarily, or with postoperative weight regain.[59] Bariatric surgery may also facilitate remission of diabetic microvascular complications.[60,61]

Impact on Cardiovascular Risk Profile

Obesity is associated with an increased risk of cardiovascular disease and increased cardiovascular mortality. Reducing this risk by pharmacologically targeting cardiovascular risk factors is effective, but also challenging, and usually involves evidenced-based multidrug regimens requiring high patient compliance. Weight loss of more than 10% may be an effective risk-reduction strategy,[62] but high rates of nonresponders to conventional weight management strategies have been disappointing. Bariatric surgery, by achieving significant and sustainable weight loss, has been shown to positively affect cardiovascular risk, by inducing resolution or improvement in cardiovascular disease risk factors, including T2D, hypertension, and dyslipidemia.[21,63] Indeed, a systematic review of 52 studies involving 16,867 patients who have undergone bariatric surgery demonstrated a reduction of 40% in Framingham risk (10-year cardiovascular disease risk score) following bariatric surgery, resolution, or improvement of 60% to 75% in traditional cardiovascular risk factors (T2DM, hypertension, and dyslipidemia) and significant reduction in novel risk factors, such as C-reactive protein and endothelial function.[63] No pharmacologic treatment has been shown to have so many patients that respond with such a marked positive impact on cardiovascular risk profile.

Impact on Other Obesity Complications

Bariatric surgery positively affects many other weight-related conditions, including obstructive sleep apnea, nonalcoholic steatohepatitis, gastroesophageal reflux disease, arthritis and back pain, urinary incontinence, gout, thyroid and parathyroid function, subfertility, asthma, and others (**Fig. 2**).[64] There is emerging evidence that bariatric surgery may reduce the incidence of cancer, with a stronger protective effect reported in women than men.[6,65] The mechanisms underlying the reduced risk of cancer after bariatric surgery are unclear, but may involve mediation of inflammatory pathways and attenuation of obesity-associated hyperinsulinism.

Impact on Mortality

Several nonrandomized studies have demonstrated that bariatric surgery significantly reduces mortality. The SOS study showed a 30% decrease in mortalities after 10 years of follow-up, mainly from decreases in deaths due to cancer and myocardial infarction.[8] Interestingly, the only predictor of mortality benefit was fasting insulin levels above the median. Similar results were reported by Adams and colleagues,[9] showing a 40% reduction in mortalities for the entire group, but a 92% reduction in mortality for patients with diabetes. Again, the benefit was driven by reduction in death due to cancer and cardiovascular disease. A recent systematic review and meta-analysis has identified 8 studies that reported on long-term mortality, involving 23,647 operated patients and 89,628 nonoperated obese controls. These

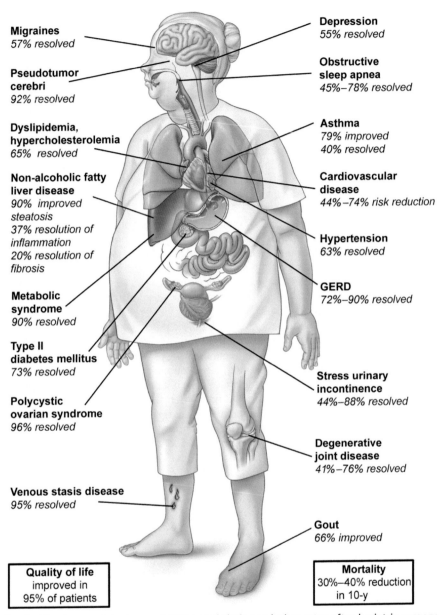

Migraines
57% resolved

**Pseudotumor
cerebri**
92% resolved

**Dyslipidemia,
hypercholesterolemia**
65% resolved

**Non-alcoholic fatty
liver disease**
*90% improved
steatosis
37% resolution of
inflammation
20% resolution of
fibrosis*

**Metabolic
syndrome**
90% resolved

**Type II
diabetes mellitus**
73% resolved

**Polycystic
ovarian syndrome**
96% resolved

Venous stasis disease
95% resolved

Quality of life
improved in
95% of patients

Depression
55% resolved

**Obstructive
sleep apnea**
45%–78% resolved

Asthma
*79% improved
40% resolved*

**Cardiovascular
disease**
44%–74% risk reduction

Hypertension
63% resolved

GERD
72%–90% resolved

**Stress urinary
incontinence**
44%–88% resolved

**Degenerative
joint disease**
41%–76% resolved

Gout
66% improved

Mortality
30%–40% reduction
in 10-y

Fig. 2. Obesity-associated comorbidities and their resolution rates after bariatric surgery. GERD, gastroesophageal reflux disease. (Reprinted with permission, Cleveland Clinic Center for Medical Art & Photography © 2017. All Rights Reserved.)

data showed a reduction of 41% in all-cause mortality after bariatric surgery. Furthermore, bariatric surgery patients were 0.42 times less likely and 0.47 times less likely as nonoperated obese controls to die from cardiovascular diseases and cancer, respectively.[66]

OUTCOMES OF BARIATRIC SURGERY: RISKS
Perioperative Mortality and Morbidity

Over the last 2 decades, the safety of bariatric surgery has been greatly improved and well documented. Developments in surgical innovations, in the medical device industry, coupled with increased experience in minimally invasive surgery have enabled this. In addition, advances in surgical technique and implementation of enhanced recovery after surgery programs have contributed to reduced operative time, length of stay, and complications. The rate of conversion to open surgery is now 1%, occurring most often in the setting of revisional surgery or for complex malabsorptive procedures.[67]

Short-term mortality after bariatric surgery is low, ranging from 0.04% to 0.3%.[68] In a meta-analysis of published mortality data after bariatric surgery, Buchwald and colleagues[69] reported an overall 30-day postoperative mortality of 0.28% (n = 84,931), and total mortality from 30 days to 2 years was 0.35% (n = 19,928). The Longitudinal Assessment of Bariatric Surgery (LABS) study subsequently reported a similarly low 30-day mortality (0.3%) among 4776 patients.[70] More recently, a population-based, nationwide study from Finland reported 30-day, 90-day, and 1-year mortalities following bariatric surgery compared with mortalities after other common operations (cholecystectomy, hysterectomy, prostatectomy, knee and hip arthroplasty, colorectal and gastric resections, coronary artery bypass graft). This study demonstrated that mortality within the first year after surgery was lowest for bariatric surgery in comparison to these other procedures.[68]

Early and long-term complications after bariatric surgery are lower than might be expected for this medically comorbid population; the LABS consortium reported a 4.3% incidence of major adverse events in the early postoperative period.[70] Although these reports are encouraging, a few complications associated with bariatric surgery are potentially fatal and merit careful consideration. These complications include sepsis from an anastomotic dehiscence, shock secondary to postoperative hemorrhage, or cardiopulmonary events in this high-risk group. The leading cause of death after bariatric surgery is thromboembolic disease, with an incidence of 0.34%.[71,72] Perhaps the most dreaded complication is sepsis secondary to an anastomotic or staple line leak, with rates ranging from 1% to 2% for primary gastric bypass and sleeve gastrectomy.[73–75] Early identification and an aggressive approach to management of leaks improve the outcome. Conservative management is only indicated for leaks that are controlled by a surgical drain, in a hemodynamically stable patient. Otherwise, a prompt and aggressive surgical approach is recommended.[76] Early postoperative bleeding complicates 1% to 4% of bariatric surgeries. Most postoperative bleeds can be treated nonoperatively with volume resuscitation and blood transfusions, but any evidence of hemodynamic instability necessitates surgical intervention.[77,78] Other complications unique to the most commonly performed bariatric procedure (RYGB) are illustrated in **Table 2**.

Several risk factors for postoperative morbidity and mortality have been identified; these include male gender, age greater than 50 years, congestive heart failure, peripheral vascular disease, and renal impairment.[79,80] Although these factors may increase risk, they do not necessarily preclude an individual from bariatric surgery and need to be considered in the individual clinical context.

Late Complications of Bariatric Surgery

Long-term complications of bariatric surgery are unique to the specific procedure. Operations such as gastric bypass, which has a narrow gastrojejunal anastomosis,

Table 2
Complications associated with Roux-En-Y gastric bypass

Frequency	Mild	Moderate	Severe
>5%	Nausea and vomiting without consequence, up to 100%	Anastomotic ulcer (8%) Anastomotic stricture (7%) Malnutrition of vitamins or minerals (up to 50%) Dumping syndrome (up to 75%)	Nausea and vomiting leading to dehydration and requiring readmission (~5%) Reoperation (for any reason, <5%)
1–5%	Self-limiting impairment in renal function (2%)	Abdominal hemorrhage or anemia without a clear source, requiring blood transfusion (5%) Pneumonia (4%) Herniation or small bowel obstruction (4%) Wound infection (3%) Arrhythmia without hemodynamic instability (2%) Gallstones (symptomatic in 2%)	Reoperation for abdominal hemorrhage (2%) Anastomotic leak (1%)
<1%			Unstable arrhythmia, myocardial infarction, or cardiac arrest (<1%) Pulmonary embolus, respiratory failure, or other potentially fatal medical complication (0.5%) Overall risk of surgical mortality approximately 0.3%

are susceptible to stricture formation leading to partial or complete luminal obstruction either in the acute setting secondary to edema or in the long term due to fibrosis and scar tissue formation. Complicating up to 8% of laparoscopic RYGB cases, and usually presenting in the first postoperative month, anastomotic strictures can often be managed endoscopically with balloon dilatations, rarely complicated by perforation.[81,82] Obstructive symptoms following gastric banding are usually the result of band slippage or overinflation and are often easily corrected by band adjustment in the clinic. Obstructive symptoms following sleeve gastrectomy usually present immediately following surgery and may indicate an excessively "tight" sleeve exacerbated by postoperative edema. As the edema resolves, symptom resolution usually ensues. Another frequently reported delayed complication of bariatric surgery, usually presenting later in the postoperative course, is ulceration in proximity to the gastrojejunal anastomosis of a gastric bypass or BPD. These "marginal ulcers" are consequent to exposure of the unprotected jejunal mucosa to gastric acidity, and the incidence is reported to be approximately 7%. Medical treatment with proton-pump inhibitors is sufficient for most cases, although there is a select group of patients who continue to suffer from symptomatic, nonhealing ulcers, despite appropriate medical treatment, who require surgical intervention (resection and revision of the ulcerated gastrojejunal anastomosis).[83] Incisional and internal herniation can complicate both open and laparoscopic bariatric procedures. The reported incidence for internal herniation ranges from 2.5% to 6.2% (4% on average); given that presenting symptoms and clinical signs associated with this phenomenon may be subtle and the potential for life-threatening bowel ischemia to occur because of the problem, a high index of suspicion is critical for early diagnosis and timely intervention.[84–86] Abdominal computed tomography is the most sensitive investigation for the identification of an internal hernia, often demonstrating the classic "swirl" sign of the herniated bowel mesentery. Prompt surgical exploration, reduction of the hernia, and resection of any nonviable bowel, and closure of the internal hernia space, are the mainstays of treatment.

Gastric band patients are predisposed to developing several band-related complications, including band slippage, band erosion, and significant esophageal dysmotility, resulting in reintervention rates as high as 48%.[87,88]

Special attention must always be given to the nutritional status of patients following bariatric procedures, particularly after malabsorptive operations. Deficiency of essential vitamins and minerals is highly likely following RYGB and BPD, and on rare occasions, may be life threatening, as with thiamine deficiency encephalopathy. The multidisciplinary team managing bariatric patients must be mindful of micronutrient deficiencies, and dietary supplementation following these procedures is essential. Lifelong supplementation of vitamins D and B12, folic acid, iron, and calcium, among others, is recommended.[89] Scheduled surveillance of the nutritional parameters by blood tests is recommended on a regular basis, at 3-month intervals for the first postoperative year, 6 monthly for the second postoperative year, and annually thereafter.[90]

Another diet-related problem after bariatric surgery, specifically after gastric bypass, is dumping syndrome, which occurs immediately after eating in approximately 50% of patients after RYGB at some stage postoperatively.[91] It is characterized by symptoms such as nausea, tremors, sweating, diarrhea, dizziness, flushing, tachycardia, and occasionally syncope, resulting from the ingestion of food containing large quantities of refined sugars and from food eaten too quickly. Although this was initially considered a desirable deterrent from such behaviors, particularly in patients who are partial to sweets, no association between symptoms and weight loss has ever been shown. Moreover, dumping syndrome can be very problematic in approximately 1% of patients.[92] Another group of patients suffer with postprandial hyperinsulinemic hypoglycemia with neuroglycopenia potentially due to changes in the gut hormonal milieu.[93] Strict dietary alteration is required, with patients eating more low glycemic index carbohydrates and protein and avoiding any medium or high glycemic index carbohydrates. Patients may require a trial of diazoxide, octreotide, or calcium-channel antagonists, among other drugs,[94] whereas GLP-1 analogues have also recently been tested as partial agonists.

Other late complications of bariatric surgery, related to significant weight loss, include gallstone formation (approximately 10% of patients), hair thinning, and excess skin. The latter can significantly affect body image and satisfaction with the surgical outcome. In addition to the aesthetic problem, it can lead to functional problems, dermatoses, and difficulties in maintaining satisfactory personal hygiene. Treatment is mainly with body contouring surgery, for which there are guidelines from international Plastic and Reconstructive Surgery associations.[95] The most troublesome complication is nonspecific abdominal pain, which can occur in 5% to 10% of patients.[53] Although the symptoms are real, the diagnosis and treatment can be very challenging.

SUMMARY

In addition to achieving substantial and durable weight loss, bariatric surgery is associated with favorable metabolic effects far beyond those achieved by lifestyle modifications and pharmacologic treatments. Perioperative morbidity and mortality have decreased significantly over the last decade such that the safety profile of bariatric surgery is better than many well-accepted procedures, such as cholecystectomy and hysterectomy. In fact, the 0.3% mortality risk of bariatric surgery is one-tenth that of coronary artery bypass surgery with significantly greater improvement in long-term mortality. Much of the improvement in perioperative morbidity and mortality can be attributed to advances in laparoscopic surgery as well as establishment of a nationwide center of excellence network and required outcome reporting. The current extensive evidence demonstrating the safety and efficacy of bariatric surgery supports it as the current standard of care for treatment of severe obesity and its related complications.

REFERENCES

1. Henkel DS, Mora-Pinzon M, Remington PL, et al. Trends in the prevalence of severe obesity and bariatric surgery access: a state-level analysis from 2011 to 2014. J Laparoendosc Adv Surg Tech A 2017;27(7):669–75.
2. Picot J, Jones J, Colquitt JL, et al. The clinical effectiveness and cost-effectiveness of bariatric (weight loss) surgery for obesity: a systematic review and economic evaluation. Health Technol Assess 2009;13(41):1–190, 215–357, iii–iv.
3. Fisher BL, Schauer P. Medical and surgical options in the treatment of severe obesity. Am J Surg 2002;184:9S–16S.
4. Mingrone G, Panunzi S, De Gaetano A, et al. Bariatric-metabolic surgery versus conventional medical treatment in obese patients with type 2 diabetes: 5 year follow-up of an open-label, single-centre, randomised controlled trial. Lancet 2015;386:964–73.
5. Schauer PR, Bhatt DL, Kirwan JP, et al. Bariatric surgery versus intensive medical therapy for diabetes—5-year outcomes. N Engl J Med 2017;376:641–51.
6. Sjöström L, Gummesson A, Sjöström CD, et al. Effects of bariatric surgery on cancer incidence in obese patients in Sweden (Swedish Obese Subjects Study): a prospective, controlled intervention trial. Lancet Oncol 2009;10:653–62.
7. Sjostrom L, Lindroos AK, Peltonen M, et al. Lifestyle, diabetes, and cardiovascular risk factors 10 years after bariatric surgery. N Engl J Med 2004;351:2683–93.
8. Sjöström L, Narbro K, Sjöström CD, et al. Effects of bariatric surgery on mortality in Swedish obese subjects. N Engl J Med 2007;357:741–52.
9. Adams TD, Gress RE, Smith SC, et al. Long-term mortality after gastric bypass surgery. N Engl J Med 2007;357:753–61.
10. Rubino F, Shukla A, Pomp A, et al. Bariatric, metabolic, and diabetes surgery: what's in a name? Ann Surg 2014;259:117–22.
11. Buchwald H, Estok R, Fahrbach K, et al. Weight and type 2 diabetes after bariatric surgery: systematic review and meta-analysis. Am J Med 2009;122:248–56.e5.
12. Mahawar KK, Sharples AJ. Contribution of malabsorption to weight loss after Roux-en-Y gastric bypass: a systematic review. Obes Surg 2017;27(8):2194–206.
13. Pournaras DJ, Le Roux CW. The effect of bariatric surgery on gut hormones that alter appetite. Diabetes Metab 2009;35:508–12.

14. Gastrointestinal surgery for severe obesity. National Institutes of Health consensus development conference statement. Am J Clin Nutr 1992;55:615S–9S.

15. Rubino F, Nathan DM, Eckel RH, et al. Metabolic surgery in the treatment algorithm for type 2 diabetes: a joint statement by international diabetes organizations. Diabetes Care 2016;39:861–77.

16. Breznikar B, Dinevski D. Bariatric surgery for morbid obesity: pre-operative assessment, surgical techniques and post-operative monitoring. J Int Med Res 2009;37:1632–45.

17. Esteban Varela J, Nguyen NT. Laparoscopic sleeve gastrectomy leads the U.S. utilization of bariatric surgery at academic medical centers. Surg Obes Relat Dis 2015;11:987–90.

18. Espinet-Coll E, Nebreda-Durán J, Gómez-Valero JA, et al. Current endoscopic techniques in the treatment of obesity. Rev Esp Enferm Dig 2012;104:72–87.

19. Gersin KS, Rothstein RI, Rosenthal RJ, et al. Open-label, sham-controlled trial of an endoscopic duodenojejunal bypass liner for preoperative weight loss in bariatric surgery candidates. Gastrointest Endosc 2010;71:976–82.

20. Buchwald H, Avidor Y, Braunwald E, et al. Bariatric surgery: a systematic review and meta-analysis. JAMA 2004;292:1724–37.

21. Vest AR, Heneghan HM, Agarwal S, et al. Bariatric surgery and cardiovascular outcomes: a systematic review. Heart 2012;98:1763–77.

22. Garb J, Welch G, Zagarins S, et al. Bariatric surgery for the treatment of morbid obesity: a meta-analysis of weight loss outcomes for laparoscopic adjustable gastric banding and laparoscopic gastric bypass. Obes Surg 2009;19:1447–55.

23. Himpens J, Dobbeleir J, Peeters G. Long-term results of laparoscopic sleeve gastrectomy for obesity. Ann Surg 2010;252:319–24.

24. Patel S, Szomstein S, Rosenthal RJ. Reasons and outcomes of reoperative bariatric surgery for failed and complicated procedures (excluding adjustable gastric banding). Obes Surg 2011;21:1209–19.

25. Chevallier J, Paita M, Rodde-Dunet MH, et al. Predictive factors of outcome after gastric banding: a nationwide survey on the role of center activity and patients' behavior. Ann Surg 2007;246:1034–9.

26. Khoursheed MA, Al-Bader IA, Al-asfar FS, et al. Revision of failed bariatric procedures to Roux-en-Y gastric bypass (RYGB). Obes Surg 2011;21:1157–60.

27. Sharples AJ, Charalampakis V, Daskalakis M, et al. Systematic review and meta-analysis of outcomes after revisional bariatric surgery following a failed adjustable gastric band. Obes Surg 2017;27:2522–36.

28. Brolin RE, Cody RP. Weight loss outcome of revisional bariatric operations varies according to the primary procedure. Ann Surg 2008;248:227–32.

29. Spyropoulos C, Kehagias I, Panagiotopoulos S, et al. Revisional bariatric surgery: 13-year experience from a tertiary institution. Arch Surg 2010;145:173–7.

30. Courcoulas AP, Belle SH, Neiberg RH, et al. Three-Year Outcomes of Bariatric Surgery vs Lifestyle Intervention for Type 2 Diabetes Mellitus Treatment: A Randomized Clinical Trial. JAMA Surg 2015;150:931–40.

31. Courcoulas AP, Goodpaster BH, Eagleton JK, et al. Surgical vs medical treatments for type 2 diabetes mellitus: a randomized clinical trial. JAMA Surg 2014;149:707–15.

32. Ding SA, Simonson DC, Wewalka M, et al. Adjustable gastric band surgery or medical management in patients with type 2 diabetes: a randomized clinical trial. J Clin Endocrinol Metab 2015;100:2546–56.

33. Cummings DE, Arterburn DE, Westbrook EO, et al. Gastric bypass surgery vs intensive lifestyle and medical intervention for type 2 diabetes: the CROSS-ROADS randomised controlled trial. Diabetologia 2016;59:945–53.

34. Petry TZ, Fabbrini E, Otoch JP, et al. Effect of duodenal-jejunal bypass surgery on glycemic control in type 2 diabetes: a randomized controlled trial. Obesity (Silver Spring) 2015;23:1973–9.

35. Mingrone G, Panunzi S, De Gaetano A, et al. Bariatric surgery versus conventional medical therapy for type 2 diabetes. N Engl J Med 2012;366:1577–85.

36. Schauer PR, Bhatt DL, Kirwan JP, et al. Bariatric surgery versus intensive medical therapy for diabetes-3-year outcomes. N Engl J Med 2014;370:2002–13.

37. Schauer PR, Kashyap SR, Wolski K, et al. Bariatric surgery versus intensive medical therapy in obese patients with diabetes. N Engl J Med 2012;366:1567–76.

38. Halperin F, Ding SA, Simonson DC, et al. Roux-en-Y gastric bypass surgery or lifestyle with intensive medical management in patients with type 2 diabetes: feasibility and 1-year results of a randomized clinical trial. JAMA Surg 2014; 149:716–26.

39. Reis LO, Favaro WJ, Barreiro GC, et al. Erectile dysfunction and hormonal imbalance in morbidly obese male is reversed after gastric bypass surgery: a prospective randomized controlled trial. Int J Androl 2010;33:736–44.

40. Ikramuddin S, Korner J, Lee WJ, et al. Durability of addition of Roux-en-Y gastric bypass to lifestyle intervention and medical management in achieving primary treatment goals for uncontrolled type 2 diabetes in mild to moderate obesity: a randomized control trial. Diabetes Care 2016;39:1510–8.

41. Ikramuddin S, Korner J, Lee WJ, et al. Roux-en-Y gastric bypass vs intensive medical management for the control of type 2 diabetes, hypertension, and hyperlipidemia: the Diabetes Surgery Study randomized clinical trial. JAMA 2013;309: 2240–9.

42. Liang Z, Wu Q, Chen B, et al. Effect of laparoscopic Roux-en-Y gastric bypass surgery on type 2 diabetes mellitus with hypertension: a randomized controlled trial. Diabetes Res Clin Pract 2013;101:50–6.

43. Dixon JB, O'Brien PE, Playfair J, et al. Adjustable gastric banding and conventional therapy for type 2 diabetes: a randomized controlled trial. JAMA 2008; 299:316–23.

44. Dixon JB, Schachter LM, O'Brien PE, et al. Surgical vs conventional therapy for weight loss treatment of obstructive sleep apnea: a randomized controlled trial. JAMA 2012;308:1142–9.

45. O'Brien PE, Dixon JB, Laurie C, et al. Treatment of mild to moderate obesity with laparoscopic adjustable gastric banding or an intensive medical program: a randomized trial. Ann Intern Med 2006;144:625–33.

46. O'Brien PE, Sawyer SM, Laurie C, et al. Laparoscopic adjustable gastric banding in severely obese adolescents: a randomized trial. JAMA 2010;303:519–26.

47. Heindorff H, Hougaard K, Larsen PN. Laparoscopic adjustable gastric band increases weight loss compared to dietary treatment: a randomized study. Obes Surg 1997;7.

48. Mingrone G, Panunzi S, De Gaetano A, et al. Bariatric surgery versus conventional medical therapy for type 2 diabetes. N Engl J Med 2012;366:1577–85.

49. Dixon J, O'Brien PE, Playfair J, et al. Adjustable gastric banding and conventional therapy for type 2 diabetes: a randomized controlled trial. JAMA 2008;299: 316–23.

50. Gloy VL, Briel M, Bhatt DL, et al. Bariatric surgery versus non-surgical treatment for obesity: a systematic review and meta-analysis of randomised controlled trials. BMJ 2013;347:f5934.

51. Carlsson LM, Peltonen M, Ahlin S, et al. Bariatric surgery and prevention of type 2 diabetes in Swedish obese subjects. N Engl J Med 2012;367:695–704.

52. Sjostrom L, Peltonen M, Jacobson P, et al. Association of bariatric surgery with long-term remission of type 2 diabetes and with microvascular and macrovascular complications. JAMA 2014;311:2297–304.

53. Schauer PR, Burguera B, Ikramuddin S, et al. Effect of laparoscopic Roux-en Y gastric bypass on type 2 diabetes mellitus. Ann Surg 2003;238:467–84 [discussion: 484–65].

54. Cummings DE, Overduin J, Shannon MH, et al, ABS Consensus Conference. Hormonal mechanisms of weight loss and diabetes resolution after bariatric surgery. Surg Obes Relat Dis 2005;1:358–68.

55. Rubino F, Forgione A, Cummings DE, et al. The mechanism of diabetes control after gastrointestinal bypass surgery reveals a role of the proximal small intestine in the pathophysiology of type 2 diabetes. Ann Surg 2006;244:741–9.

56. Anhe FF, Varin TV, Schertzer JD, et al. The gut microbiota as a mediator of metabolic benefits after bariatric surgery. Can J Diabetes 2017;41(4):439–47.

57. Hayes MT, Hunt LA, Foo J, et al. A model for predicting the resolution of type 2 diabetes in severely obese subjects following Roux-en Y gastric bypass surgery. Obes Surg 2011;21:910–6.

58. Khanna V, Malin SK, Bena J, et al. Adults with long-duration type 2 diabetes have blunted glycemic and beta-cell function improvements after bariatric surgery. Obesity (Silver Spring) 2015;23:523–6.

59. DiGiorgi M, Rosen DJ, Choi JJ, et al. Re-emergence of diabetes after gastric bypass in patients with mid- to long-term follow-up. Surg Obes Relat Dis 2010; 6:249–53.

60. Iaconelli A, Panunzi S, De Gaetano A, et al. Effects of bilio-pancreatic diversion on diabetic complications: a 10-year follow-up. Diabetes Care 2011;34:561–7.

61. Miras AD, Chuah LL, Khalil N, et al. Type 2 diabetes mellitus and microvascular complications 1 year after Roux-en-Y gastric bypass: a case-control study. Diabetologia 2015;58:1443–7.

62. Gregg EW, Jakicic JM, Blackburn G, et al, Look AHEAD Research Group. Association of the magnitude of weight loss and changes in physical fitness with long-term cardiovascular disease outcomes in overweight or obese people with type 2 diabetes: a post-hoc analysis of the Look AHEAD randomised clinical trial. Lancet Diabetes Endocrinol 2016;4:913–21.

63. Heneghan HM, Meron-Eldar S, Brethauer SA, et al. Effect of bariatric surgery on cardiovascular risk profile. Am J Cardiol 2011;108:1499–507.

64. Schauer PR, Ikramuddin S, Gourash W, et al. Outcomes after laparoscopic Roux-en-Y gastric bypass for morbid obesity. Ann Surg 2000;232:515–29.

65. Ashrafian H, Ahmed K, Rowland SP, et al. Metabolic surgery and cancer: protective effects of bariatric procedures. Cancer 2011;117:1788–99.

66. Cardoso L, Rodrigues D, Gomes L, et al. Short- and long-term mortality after bariatric surgery: a systematic review and meta-analysis. Diabetes Obes Metab 2017;19(9):1223–32.

67. Sundbom M. Laparoscopic revolution in bariatric surgery. World J Gastroenterol 2014;20:15135–43.

68. Bockelman C, Hahl T, Victorzon M. Mortality following bariatric surgery compared to other common operations in finland during a 5-year period (2009-2013). A Nationwide Registry Study. Obes Surg 2017;27:2444–51.

69. Buchwald H, Estok R, Fahrbach K, et al. Trends in mortality in bariatric surgery: a systematic review and meta-analysis. Surgery 2007;142(4):621–32 [discussion: 632–5].

70. Flum DR, Belle SH, King WC, et al. Perioperative safety in the longitudinal assessment of bariatric surgery. N Engl J Med 2009;361:445–54.

71. Morino M, Toppino M, Forestieri P, et al. Mortality after bariatric surgery: analysis of 13,871 morbidly obese patients from a national registry. Ann Surg 2007;246: 1002–7 [discussion: 1007–9].

72. Poulose BK, Griffin MR, Zhu Y, et al. National analysis of adverse patient safety for events in bariatric surgery. Am Surg 2005;71:406–13.

73. Brethauer SA, Hammel JP, Schauer PR. Systematic review of sleeve gastrectomy as staging and primary bariatric procedure. Surg Obes Relat Dis 2009;5:469–75.

74. Podnos YD, Jimenez JC, Wilson SE, et al. Complications after laparoscopic gastric bypass: a review of 3464 cases. Arch Surg 2003;138:957–61.

75. Tice JA, Karliner L, Walsh J, et al. Gastric banding or bypass? A systematic review comparing the two most popular bariatric procedures. Am J Med 2008; 121:885–93.

76. Jacobsen HJ, Nergard BJ, Leifsson BG, et al. Management of suspected anastomotic leak after bariatric laparoscopic Roux-en-y gastric bypass. Br J Surg 2014;101:417–23.

77. Heneghan HM, Meron-Eldar S, Yenumula P, et al. Incidence and management of bleeding complications after gastric bypass surgery in the morbidly obese. Surg Obes Relat Dis 2011;8(6):729–35.

78. Nguyen NT, Rivers R, Wolfe BM. Early gastrointestinal hemorrhage after laparoscopic gastric bypass. Obes Surg 2003;13:62–5.

79. Nguyen NT, Masoomi H, Laugenour K, et al. Predictive factors of mortality in bariatric surgery: data from the Nationwide Inpatient Sample. Surgery 2011;150: 347–51.

80. Nguyen NT, Nguyen B, Smith B, et al. Proposal for a bariatric mortality risk classification system for patients undergoing bariatric surgery. Surg Obes Relat Dis 2013;9:239–46.

81. Carrodeguas L, Szomstein S, Zundel N, et al. Gastrojejunal anastomotic strictures following laparoscopic Roux-en-Y gastric bypass surgery: analysis of 1291 patients. Surg Obes Relat Dis 2006;2:92–7.

82. Yimcharoen P, Heneghan H, Chand B, et al. Successful management of gastrojejunal strictures after gastric bypass: is timing important? Surg Obes Relat Dis 2012;8:151–7.

83. Gumbs AA, Duffy AJ, Bell RL. Incidence and management of marginal ulceration after laparoscopic Roux-Y gastric bypass. Surg Obes Relat Dis 2006;2:460–3.

84. Bauman RW, Pirrello JR. Internal hernia at Petersen's space after laparoscopic Roux-en-Y gastric bypass: 6.2% incidence without closure–a single surgeon series of 1047 cases. Surg Obes Relat Dis 2009;5:565–70.

85. Facchiano E, Leuratti L, Veltri M, et al. Laparoscopic management of internal hernia after Roux-en-Y gastric bypass. Obes Surg 2016;26:1363–5.

86. Nimeri AA, Maasher A, Al Shaban T, et al. Internal hernia following laparoscopic Roux-en-Y gastric bypass: prevention and tips for intra-operative management. Obes Surg 2016;26:2255–6.

87. Arapis K, Tammaro P, Parenti LR, et al. Long-term results after laparoscopic adjustable gastric banding for morbid obesity: 18-year follow-up in a single university unit. Obes Surg 2017;27:630–40.
88. Ibrahim AM, Thumma JR, Dimick JB. Reoperation and medicare expenditures after laparoscopic gastric band surgery. JAMA Surg 2017;152(9):835–42.
89. Toh SY, Zarshenas N, Jorgensen J. Prevalence of nutrient deficiencies in bariatric patients. Nutrition 2009;25:1150–6.
90. Parrott J, Frank L, Rabena R, et al. American Society for Metabolic and Bariatric Surgery integrated health nutritional guidelines for the surgical weight loss patient 2016 update: micronutrients. Surg Obes Relat Dis 2017;13(5):727–41.
91. Hammer HF. Medical complications of bariatric surgery: focus on malabsorption and dumping syndrome. Dig Dis 2012;30:182–6.
92. Marsk R, Jonas E, Rasmussen F, et al. Nationwide cohort study of post-gastric bypass hypoglycaemia including 5,040 patients undergoing surgery for obesity in 1986-2006 in Sweden. Diabetologia 2010;53:2307–11.
93. Malik S, Mitchell JE, Steffen K, et al. Recognition and management of hyperinsulinemic hypoglycemia after bariatric surgery. Obes Res Clin Pract 2016;10:1–14.
94. Cui Y, Elahi D, Andersen DK. Advances in the etiology and management of hyperinsulinemic hypoglycemia after Roux-en-Y gastric bypass. J Gastrointest Surg 2011;15:1879–88.
95. Soldin M, Mughal M, Al-Hadithy N, et al. National commissioning guidelines: body contouring surgery after massive weight loss. J Plast Reconstr Aesthet Surg 2014;67:1076–81.

Maintenance of Lost Weight and Long-Term Management of Obesity

Kevin D. Hall, PhD[a],*, Scott Kahan, MD, MPH[b,c]

KEYWORDS

- Obesity treatment • Weight loss • Weight maintenance • Behavioral counseling
- Appetite • Physiology

KEY POINTS

- Long-term maintenance of lost weight is the primary challenge of obesity treatment.
- Biological, behavioral, and environmental factors conspire to resist weight loss and promote regain.
- Treatment of obesity requires ongoing attention and support, and weight maintenance–specific counseling, to improve long-term weight management.
- The magnitude of long-term weight loss typically achieved is usually lower than patient and health care provider expectations. However, even small amounts of sustained weight loss lead to clinical health improvements and risk factor reductions.

INTRODUCTION

Robert is a 47-year-old patient who initially weighed 120 kilograms. He lost 40 kilograms 3 years ago by carefully following your guidance to decrease his caloric intake to 1500 calories per day and exercise 6 days weekly. Today he comes in for his annual physical examination. You were excited to hear about his continued progress and see how much more he's lost, but you felt immediately dejected to see that he had regained almost 30 kilograms. "I don't know what to do...the weight keeps coming

Funding: This research was supported by the Intramural Research Program of the NIH, National Institute of Diabetes & Digestive & Kidney Diseases.
Conflicts of Interest: K.D. Hall has received funding from the Nutrition Science Initiative to investigate the effects of ketogenic diets on human energy expenditure. K.D. Hall also has a patent on a method of personalized dynamic feedback control of body weight (US Patent No 9,569,483; assigned to the National Institutes of Health). S. Kahan has no relevant disclosures.
[a] National Institute of Diabetes and Digestive and Kidney Diseases, 12A South Drive, Room 4007, Bethesda, MD 20892, USA; [b] Johns Hopkins Bloomberg School of Public Health, Baltimore, MD, USA; [c] George Washington University School of Medicine, 1020 19th Street NW, Suite 450, Washington, DC 20036, USA
* Corresponding author.
E-mail address: kevinh@niddk.nih.gov

Med Clin N Am 102 (2018) 183–197
https://doi.org/10.1016/j.mcna.2017.08.012
0025-7125/18/Published by Elsevier Inc.

medical.theclinics.com

back on. I keep trying, but there must be something wrong. I'm sure my metabolism is in the dumps. It feels like every moment of the day I can't help but think about food—it was never like this before I lost the weight. And no matter how hard I try to stop eating after one serving, I just can't seem to do it anymore." Feeling defeated, he says, "I don't even know what's the point of doing this anymore!" Frustrated, you remind him that he was able to do it just fine when he was losing weight initially, and he just needs to keep working hard at it. "I know it's not easy, but I can't help you unless you're willing to help yourself. You just need to work harder and take control of this again." You feel for him, but you know that you need to be stern to get him past this backsliding. Hoping to motivate him, you remind him how bad he will feel if he regains more weight, and you tell him to make a follow-up appointment for 6 months and warn him that if he doesn't turn things around quickly he will have to restart his blood pressure medications.

Substantial weight loss is possible across a range of treatment modalities, but long-term sustenance of lost weight is much more challenging, and weight regain is typical.[1–3] In a meta-analysis of 29 long-term weight loss studies, more than half of the lost weight was regained within 2 years, and by 5 years more than 80% of lost weight was regained (**Fig. 1**).[4] Indeed, previous failed attempts at achieving durable weight loss may have contributed to the recent decrease in the percentage of people with obesity who are trying to lose weight,[5] and many now believe that weight loss is a futile endeavor.[6]

Here, the authors describe their current understanding of the factors contributing to weight gain, physiologic responses that resist weight loss, behavioral correlates of successful maintenance of lost weight, as well as the implications and recommendations for long-term clinical management of patients with obesity.

WHY IS IT SO DIFFICULT TO LOSE WEIGHT AND KEEP IT OFF?
The Obesogenic Environment

Long-term weight management is extremely challenging because of interactions between our biology, behavior, and the obesogenic environment. The increase in obesity prevalence over the past several decades has been mirrored by industrialization of the food system,[7] involving increased production and marketing of inexpensive, highly processed foods[8–10] with supernormal appetitive properties.[11,12] Ultraprocessed foods[13] now contribute most of the calories consumed in America,[14] and their overconsumption has been implicated as a causative factor in weight gain.[15] Such foods are typically more calorically dense and far less healthy than unprocessed foods, such as fruits, vegetables, and fish.[16] Food has progressively become cheaper[17]; fewer people prepare meals at home,[18,19] and more food is consumed in

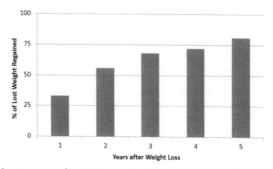

Fig. 1. Average time course of weight regain after a weight loss intervention. (*Data from* Anderson JW, Konz EC, Frederich RC, et al. Long-term weight-loss maintenance: a meta-analysis of US studies. Am J Clin Nutr 2001;74(5):579–84.)

restaurants.[18] In addition, changes in the physical activity environment have made it more challenging to be active throughout the day. Occupations have become more sedentary,[20] and suburban sprawl necessitates vehicular transportation rather than walking to work or school as had been common in the past. Taken together, changes in the food and physical activity environments tend to drive individuals toward increased intake, decreased activity, and ultimately, weight gain.

Physiologic Responses to Weight Loss

Outdated guidance to physicians and their patients gives the mistaken impression that relatively modest diet changes will consistently and progressively result in substantial weight loss at a rate of one pound (about half of a kilogram) for every 3500 kcal of accumulated dietary calorie deficit.[21–24] For example, cutting just a couple of cans of soda (~300 kcal) from one's daily diet was thought to lead to about *14 kilograms* of weight loss in a year, *27 kilograms* in 2 years, and so on. Failure to achieve and maintain substantial weight loss over the long term is then simply attributed to poor adherence to the prescribed lifestyle changes, thereby potentially further stigmatizing the patient as lacking in willpower, motivation, or fortitude to lose weight.[25]

It is now known that the simple calculations underlying the old weight loss guidelines are fatally flawed because they fail to consider declining energy expenditure with weight loss.[26] More realistic calculations of expected weight loss for a given change in energy intake or physical activity are provided by a Web-based tool called the NIH Body Weight Planner (http://BWplanner.niddk.nih.gov) that uses a mathematical model to account for dynamic changes in human energy balance.[27]

In addition to adaptations in energy expenditure with weight loss, body weight is regulated by negative feedback circuits that influence food intake.[28,29] Weight loss is accompanied by persistent endocrine adaptations[30] that increase appetite and decrease satiety,[31] thereby resisting continued weight loss and conspiring against long-term weight maintenance.

EXPLAINING THE WEIGHT PLATEAU

The overlapping physiologic changes that occur with weight loss help explain the near-ubiquitous weight loss time course: early weight loss that stalls after several months, followed by progressive weight regain.[32] Different interventions result in varying degrees of weight loss and regain, but the overall time courses are similar. As people progressively lose more and more weight, they fight an increasing battle against the biological responses that oppose further weight loss.

Appetite changes likely play a more important role than slowing metabolism in explaining the weight loss plateau because the feedback circuit controlling long-term calorie intake has greater overall strength than the feedback circuit controlling calorie expenditure. Specifically, it has been estimated that for each kilogram of lost weight, calorie expenditure decreases by about 20 to 30 kcal/d, whereas appetite increases by about 100 kcal/d above the baseline level before weight loss.[31] Despite these known physiologic changes, the typical response of the patient is to blame themselves as lazy or lacking in willpower, sentiments that are often reinforced by health care providers, as in the example of Robert, above.

Using a validated mathematical model of human energy metabolism,[27,31] **Fig. 2** illustrates the simulated energy balance dynamics underlying the weight loss time courses of two hypothetical 90-kg women who either regain (blue curves) or maintain (red curves) much of their lost weight after reaching a plateau within the first year of a diet intervention. In both women, large decreases in calorie intake at the start of the

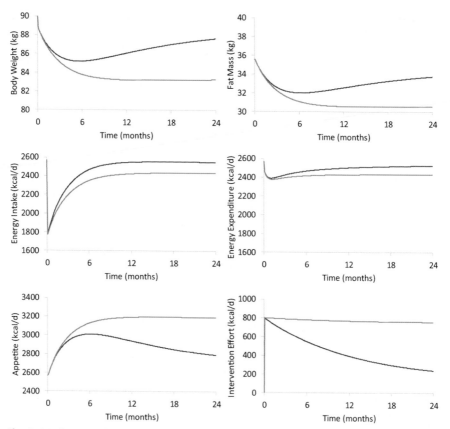

Fig. 2. Mathematical model simulations of body weight, fat mass, energy intake, energy expenditure, appetite, and intervention effort for two hypothetical women participating in a weight loss program. The curves in blue depict the typical weight loss, plateau, and re-gain trajectory, whereas the red curves show successful weight loss maintenance.

intervention result in rapid loss of weight and body fat leading to a modest decrease in calorie expenditure that contributes to slowing weight loss. However, the exponential increase in calorie intake from its initially reduced value is the primary factor that halts weight loss within the first year. In contrast to the modest drop in calorie expenditure of less than 200 kcal/d at the weight plateau, appetite has risen by 400 to 600 kcal/d and energy intake has increased by 600 to 700 kcal/d since the start of the intervention.

These mathematical model results contrast with patients' reports of eating approx-imately the same diet after the weight plateau that was previously successful during the initial phases of weight loss.[33] Although self-reported diet measurements are noto-riously inaccurate and imprecise,[34–36] it is entirely possible that patients truly believe they are sticking with their diet despite not losing any more weight or even regaining weight.

The patient's perception of ongoing diet maintenance despite no further weight loss may arise because the physiologic regulation of appetite occurs in brain regions that operate below the patient's conscious awareness.[37] Thus, signals to the brain that increase appetite with weight loss could introduce subconscious biases, such as portion sizes creeping upwards over time. Such a slow drift upwards in energy intake would be difficult to detect given the large 20% to 30% fluctuations in energy intake from day to day.[38,39] Furthermore, a relatively persistent effort is required to avoid overeating to match the increased appetite that grows in proportion to the weight lost.[31] For example, the simulated patient who plateaus at ~6 months and then maintains weight loss (see **Fig. 2**, red curves) sustains more than 95% of their intervention effort as defined by the difference between their appetite (what their body wants to be eating) and their actual calorie intake. Even the simulated patient who experiences weight regain (see **Fig. 2**, blue curves) maintains ~70% of their initial intervention effort until the plateau. Perhaps self-reported diet maintenance before and after the weight plateau is more representative of the patients' relatively persistent effort to avoid overeating in response to their increased appetite.[31] New technologies using repeated weight monitoring can be used to calculate changes in calorie intake and effort over time[40] and help guide individuals participating in a weight loss intervention.[41–44]

WEIGHT REGAIN VERSUS MAINTENANCE

From a purely calorie balance perspective, a patient who maintains lost weight after the first year of an intervention (see **Fig. 2**, red curves) may be eating only about 100 kcal/d fewer than a patient who experiences long-term weight regain (see **Fig. 2**, blue curves). However, such a small difference in food intake behavior is somewhat misleading considering that prevention of weight regain requires about 300 to 500 kcal/d of increased persistent effort to counter the ongoing slowing of metabolism and increased appetite associated with the lost weight. The more typical pattern of long-term weight regain is characterized by a waning effort to sustain the intervention.

There are likely many factors that account for the ability of some patients to achieve and maintain large weight losses over the long term, whereas others experience substantial weight regain. Unraveling the biological, psychosocial, educational, and environmental determinants of such individual variability will be an active area of obesity research for the foreseeable future.[45]

THE ROLE OF DIET COMPOSITION

Altering dietary macronutrient composition could theoretically influence overall calorie intake or expenditure resulting in a corresponding change in body weight. Alternatively, manipulation of diet composition can result in differences in the endocrine status in a way that could theoretically influence the propensity to accumulate body fat or affect subjective hunger or satiety. These possibilities do not violate the laws of thermodynamics because any change in the body's overall energy stores (ie, fat mass) must be accompanied by changes in calorie intake or expenditure. Therefore, it is theoretically possible that a particular diet could result in an advantageous endocrine or metabolic state that promotes weight loss. This promise provides fodder for the diet industry and false hope to the patient with obesity because it implies that if they simply choose the right diet, then long-lasting weight loss can be easily achieved.

In recent years, there has been a reemergence of low-carbohydrate, high-fat diets as popular weight loss interventions. Such diets have been claimed to reverse the metabolic and endocrine derangements resulting from following advice to consume low-fat, high-carbohydrate diets that allegedly caused the obesity epidemic. Specifically, the so-called "carbohydrate-insulin model of obesity" posits that diets high in carbohydrates are particularly fattening because they increase the secretion of insulin and thereby drive fat accumulation in adipose tissue and away from oxidation by metabolically active tissues. Altered fat partitioning thereby results in a state of "cellular starvation" leading to adaptive increases in hunger, and suppression of energy expenditure.[46] Therefore, the carbohydrate-insulin model implies that reversing these processes by eating a low-carbohydrate, high-fat diet should result in effortless weight loss.[47] Unfortunately, important aspects of the carbohydrate-insulin model have failed experimental interrogation[48] and, for all practical purposes, "a calorie is a calorie" when it comes to body fat and energy expenditure differences between controlled isocaloric diets widely varying in the ratio of carbohydrate to fat.[49] Nevertheless, low-carbohydrate, high-fat diets may lead to spontaneous reduction in calorie intake and increased weight loss, especially over the short term.[50–52] Meta-analyses of long-term studies have suggested that low-fat weight loss diets are slightly inferior to low-carbohydrate diets,[53] but the average differences between diets is too small to be clinically significant.[54] Furthermore, the similarity of the mean weight loss patterns between diet groups in randomized weight loss trials strongly suggests that there is no generalizable advantage of one diet over another when it comes to long-term calorie intake or expenditure.[33]

In contrast to the near equivalency of dietary carbohydrate and fat, dietary protein is known to positively influence body composition during weight loss[55,56] and has a small positive effect on resting metabolism.[57] Diets with higher protein may also offer benefits for maintaining weight loss,[58] particularly when the overall diet has a low glycemic index.[59] Improved weight loss maintenance with higher protein diets might be partially mediated by protein's greater effect on satiety compared with carbohydrate and fat[55,56] along with the possibility of increased overall energy expenditure.[60] More research is needed to better understand whether these potentially positive attributes of higher protein diets outweigh concerns that such diets mitigate improvements in insulin sensitivity that are typically achieved with weight loss using lower protein diets.[61]

Whereas long-term diet trials have not resulted in clear superiority of one diet over another with respect to average weight loss, within each diet group there is a high degree of individual variability, and anecdotal success stories abound for a wide range of weight loss diets.[33] Some of this variability may be due to interactions between diet type and patient genetics[62,63] or baseline physiology such as insulin sensitivity.[64–67] Such interactions offer the promise of personalized diets that optimize the patient's chances for long-term weight loss success.[45,63] Unfortunately, diet-biology interactions for weight loss have not always been reproducible[68,69] and likely explain only a fraction of the individual variability.

It is certainly possible that the patients who successfully lost weight on one diet would have been equally successful had they been assigned to an alternative diet. In other words, long-term success with a weight loss diet may have less to do with biology than factors such as the patient's food environment, socioeconomics, medical comorbidities, and social support, as well as practical factors, such as developing cooking skills and managing job requirements. Such nonbiological factors likely play a strong role in determining whether diet adherence is sustainable.

CLINICAL RECOMMENDATIONS FOR LONG-TERM WEIGHT MANAGEMENT COUNSELING

Given the physiologic and environmental obstacles to long-term maintenance of lost weight described above, the authors offer the following recommendations for clinical practice and then present an alternative preferable depiction of the opening case example.

Long-Term Benefits Require Long-Term Attention

Long-term behavioral changes and obesity management require ongoing attention. Even the highest-quality short-term interventions are unlikely to yield continued positive outcomes without persisting intervention and support. Several studies show that ongoing interaction with health care providers or in group settings significantly improves weight maintenance and long-term outcomes, compared with treatments that end after a short period of time (**Fig. 3**).[70,71] The importance of long-term intervention has been codified in the obesity treatment guidelines, which state that weight loss interventions should include long-term comprehensive weight loss maintenance programs that continue for at least 1 year.[72]

With respect to the case study at the start of this article, the physician should not expect ongoing weight loss without ongoing support and interaction. Rather than asking Robert to turn things around on his own, the physician has an opportunity to reengage with Robert to offer guidance and support in a more intensive and regular manner than sending him off on his own for 6 months, or if this is not realistic in a busy primary care practice, he could refer Robert to an obesity medicine specialist, registered dietitian, or comprehensive weight management clinic, or recommend that he engage in a community weight management group, such as the Diabetes Prevention Program (now covered by Medicare for patients with prediabetes), or a commercial program, such as Weight Watchers.

Use of Weight Maintenance-Specific Counseling/Strategies

Behavioral strategies for initiation of weight loss are described Scott Kahan and colleagues' article, "The Role of Behavioral Medicine in the Treatment of Obesity in Primary Care," in this issue. Weight-loss specific behaviors associated with long-term success include frequent self-monitoring and self-weighing, reduced calorie intake, smaller and more frequent meals/snacks throughout the day, increased physical activity, consistently eating breakfast, more frequent at-home meals compared with restaurant and fast-food meals, reducing screen time, and use of portion-controlled meals or meal substitutes.[2,73–75] Weight maintenance–specific behavioral skills and strategies help patients to build insight for long-term management, anticipate struggles and prepare contingency plans, moderate behavioral fatigue, and put into perspective the inevitable lapses and relapses of any long-term engagement.

Although the research is mixed, several studies show improved weight loss outcomes in patients receiving weight maintenance–specific training, compared with

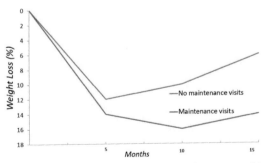

Fig. 3. Weight management programs with a focus on maintenance of lost weight demonstrate improved long-term weight loss (*red curve*) compared with programs without maintenance visits (*blue curve*). (*Data from* Perri MG, McAllister DA, Gange JJ, et al. Effects of four maintenance programs on the long-term management of obesity. J Consult Clin Psychol 1988;56(4):529–34.)

those who only receive traditional weight loss training.[76–79] Strategies are discussed later for weight maintenance–specific counseling.

Strengthen Satisfaction with Outcomes

People tend to focus on what they have not achieved, rather than what they have already accomplished. Unlike with weight loss, during which the external reward of watching the scale decrease and clinical measures (eg, lipid levels) improve can increase motivation, the extended period of weight maintenance has fewer of these explicit rewards. To support motivation and make salient satisfaction with outcomes, call attention to patients' progress, which often becomes overlooked. Providers can point to the magnitude of weight that has been kept off, putting it into context in terms of average expected weight loss (described in later discussion), as well as clinical improvements in risk factors, such as blood pressure and glycemic control. In addition, showing patients "before and after" photographs of themselves and other tangible evidence of progress helps them to build awareness of and appreciate the benefits they have already achieved, which may improve long-term persistence with weight maintenance efforts.

Relapse Prevention Training

Anticipating and managing high-risk situations for "slips" and lapses helps patients minimize lapses, get back on track, and avoid giving up. This counseling often includes self-weighing and identifying weight thresholds that signal the need for reengaging with a support team or initiating contingency strategies; proactively developing plans and practicing strategies for managing and coping with lapses; problem solving to identify challenges, formulate solutions, and evaluate options; and building strategies for non–food activities and coping mechanisms, such as engaging in hobbies or mindfulness activities, to minimize counterproductive coping mechanisms, such as emotional eating.

Cognitive Restructuring

Cycles of negative and maladaptive thoughts (eg, "What's the point…I failed again and I'll never lose weight!") and coping patterns (eg, binge eating in response to gaining a little weight) are counterproductive and demotivating. Helping patients to recognize and restructure the core beliefs and thought processes that underlie these patterns helps minimize behavioral fatigue and prevent or productively manage slips and lapses.

Developing Cognitive Flexibility

Many tendencies that promote initial weight loss are unrealistic over the long term. For example, many patients aim to make large, absolute changes in an "all-or-none" fashion via rigid rules, such as aiming for "no carbs" or very restrictive intake. Much as a sprinter can run all-out for a short race, but not for the entirety of a marathon, expecting strict, all-out efforts and clear-cut, black-and-white outcomes over the lifelong management of obesity is a recipe for frustration and failure. Instead, learning to accept that rigid expectations and "perfect" adherence to behavioral goals is unrealistic, and building cognitive flexibility to take in stride when one's plans do not go according to plan is a core competency for long-term sustainable behavioral changes and weight management.

Appeal to Patients' Deeper Motivations

External, superficial rewards are unlikely to support the long-term endurance needed for weight maintenance. For example, studies of financial rewards to incentivize behavioral changes, such as weight loss or tobacco cessation, yield initial benefits that invariably wane precipitously over time.[80,81] Whereas "white knuckling" and external, controlled motivations, such as directives from a spouse or health care provider, may lead to short-term weight loss, longer-term sustained motivation is more likely when patients take ownership of their behavioral changes and goals, and engage in them because they are deeply meaningful or enjoyable.[80,81] As an example, compared with difficulty of sticking to a strict low-fat or low-carbohydrate diet, which is often arbitrarily prescribed and of little personal significance to the patient, and therefore difficult to maintain, countless millions throughout the world rigorously stick to comparably strict kosher, halal, or vegan eating patterns, which are aligned with their religious, ethical, or other deeply held beliefs and values. Similarly, prescribing daily gym visits to someone who hates the gym environment or gym activities is unlikely to be fruitful, whereas supporting patients to find more enjoyable physical activities, such as sports or group dance-exercise classes, increases the likelihood of continuing over time.

Manage Expectations: Both for Patients and for Providers

Both patients and health care providers have wildly unrealistic expectations for weight loss outcomes. In one study, patients entering a diet and exercise program expected to lose 20% to 40% of their starting body weight, amounts that can only realistically be achieved by bariatric surgery.[82] Physician expectations are similarly inflated: in a survey of primary care physicians, acceptable behavioral weight loss was considered to be a loss of 21% of initial body weight.[83] In contrast, numerous studies show that diet, exercise, and behavioral counseling, in the best of cases, only leads to 5% to 10% average weight loss, and few patients with significantly elevated initial weights achieve and maintain an "ideal" body weight. From a cognitive psychology perspective, a waning intervention effort may be due to disappointment in the degree of weight loss actually achieved,[82] leading the patient to conclude that the effort is not worth the achieved benefits.[84]

Although the published data are mixed on whether unrealistic outcomes will deter weight loss success, it stands to reason that excessive discrepancies between expectations and actual outcomes would be demoralizing and increase negative thoughts and self-blame (which itself is associated with numerous negative health outcomes[85]) and may diminish long-term persistence for continued behavioral change and weight loss maintenance. The authors recommend advising patients about the physiologic challenges of long-term weight loss and the degree of weight loss that can be realistically expected from behavioral interventions. At minimum, there is no known harm of offering this insight and being frank with patients about expectations, and it may help them navigate the minefield of unscrupulous diet programs that promise miraculous outcomes.

Nonetheless, positive outcomes of behavioral counseling extend beyond weight loss. Despite the modest weight losses associated with behavioral interventions, small weight losses can lead to impressive health improvements and risk factor reductions. In the Diabetes Prevention Program, 7% weight loss over 6 months led to 58% reduction in development of diabetes, despite half the weight being regained over 3 years.[86] In the Look Ahead trial, 6% weight loss over 8 years yielded improvements in a range of cardiovascular risk factors, including glycemic control and lipids, as well as less medication usage, and reduced hospitalizations and health care costs.[87,88]

Although losing weight is important for improved health, people's motivations for seeing the scale go down are all too often driven by cultural norms for thinness and health care provider-imposed weight loss directives. These external motivations can move the weight loss needle in the short run, but they rarely lead to long-lasting determination. As described in the section above, long-term management is improved when motivations are aligned with personal values and preferences. Helping patients shift their locus of motivation from weight loss alone to intrinsically meaningful areas, such as health improvement, can improve long-term weight and behavioral outcomes.[89]

Escalate Treatment as Needed

For patients that do not achieve sufficient weight loss or health improvements with basic counseling in primary care settings, there are several opportunities to intensify therapy. Consider referral to a registered dietitian, obesity medicine physician, or comprehensive weight management clinic, as well as targeted specialists (such as a behavioral psychologist for patients with binge eating disorder or body dysmorphia). For patients with body mass index (BMI) greater than 30 kg/m^2 (or 27–30 kg/m^2 with obesity-related comorbid conditions), obesity pharmacotherapy leads to as much as 15% weight loss in responders, with weight loss being maintained in several studies for several years.[90–92] For patients with BMI greater than 40 kg/m^2 (or 35–40 kg/m^2 with comorbidities), bariatric surgery is a well-studied and valuable option that leads to large, sustainable weight losses in most patients.[93]

Using the principles discussed above, a more productive encounter in response to Robert's presentation might go like this:

Physician: "I understand, and I know it's challenging. It sounds like you're feeling frustrated because you've worked so hard and you feel like you've got nothing to show for it."

He nods and says, "Exactly. What's the point of doing this anymore?"

Physician: "From my view, the evidence we have shows something different: You're actually doing quite well in the scheme of things. I actually see quite a lot of progress for your efforts. You're down 25 lbs, right? That's almost 10% down from where you started…that's impressive. Few people lose that much weight and keep it off for 3 years. Studies show that even under the best of circumstances with aggressive counseling, average weight loss is between 5% to 10% of starting body weight; so you're doing better than most! You've been able to get off several blood pressure medications and you no longer take the pain medicine for your back and knees. And, we know from studies that losing just 7%, even if part of it is regained over the years, lowers the risk of diabetes by 60%!" His eyes widen. "Weight goes up and down, and our bodies fight back against weight loss, so this is never easy. Some regain and relapse is inevitable, just like in other areas of life." He takes a deep breath and clearly seems more engaged and hopeful. "So let's figure out how we can move forward and keep getting the benefits, and I'll be here with you to help along the way. Let's agree on a couple of next steps, and we'll meet again in a few weeks to see how it's going. If we need, we can also consider additional strategies or treatments."

SUMMARY

The degree of weight loss and its maintenance should not be the sole metric of obesity treatment success. Rather, physicians should support and encourage patients to make sustainable improvements in their diet quality and physical activities if these behaviors fail to meet national guidelines.[94,95] Such lifestyle changes over the long term will likely improve the health of patients even in the absence of major weight loss.[96]

REFERENCES

1. Loveman E, Frampton GK, Shepherd J, et al. The clinical effectiveness and cost-effectiveness of long-term weight management schemes for adults: a systematic review. Health Technol Assess 2011;15(2):1–182.

2. Wing RR, Phelan S. Long-term weight loss maintenance. Am J Clin Nutr 2005; 82(1 Suppl):222S–5S.
3. Wu T, Gao X, Chen M, et al. Long-term effectiveness of diet-plus-exercise interventions vs. diet-only interventions for weight loss: a meta-analysis. Obes Rev 2009;10(3):313–23.
4. Anderson JW, Konz EC, Frederich RC, et al. Long-term weight-loss maintenance: a meta-analysis of US studies. Am J Clin Nutr 2001;74(5):579–84.
5. Snook KR, Hansen AR, Duke CH, et al. Change in percentages of adults with overweight or obesity trying to lose weight, 1988-2014. JAMA 2017;317(9):971–3.
6. Mann T, Tomiyama AJ, Westling E, et al. Medicare's search for effective obesity treatments: diets are not the answer. Am Psychol 2007;62(3):220–33.
7. Stuckler D, McKee M, Ebrahim S, et al. Manufacturing epidemics: the role of global producers in increased consumption of unhealthy commodities including processed foods, alcohol, and tobacco. PLoS Med 2012;9(6):e1001235.
8. Swinburn BA, Sacks G, Hall KD, et al. The global obesity pandemic: shaped by global drivers and local environments. Lancet 2011;378(9793):804–14.
9. Blatt H. America's food: what you don't know about what you eat. Cambridge: The MIT Press; 2008.
10. Roberts P. The end of food. New York: Houghton Mifflin Harcourt Publishing Company; 2008.
11. Kessler DA. The end of overeating: controlling the insatiable American appetite. New York: Rodale Inc; 2009.
12. Moss M. Salt, sugar, fat: how the food giants hooked us. New York: Random House; 2013.
13. Monteiro CA, Levy RB, Claro RM, et al. A new classification of foods based on the extent and purpose of their processing. Cad Saude Publica 2010;26(11): 2039–49.
14. Martinez Steele E, Baraldi LG, Louzada ML, et al. Ultra-processed foods and added sugars in the US diet: evidence from a nationally representative cross-sectional study. BMJ open 2016;6(3):e009892.
15. Mendonca RD, Pimenta AM, Gea A, et al. Ultraprocessed food consumption and risk of overweight and obesity: the University of Navarra Follow-Up (SUN) cohort study. Am J Clin Nutr 2016;104(5):1433–40.
16. Kahan S, Cheskin LJ. Obesity and eating behaviors and behavior change. In: Kahan S, Gielen AC, Fagen PJ, et al, editors. Health behavior change in populations. Baltimore (MD): Johns Hopkins University Press; 2014. p. 233–61.
17. Putnam J. Major trends in the U.S. food supply, 1909-99. Food Rev 2000;23(1): 8–15.
18. Lin BH, Guthrie J. Nutritional quality of food prepared at home and away from home. U.S. Department of Agriculture; 2012. p. EIB-105.
19. Smith LP, Ng SW, Popkin BM. Trends in US home food preparation and consumption: analysis of national nutrition surveys and time use studies from 1965-1966 to 2007-2008. Nutr J 2013;12:45.
20. Church TS, Thomas DM, Tudor-Locke C, et al. Trends over 5 decades in U.S. occupation-related physical activity and their associations with obesity. PLoS One 2011;6(5):e19657.
21. Guth E. JAMA patient page. Healthy weight loss. JAMA 2014;312(9):974.
22. NHLBI. Aim for a healthy weight. National Institutes of Health. National Heart, Lung and Blood Institute; 2005. p. 05-5213.
23. NHLBI obesity education initiative expert panel on the identification E, and treatment of overweight and obesity in adults. The practical guide: identification,

evaluation, and treatment of overweight and obesity in adults. National Heart, Lung, and Blood Institute; 2000.

24. NHS. Your weight your health: how to take control of your weight. London: National Health Service, Department of Health; 2006. p. 274537.

25. Puhl RM, Heuer CA. The stigma of obesity: a review and update. Obesity (Silver Spring) 2009;17(5):941–64.

26. Rosenbaum M, Hirsch J, Gallagher DA, et al. Long-term persistence of adaptive thermogenesis in subjects who have maintained a reduced body weight. Am J Clin Nutr 2008;88(4):906–12.

27. Hall KD, Sacks G, Chandramohan D, et al. Quantification of the effect of energy imbalance on bodyweight. Lancet 2011;378(9793):826–37.

28. Greenway FL. Physiological adaptations to weight loss and factors favouring weight regain. Int J Obes (lond) 2015;39(8):1188–96.

29. Ochner CN, Tsai AG, Kushner RF, et al. Treating obesity seriously: when recommendations for lifestyle change confront biological adaptations. Lancet Diabetes Endocrinol 2015;3(4):232–4.

30. Sumithran P, Prendergast LA, Delbridge E, et al. Long-term persistence of hormonal adaptations to weight loss. N Engl J Med 2011;365(17):1597–604.

31. Polidori D, Sanghvi A, Seeley RJ, et al. How strongly does appetite counter weight loss? Quantification of the feedback control of human energy intake. Obesity (Silver Spring) 2016;24(11):2289–95.

32. Franz MJ, VanWormer JJ, Crain AL, et al. Weight-loss outcomes: a systematic review and meta-analysis of weight-loss clinical trials with a minimum 1-year follow-up. J Am Diet Assoc 2007;107(10):1755–67.

33. Freedhoff Y, Hall KD. Weight loss diet studies: we need help not hype. Lancet 2016;388(10047):849–51.

34. Dhurandhar NV, Schoeller DA, Brown AW, et al. Energy balance measurement: when something is not better than nothing. Int J Obes 2014;39(7):1109–13.

35. Schoeller DA. How accurate is self-reported dietary energy intake? Nutr Rev 1990;48(10):373–9.

36. Winkler JT. The fundamental flaw in obesity research. Obes Rev 2005;6(3):199–202.

37. Berthoud HR, Munzberg H, Morrison CD. Blaming the brain for obesity: integration of hedonic and homeostatic mechanisms. Gastroenterology 2017;152(7):1728–38.

38. Chow CC, Hall KD. Short and long-term energy intake patterns and their implications for human body weight regulation. Physiol Behav 2014;134:60–5.

39. Kim WW, Kelsay JL, Judd JT, et al. Evaluation of long-term dietary intakes of adults consuming self-selected diets. Am J Clin Nutr 1984;40(6 Suppl):1327–32.

40. Sanghvi A, Redman LA, Martin CK, et al. Validation of an inexpensive and accurate mathematical method to measure long-term changes in free-living energy intake. Am J Clin Nutr 2015;102(2):353–8.

41. Brady I, Hall KD. Dispatch from the field: is mathematical modeling applicable to obesity treatment in the real world? Obesity (Silver Spring) 2014;22(9):1939–41.

42. Hall KD, inventor; National Institutes of Health, assignee. Personalized dynamic feedback control of body weight. US patent 9,569,483. 02/14/2017, 2013.

43. Martin CK, Gilmore LA, Apolzan JW, et al. Smartloss: a personalized mobile health intervention for weight management and health promotion. JMIR Mhealth and Uhealth 2016;4(1):e18.

44. Martin CK, Miller AC, Thomas DM, et al. Efficacy of SmartLoss, a smartphone-based weight loss intervention: results from a randomized controlled trial. Obesity (Silver Spring) 2015;23(5):935–42.

45. MacLean PS, Wing RR, Davidson T, et al. NIH working group report: innovative research to improve maintenance of weight loss. Obesity (Silver Spring) 2015; 23(1):7–15.

46. Ludwig DS, Friedman MI. Increasing adiposity: consequence or cause of over-eating? JAMA 2014;311(21):2167–8.

47. Ludwig DS. Always hungry? Conquer cravings, retrain your fat cells and lose weight permanently. New York: Grand Central Life & Style; 2016.

48. Hall KD. A review of the carbohydrate-insulin model of obesity. Eur J Clin Invest 2017;71(3):323–6.

49. Hall KD, Guo J. Obesity energetics: body weight regulation and the effects of diet composition. Gastroenterology 2017;152(7):1718–27.e3.

50. Foster GD, Wyatt HR, Hill JO, et al. A randomized trial of a low-carbohydrate diet for obesity. N Engl J Med 2003;348(21):2082–90.

51. Gardner CD, Kiazand A, Alhassan S, et al. Comparison of the Atkins, Zone, Or-nish, and LEARN diets for change in weight and related risk factors among over-weight premenopausal women: the A TO Z weight loss study: a randomized trial. JAMA 2007;297(9):969–77.

52. Samaha FF, Iqbal N, Seshadri P, et al. A low-carbohydrate as compared with a low-fat diet in severe obesity. N Engl J Med 2003;348(21):2074–81.

53. Tobias DK, Chen M, Manson JE, et al. Effect of low-fat vs. other diet interventions on long-term weight change in adults: a systematic review and meta-analysis. Lancet Diabetes Endocrinol 2015;3(12):968–79.

54. Hall KD. Prescribing low-fat diets: useless for long-term weight loss? Lancet Diabetes Endocrinol 2015;3(12):920–1.

55. Leidy HJ, Clifton PM, Astrup A, et al. The role of protein in weight loss and main-tenance. Am J Clin Nutr 2015;101:1320S–9S.

56. Westerterp-Plantenga MS, Nieuwenhuizen A, Tome D, et al. Dietary protein, weight loss, and weight maintenance. Annu Rev Nutr 2009;29:21–41.

57. Wycherley TP, Moran LJ, Clifton PM, et al. Effects of energy-restricted high-pro-tein, low-fat compared with standard-protein, low-fat diets: a meta-analysis of randomized controlled trials. Am J Clin Nutr 2012;96(6):1281–98.

58. Westerterp-Plantenga MS, Lejeune MP, Nijs I, et al. High protein intake sustains weight maintenance after body weight loss in humans. Int J Obes Relat Metab Disord 2004;28(1):57–64.

59. Larsen TM, Dalskov SM, van Baak M, et al. Diets with high or low protein content and glycemic index for weight-loss maintenance. N Engl J Med 2010;363(22): 2102–13.

60. Ebbeling CB, Swain JF, Feldman HA, et al. Effects of dietary composition on en-ergy expenditure during weight-loss maintenance. JAMA 2012;307(24):2627–34.

61. Smith GI, Yoshino J, Kelly SC, et al. High-protein intake during weight loss ther-apy eliminates the weight-loss-induced improvement in insulin action in obese postmenopausal women. Cell Rep 2016;17(3):849–61.

62. Bray GA, Siri-Tarino PW. The role of macronutrient content in the diet for weight management. Endocrinol Metab Clin North America 2016;45(3):581–604.

63. Bray MS, Loos RJ, McCaffery JM, et al. NIH working group report—using genomic information to guide weight management: from universal to precision treatment. Obesity (Silver Spring) 2016;24(1):14–22.

64. Cornier MA, Donahoo WT, Pereira R, et al. Insulin sensitivity determines the effectiveness of dietary macronutrient composition on weight loss in obese women. Obes Res 2005;13(4):703–9.

65. Ebbeling CB, Leidig MM, Feldman HA, et al. Effects of a low-glycemic load vs low-fat diet in obese young adults: a randomized trial. JAMA 2007;297(19): 2092–102.

66. McClain AD, Otten JJ, Hekler EB, et al. Adherence to a low-fat vs. low-carbohydrate diet differs by insulin resistance status. Diabetes Obes Metab 2013;15(1):87–90.

67. Pittas AG, Das SK, Hajduk CL, et al. A low-glycemic load diet facilitates greater weight loss in overweight adults with high insulin secretion but not in overweight adults with low insulin secretion in the CALERIE Trial. Diabetes Care 2005;28(12): 2939–41.

68. Gardner CD, Hauser M, Del Gobbo L, et al. Neither insulin secretion nor genotype pattern modify 12-month weight loss effects of healthy low-fat vs. healthy low-carbohydrate diets among adults with obesity. Portland (OR): EPI | Lifestyle Scientific Sessions; 2017.

69. Gardner CD, Offringa LC, Hartle JC, et al. Weight loss on low-fat vs. low-carbohydrate diets by insulin resistance status among overweight adults and adults with obesity: a randomized pilot trial. Obesity (Silver Spring) 2016;24(1): 79–86.

70. Perri MG, McAllister DA, Gange JJ, et al. Effects of four maintenance programs on the long-term management of obesity. J Consulting Clin Psychol 1988;56(4): 529–34.

71. Middleton KM, Patidar SM, Perri MG. The impact of extended care on the long-term maintenance of weight loss: a systematic review and meta-analysis. Obes Rev 2012;13(6):509–17.

72. Jensen MD, Ryan DH, Apovian CM, et al. 2013 AHA/ACC/TOS guideline for the management of overweight and obesity in adults: a report of the American College of Cardiology/American Heart Association Task Force on Practice Guidelines and The Obesity Society. Circulation 2014;129(25 Suppl 2):S102–38.

73. Pi-Sunyer X, Blackburn G, Brancati FL, et al. Reduction in weight and cardiovascular disease risk factors in individuals with type 2 diabetes: one-year results of the look AHEAD trial. Diabetes Care 2007;30(6):1374–83.

74. Thomas JG, Bond DS, Phelan S, et al. Weight-loss maintenance for 10 years in the National Weight Control Registry. Am J Prev Med 2014;46(1):17–23.

75. Wing RR, Hill JO. Successful weight loss maintenance. Annu Rev Nutr 2001;21: 323–41.

76. Perri MG, Limacher MC, Durning PE, et al. Extended-care programs for weight management in rural communities: the treatment of obesity in underserved rural settings (TOURS) randomized trial. Arch Intern Med 2008;168(21):2347–54.

77. Svetkey LP, Stevens VJ, Brantley PJ, et al. Comparison of strategies for sustaining weight loss: the weight loss maintenance randomized controlled trial. JAMA 2008;299(10):1139–48.

78. Voils CI, Olsen MK, Gierisch JM, et al. Maintenance of weight loss after initiation of nutrition training: a randomized trial. Ann Intern Med 2017;166(7):463–71.

79. Wing RR, Tate DF, Gorin AA, et al. A self-regulation program for maintenance of weight loss. N Engl J Med 2006;355(15):1563–71.

80. Halpern SD, French B, Small DS, et al. Randomized trial of four financial-incentive programs for smoking cessation. N Engl J Med 2015;372(22):2108–17.

81. Volpp KG, John LK, Troxel AB, et al. Financial incentive-based approaches for weight loss: a randomized trial. JAMA 2008;300(22):2631–7.
82. Foster GD, Wadden TA, Vogt RA, et al. What is a reasonable weight loss? Patients' expectations and evaluations of obesity treatment outcomes. J Consulting Clin Psychol 1997;65(1):79–85.
83. Phelan S, Nallari M, Darroch FE, et al. What do physicians recommend to their overweight and obese patients? J Am Board Fam Med 2009;22(2):115–22.
84. Rothman AJ. Toward a theory-based analysis of behavioral maintenance. Health Psychol 2000;19(1S):64–9.
85. Kahan S, Puhl RM. The damaging effects of weight bias internalization. Obesity (Silver Spring) 2017;25(2):280–1.
86. Knowler WC, Barrett-Connor E, Fowler SE, et al. Reduction in the incidence of type 2 diabetes with lifestyle intervention or metformin. N Engl J Med 2002; 346(6):393–403.
87. Espeland MA, Glick HA, Bertoni A, et al. Impact of an intensive lifestyle intervention on use and cost of medical services among overweight and obese adults with type 2 diabetes: the action for health in diabetes. Diabetes Care 2014; 37(9):2548–56.
88. Wing RR, Bolin P, Brancati FL, et al. Cardiovascular effects of intensive lifestyle intervention in type 2 diabetes. N Engl J Med 2013;369(2):145–54.
89. Silva MN, Vieira PN, Coutinho SR, et al. Using self-determination theory to promote physical activity and weight control: a randomized controlled trial in women. J Behav Med 2010;33(2):110–22.
90. Allison DB, Gadde KM, Garvey WT, et al. Controlled-release phentermine/topiramate in severely obese adults: a randomized controlled trial (EQUIP). Obesity (Silver Spring) 2012;20(2):330–42.
91. le Roux CW, Astrup A, Fujioka K, et al. 3 years of liraglutide versus placebo for type 2 diabetes risk reduction and weight management in individuals with prediabetes: a randomised, double-blind trial. Lancet 2017;389(10077):1399–409.
92. Torgerson JS, Hauptman J, Boldrin MN, et al. XENical in the prevention of diabetes in obese subjects (XENDOS) study: a randomized study of orlistat as an adjunct to lifestyle changes for the prevention of type 2 diabetes in obese patients. Diabetes Care 2004;27(1):155–61.
93. Sjostrom L, Peltonen M, Jacobson P, et al. Bariatric surgery and long-term cardiovascular events. JAMA 2012;307(1):56–65.
94. Promotion CfNPa. Dietary Guidelines for Americans. 2015. Available at: https://www.cnpp.usda.gov/2015-2020-dietary-guidelines-americans. Accessed July 14, 2017.
95. Promotion OoDPaH. Physical activity guidelines for Americans. 2008. Available at: https://health.gov/paguidelines/guidelines. Accessed July 14, 2017.
96. Matheson EM, King DE, Everett CJ. Healthy lifestyle habits and mortality in overweight and obese individuals. J Am Board Fam Med 2012;25(1):9–15.

Moving?

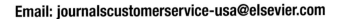

Make sure your subscription moves with you!

To notify us of your new address, find your **Clinics Account Number** (located on your mailing label above your name), and contact customer service at:

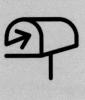

Email: journalscustomerservice-usa@elsevier.com

800-654-2452 (subscribers in the U.S. & Canada)
314-447-8871 (subscribers outside of the U.S. & Canada)

Fax number: 314-447-8029

Elsevier Health Sciences Division
Subscription Customer Service
3251 Riverport Lane
Maryland Heights, MO 63043

*To ensure uninterrupted delivery of your subscription, please notify us at least 4 weeks in advance of move.

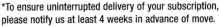

ELSEVIER